1999
YEAR BOOK OF
CARDIOLOGY®

Statement of Purpose

The YEAR BOOK Service

The YEAR BOOK series was devised in 1901 by practicing health professionals who observed that the literature of medicine and related disciplines had become so voluminous that no one individual could read and place in perspective every potential advance in a major specialty. In the final decade of the 20th century, this recognition is more acutely true than it was in 1901.

More than merely a series of books, YEAR BOOK volumes are the tangible results of a unique service designed to accomplish the following:

- to *survey* a wide range of journals of proven value
- to *select* from those journals papers representing significant advances and statements of important clinical principles
- to provide *abstracts* of those articles that are readable, convenient summaries of their key points
- to provide *commentary* about those articles to place them in perspective

These publications grow out of a unique process that calls on the talents of outstanding authorities in clinical and fundamental disciplines, trained literature specialists, and professional writers, all supported by the resources of Mosby, the world's preeminent publisher for the health professions.

The Literature Base

Mosby and its editors survey approximately 500 journals published worldwide, covering the full range of the health professions. On an annual basis, the publisher examines usage patterns and polls its expert authorities to add new journals to the literature base and to delete journals that are no longer useful as potential YEAR BOOK sources.

The Literature Survey

The publisher's team of literature specialists, all of whom are trained and experienced health professionals, examines every original, peer-reviewed article in each journal issue. More than 250,000 articles per year are scanned systematically, including title, text, illustrations, tables, and references. Each scan is compared, article by article, to the search strategies that the publisher has developed in consultation with the 270 outside experts who form the pool of YEAR BOOK editors. A given article may be reviewed by any number of editors, from one to a dozen or more, regardless of the discipline for which the paper was originally published. In turn, each editor who receives the article reviews it to determine whether the article should be included in the YEAR BOOK. This decision is based on the article's inherent quality, its probable usefulness to readers of that YEAR BOOK, and the editor's goal to represent a balanced picture of a given field in each volume of the YEAR BOOK. In addition, the editor indicates when to include figures and tables from the article to help the YEAR BOOK reader better understand the information.

Of the quarter million articles scanned each year, only 5% are selected for detailed analysis within the YEAR BOOK series, thereby assuring readers of the high value of every selection.

The Abstract

The publisher's abstracting staff is headed by a seasoned medical professional and includes individuals with training in the life sciences, medicine, and other areas, plus extensive experience in writing for the health professions and related industries. Each selected article is assigned to a specific writer on this abstracting staff. The abstracter, guided in many cases by notations supplied by the expert editor, writes a structured, condensed summary designed so that the reader can rapidly acquire the essential information contained in the article.

The Commentary

The YEAR BOOK editorial boards, sometimes assisted by guest commentators, write comments that place each article in perspective for the reader. This provides the reader with the equivalent of a personal consultation with a leading international authority—an opportunity to better understand the value of the article and to benefit from the authority's thought processes in assessing the article.

Additional Editorial Features

The editorial boards of each YEAR BOOK organize the abstracts and comments to provide a logical and satisfying sequence of information. To enhance the organization, editors also provide introductions to sections or individual chapters, comments linking a number of abstracts, citations to additional literature, and other features.

The published YEAR BOOK contains enhanced bibliographic citations for each selected article, including extended listings of multiple authors and identification of author affiliations. Each YEAR BOOK contains a Table of Contents specific to that year's volume. From year to year, the Table of Contents for a given YEAR BOOK will vary depending on developments within the field.

Every YEAR BOOK contains a list of the journals from which papers have been selected. This list represents a subset of approximately 500 journals surveyed by the publisher and occasionally reflects a particularly pertinent article from a journal that is not surveyed on a routine basis.

Finally, each volume contains a comprehensive subject index and an index to authors of each selected paper.

The 1999 Year Book Series

Year Book of Allergy, Asthma, and Clinical Immunology: Drs. Rosenwasser, Boguniewicz, Borish, Routes, Spahn, and Weber

Year Book of Anesthesiology and Pain Management®: Drs. Tinker, Abram, Chestnut, Roizen, Rothenberg, and Wood

Year Book of Cardiology®: Drs. Schlant, Collins, Gersh, Graham, Kaplan, and Waldo

Year Book of Chiropractic®: Dr. Lawrence

Year Book of Critical Care Medicine®: Drs. Parrillo, Balk, Calvin, Franklin, and Shapiro

Year Book of Dentistry®: Drs. Meskin, Berry, Jeffcoat, Leinfelder, Roser, Summitt, and Zakariasen

Year Book of Dermatology and Dermatologic Surgery™: Drs. Thiers and Lang

Year Book of Diagnostic Radiology®: Drs. Osborn, Birdwell, Dalinka, Groskin, Maynard, Pentecost, Ros, Smirniotopoulos, and Young

Year Book of Emergency Medicine®: Drs. Wagner, Dronen, Davidson, King, Niemann, and Hamilton

Year Book of Endocrinology®: Drs. Bagdade, Braverman, Fitzpatrick, Horton, Kannan, Landsberg, Molitch, Morley, Odell, Poehlman, and Rogol

Year Book of Family Practice®: Drs. Berg, Bowman, Davidson, Dexter, and Scherger

Year Book of Gastroenterology: Drs. Aliperti and Fleshman

Year Book of Hand Surgery®: Drs. Amadio and Hentz

Year Book of Medicine®: Drs. Klahr, Frishman, Malawista, Mandell, Jett, Young, Barkin, and Bagdade

Year Book of Neonatal and Perinatal Medicine®: Drs. Fanaroff, Maisels, and Stevenson

Year Book of Nephrology, Hypertension, and Mineral Metabolism: Drs. Schwab, Bennett, Emmett, Hostetter, and Moe

Year Book of Neurology and Neurosurgery®: Drs. Bradley and Gibbs

Year Book of Nuclear Medicine®: Drs. Gottschalk, Blaufox, Coleman, Strauss, and Zubal

Year Book of Obstetrics, Gynecology, and Women's Health®: Drs. Mishell, Herbst, and Kirschbaum

Year Book of Oncology®: Drs. Ozols, Eisenberg, Glatstein, Loehrer, and Urba

Year Book of Ophthalmology®: Drs. Wilson, Augsburger, Cohen, Eagle, Grossman, Laibson, Maguire, Nelson, Penne, Rapuano, Sergott, Spaeth, Tipperman, Ms. Gosfield, and Ms. Salmon

Year Book of Orthopedics®: Drs. Morrey, Beauchamp, Currier, Tolo, Trigg, and Swiontkowski

1999

The Year Book of CARDIOLOGY®

Editor in Chief

Robert C. Schlant, M.D.

Professor and Chairman, Emory University School of Medicine; Chief of Cardiology, Grady Memorial Hospital, Atlanta, Georgia

Editors

John J. Collins, Jr., M.D.

Professor of Surgery, Director, Sub-Department of Thoracic and Cardiac Surgery, Harvard Medical School; Senior Surgeon, Emeritus, Brigham and Women's Hospital, Boston, Massachusetts

Bernard J. Gersh, M.B., Ch.B., D.Phil., F.R.C.P.

Professor of Medicine, Mayo Medical School; Consultant, Cardiovascular Diseases/Internal Medicine, Mayo Clinic, Rochester, Minnesota

Thomas P. Graham, M.D.

Ann and Monroe Carell Family Professor of Pediatric Cardiology; Director, Pediatric Cardiology; Vanderbilt University Medical Center, Nashville, Tennessee

Norman M. Kaplan, M.D.

Professor of Internal Medicine, University of Texas Southwestern Medical School, Dallas, Texas

Albert L. Waldo, M.D.

The Walter H. Pritchard Professor of Cardiology and Professor of Medicine, Case Western Reserve University; Director, Clinical Cardiac Electrophysiology Program, University Hospitals of Cleveland, Cleveland, Ohio

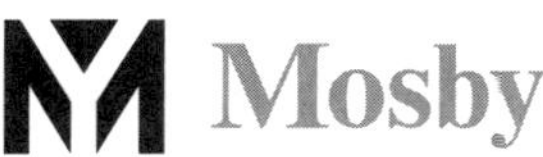

St. Louis Baltimore Boston Carlsbad Naples New York Philadelphia Portland London
Madrid Mexico City Singapore Sydney Tokyo Toronto Wiesbaden

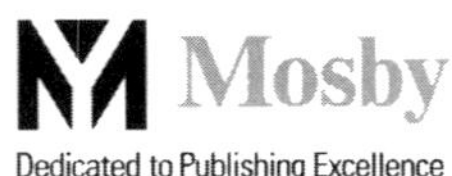

Dedicated to Publishing Excellence

Publisher: Theresa Van Schaik
Developmental Editor: Sarah A. Zagarri
Manager, Periodical Editing: Kirk Swearingen
Manuscript Editor: Pat Costigan
Project Supervisor, Production: Joy Moore
Production Assistant: Laura Bayless
Manager, Literature Services: Idelle L. Winer
Illustrations and Permissions Coordinator: Chidi C. Ukabam

1999 EDITION
Copyright © 1999 by Mosby, Inc.

Printed in the United States of America
Composition by Reed Technology and Information Services, Inc.
Printing/binding by Maple-Vail

Editorial Office:
Mosby, Inc.
11830 Westline Industrial Drive
St. Louis, MO 63146
Customer Service: customer.support@mosby.com
            www.mosby.com/Mosby/CustomerSupport/index.html
series.editorial@mosby.com

International Standard Serial Number: 0145-4145
International Standard Book Number: 0-8151-9602-4

Table of Contents

Journals Represented

Mosby and its editors survey approximately 500 journals for its abstract and commentary publications. From these journals, the editors select the articles to be abstracted. Journals represented in this YEAR BOOK are listed below.

Age and Ageing
American Heart Journal
American Journal of Cardiology
American Journal of Clinical Nutrition
American Journal of Emergency Medicine
American Journal of Hypertension
American Journal of Medicine
American Journal of Respiratory and Critical Care Medicine
American Journal of the Medical Sciences
Anesthesia and Analgesia
Annals of Internal Medicine
Annals of Surgery
Annals of Thoracic Surgery
Archives of Surgery
Arteriosclerosis, Thrombosis, and Vascular Biology
British Medical Journal
Canadian Journal of Cardiology
Chest
Circulation
Clinical Pharmacology and Therapeutics
European Heart Journal
Heart
Hypertension
Journal of Cardiac Failure
Journal of Clinical Investigation
Journal of Human Hypertension
Journal of Hypertension
Journal of Neurology, Neurosurgery and Psychiatry
Journal of Neurosurgery
Journal of Pediatrics
Journal of Thoracic and Cardiovascular Surgery
Journal of the American College of Cardiology
Journal of the American Geriatrics Society
Journal of the American Medical Association
Lancet
Mayo Clinic Proceedings
Nephrology, Dialysis, Transplantation
New England Journal of Medicine
PACE–Pacing and Clinical Electrophysiology
Pediatrics
Proceedings of the National Academy of Sciences
Radiology

STANDARD ABBREVIATIONS

The following terms are abbreviated in this edition: acquired immunodeficiency syndrome (AIDS), cardiopulmonary resuscitation (CPR), central nervous system

(CNS), cerebrospinal fluid (CSF), computed tomography (CT), deoxyribonucleic acid (DNA), electrocardiography (ECG), health maintenance organization (HMO), human immunodeficiency virus (HIV), intensive care unit (ICU), intramuscular (IM), intravenous (IV), magnetic resonance (MR) imaging (MRI), and ribonucleic acid (RNA).

NOTE

The YEAR BOOK OF CARDIOLOGY is a literature survey service providing abstracts of articles published in the professional literature. Every effort is made to assure the accuracy of the information presented in these pages. Neither the editors nor the publisher of the YEAR BOOK OF CARDIOLOGY can be responsible for errors in the original materials. The editors' comments are their own opinions. Mention of specific products within this publication does not constitute endorsement.

To facilitate the use of the YEAR BOOK OF CARDIOLOGY as a reference tool, all illustrations and tables included in this publication are now identified as they appear in the original article. This change is meant to help the reader recognize that any illustration or table appearing in the YEAR BOOK OF CARDIOLOGY may be only one of many in the original article. For this reason, figure and table numbers will often appear to be out of sequence within the YEAR BOOK OF CARDIOLOGY.

Introduction

This 1999 YEAR BOOK OF CARDIOLOGY is the 39th in the series. Each of our six editors has carefully selected and provided comments on important, clinically relevant articles in cardiology.

All the editors again thank the staff at Mosby, Inc., for their assistance, understanding, and especially patience. We are particularly indebted to Ms. Sarah Zagarri.

Robert C. Schlant, M.D.

1 Hypertension

Introduction

A major theme running through the literature relating to hypertension over the past year is the continued inadequacy of current control of the disease. As documented in the sixth report of the Joint National Committee,[1] only 27% of persons in the United States with hypertension have blood pressures below 140/90 mm Hg. Even worse control rates have been reported from Canada and England, where national health services would be assumed to better be able to manage a chronic condition.

The underlying problem is the asymptomatic nature of hypertension, which requires therapy for a lifetime but provides no immediate obvious benefit and often introduces bothersome side effects and considerable financial costs. As I have repeatedly observed,[2] we and our patients would be more likely to achieve better success if untreated hypertension hurt, not a great deal but enough, to remind the patient of the need to take medication to obtain relief.

Even when treated to levels that have previously been thought to be adequate, hypertensives continue to suffer an increased prevalence of stroke, myocardial infarction, and heart failure.[3, 4] Therefore, we must not only push therapy to below 140/90 mm Hg in high-risk patients, but we must correct the commonly coexisting major risk factors—dyslipidemia, smoking, and diabetes. Moreover, we must identify the high prevalence of hypertension and these other risk factors in the siblings of patients with documented coronary disease that appears below age 60.[5] Only primary prevention offers the hope for meaningful reversal of the high rates of cardiovascular disease in our population.

Norman M. Kaplan, M.D.

References

1. The sixth report of the Joint National Committee on prevention, detection, evaluation and treatment of high blood pressure. *Arch Intern Med* 157:2413-2446, 1997.
2. Kaplan NM: Hypertension in the population at large, in *Clinical Hypertension*, ed 7. Baltimore, Md, Williams & Wilkins, 1998, pp 19-39.
3. Andersson OK, Almgren T, Persson B, et al: Survival in treated hypertension: Follow up study after two decades. *BMJ* 317:167-171, 1998.
4. Alderman MH, Cohen H, Madhavan S: Epidemiology of risk in hypertensives. *Am J Hypertens* 11:874-876, 1998.

5. Yanek LR, Moy TF, Blumenthal RS, et al: Hypertension among siblings of persons with premature coronary heart disease. *Hypertension* 32:123-128, 1998.

Diagnosis and Monitoring

Blood Pressure Screening, Management and Control in England: Results From the Health Survey for England 1994

Colhoun HM, Dong W, Poulter NR (Univ College London Med School; Imperial College School of Medicine, London)
J Hypertens 16:747-752, 1998

1-1

Introduction.—Recent U.S. studies have suggested improvements in the awareness, treatment, and control of hypertension. By contrast, data from the United Kingdom continue to suggest low rates of hypertension treatment and control. The awareness, treatment, and control of hypertension in England was retrospectively analyzed using data from a cross-sectional nationwide survey.

Methods.—The study included a random sample of 12,116 adult participants in the 1994 Health Survey for England, which was a representative sample of the population. Information provided by these subjects was analyzed to assess the prevalence of awareness, treatment, and control of hypertension. The prevalences of other cardiovascular disease risk factors were determined as well. Among subjects receiving antihypertensive treatment, the number and types of drugs used were analyzed.

Results.—When hypertension was described as either a systolic blood pressure of 160 mm Hg or more, a diastolic blood pressure of 95 mm Hg

TABLES 2, 3.—Awareness, Treatment, and Control of Blood
Pressure Among English Adults With Two Different
Thresholds Defining Hypertension*

	BP > 160/95 Total†	BP > 140/90 Total†
Men	1,044	2,322
Women	1,315	2,262
Total	2,359	4,584
Awareness (%)		
Men	60.0	33.4
Women	65.8	46.0
Total	63.2	39.6
Treatment (%)		
Men	44.8	20.2
Women	54.4	31.6
Total	50.1	25.8
Control (%)		
Men	26.7	4.7
Women	31.8	7.1
Total	29.6	5.9

*Hypertension is described as blood pressure higher than 160/95(Column 2) or 140/90(Column 3) or a subject's being administered antihypertensive medication.
†Values are expressed as numbers or percentages where indicated.
(Modified from Colhoun HM, Dong W, Poulter NR: Blood pressure screening, management and control in England: Results from the Health Survey for England 1994. *J Hypertens* 16:747-752, 1998.)

or more, or the use of antihypertensive drug therapy, the prevalence of awareness of hypertension was 63%. When the definition was changed to a systolic blood pressure of 140 mm Hg or more or diastolic blood pressure of 90 mm Hg or more, this figure decreased to 40%. At the higher threshold, 50% of hypertensive patients were receiving treatment and 30% had their blood pressure under control; at the lower cutoff point, these values were 26% and 6%, respectively (Tables 2 and 3[combined]). Sixty percent of patients receiving antihypertensive therapy were receiving a single drug. The most frequently used agents were diuretics and β-blockers.

Conclusions.—In the English population, awareness, treatment, and control of hypertension are significantly lower than in the United States. At the higher cutoff point studied, most patients with hypertension are aware of their condition; however, half of these are untreated, and many treated patients do not have their blood pressure under control. Improving the treatment and control of hypertension in the English population could lead to further reductions in cardiovascular disease mortality.

▶ As noted in Abstract 1–44, control rates for hypertension in the United States are low, even under the best of circumstances. Reasons for the poor rates could include poor access to medical care and the high cost of antihypertensive drugs. However, the even worse control rates in England shown in this paper for a level of 140/90 suggest that neither of these factors likely are important, because, under their National Health Service, access is easy and drugs cost little.

It is important to recognize another discrepancy between the United States and England: the English generally do not diagnose or treat levels of blood pressure between 140/90 (the usual level accepted by U.S. practitioners) and 160/95. Therefore, if their control rates for 160/95 are used, their success rate is quite similar to ours.

I believe we are closer to the needs of patients than are the more conservative English. Everyone, here and elsewhere, must recognize the difficulty of keeping asymptomatic patients on long-term (lifelong) daily therapy that provides no obvious benefit and may make the patient feel worse. Oh, if hypertension only hurt a little and the pain would go away when the blood pressure went down, we and our patients would be much better off.

N.M. Kaplan, M.D.

Trends in Hypertension Prevalence, Treatment, and Control: In a Well-Defined Older Population
Barker WH, Mullooly JP, Linton KLP (Univ of Rochester, NY; Kaiser Permanente Ctr for Health Research, Portland, Ore)
Hypertension 31:552–559, 1998   1–2

Background.—The risk of hypertension-related cardiovascular conditions is highest among patients older than 65 years. Although the benefits of treating hypertension are well documented, these studies included relatively few patients older than 65 years. This situation has led to doubt regarding the necessity and safety of treating high blood pressure in the elderly. Trends in the prevalence, treatment, and control of hypertension in patients aged 65 and older were retrospectively studied.

Methods.—Random samples of 400 to 500 HMO members aged 65 years or older were analyzed at 4 periods: 1967, 1974, 1981, and 1988. The medical records included an initial ambulatory blood pressure measurement in more than 90% of patients in each period. The study definition of hypertension was a systolic blood pressure (SBP) of 160 mm Hg or greater, a diastolic blood pressure (DBP) of 95 or greater, or treatment with antihypertensive drugs.

Results.—Across the 4 periods, the prevalence of hypertension ranged from 44% to 53%. At the same time, the proportion of hypertensive patients receiving treatment increased from 25% to 60%, while the proportion receiving treatment and with controlled blood pressure increased from 8% to 34%. Overall, mean blood pressure in the elderly samples decreased from 155/85 mm Hg in 1967 to 144/81 mm Hg in 1988. There was no change over time in the proportion of patients with isolated systolic hypertension, defined as an SBP of 160 mm Hg or greater with a DBP of less than 90 mm Hg: 12% to 14%. During the 1980s, the use of β-blockers and other new antihypertensive drugs increased as the use of diuretics and adrenergic antagonist drugs decreased.

Conclusions.—A reduction in the prevalence of hypertension was demonstrated among patients aged 65 years and older from the late 1960s through the later 1980s. At the same time, the percentage of treated hypertensive patients and the proportion of patients with controlled hypertension increased. The findings are comparable to recent data on trends in hypertension among younger adults. However, favorable trends are delayed among the elderly, with a high proportion of the elderly continuing to have uncontrolled hypertension.

▶ There's both good news and bad news in this survey of samples of patients older than 65 years enrolled in the Kaiser Permanente health plan. The good news is that the percentage of patients being treated for hypertension rose from 25% in 1967 to 60% in 1988 and the percentage of well-controlled hypertensives rose from 8% to 34%. The bad news is obvious: the majority remained uncontrolled.

These data are similar to the recently published figures from the third National Health and Nutrition Examination Survey (NHANES III), obtained from 1991 to 1994 from a cross-section of the entire adult U.S. population.[1] The NHANES III found that about half of hypertensives are being treated, but only 27% are under good control.

Obviously, we have a long way to go to adequately protect the highly vulnerable and fast-growing elderly hypertensive population.

N.M. Kaplan, M.D.

Reference

1. The sixth report of the Joint National Committee on detection, evaluation and treatment of high blood pressure (JNCV). *Arch Intern Med* 157:2413-2446, 1997.

Limitations of the Difference Between Clinic and Daytime Blood Pressure as a Surrogate Measure of the "White-Coat" Effect

Parati G, for the Syst-Eur Investigators (Univ of Milan, Italy; et al)
J Hypertens 16:23-29, 1998

1–3

Introduction.—Measurements of blood pressure taken by a doctor may cause an alerting reaction and an increase in the heart rate and blood pressure of the patient. This "white-coat effect" can lead to a mistaken diagnosis of hypertension or an incorrect estimate of the response to antihypertensive treatment. To circumvent this, the patient takes a daytime average blood pressure with noninvasive ambulatory blood pressure monitoring, and this is compared to the clinic measurement. The reproducibility of this difference and its relationship with clinic and average ambulatory daytime blood pressure levels were assessed.

Methods.—There were 783 outpatients with systolic and diastolic essential hypertension aged a mean of 50.8 years participating in standardized trials of antihypertensive drugs and 506 elderly patients with isolated systolic hypertension, participating in the European Syst-Eur trial aged a mean of 71 years. These patients had their clinic and ambulatory blood pressures measured, and the reproducibility of this difference was assessed.

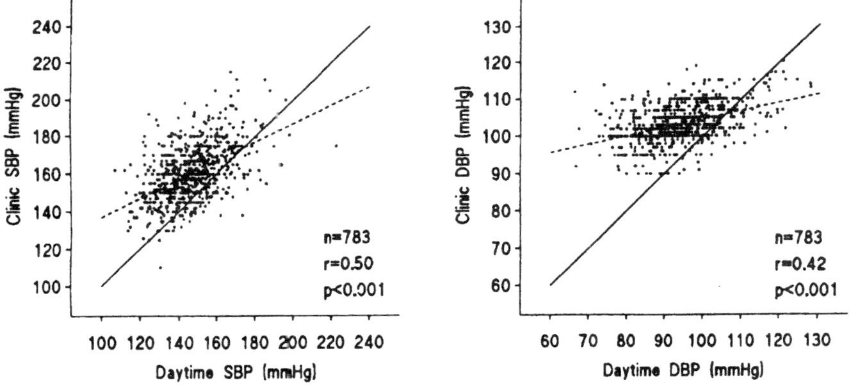

FIGURE 1.—Relationship between clinic and daytime blood pressures for 783 patients with mild or moderate essential hypertension. Individual data for systolic blood pressure (*SBP*) and diastolic blood pressure (*DBP*) are shown separately. Continuous lines represent the identity and the dashed lines the regression lines for relationships between clinic and daytime blood pressures. (Courtesy of Parati G, for the Syst-Eur Investigators: Limitations of the difference between clinic and daytime blood pressure as a surrogate measure of the "White-coat" effect. *J Hypertens* 16:23-29, 1998.)

Results.—For the essential systolic and diastolic hypertensive patient, the mean clinic minus daytime blood pressure difference was 13.6 mm Hg for systolic and 9.1 mm Hg for diastolic blood pressure (Fig 1). For the elderly patients with isolated systolic hypertension, the difference was 21.2 mm Hg for systolic and 1.3 mm Hg for diastolic blood pressure. Regarding the heart rate, little or no systematic clinic minus daytime difference could be observed. For 108 (13.8%) essential systolic and diastolic hypertensive patients and 128 (25.3%) isolated systolic hypertensives, the reproducibility of the clinic minus daytime blood pressure difference was invariably lower than that of both daytime and clinic blood pressure values. For increasing levels of clinic blood pressure, the clinic minus daytime blood pressure difference was progressively higher. For higher levels of ambulatory daytime blood pressure, the clinic minus daytime blood pressure difference was progressively lower.

Conclusion.—There is limited reproducibility with the clinic minus daytime blood pressure difference. Reproducibility depends on daytime mean blood pressure and on clinic blood pressure and is a function of the blood pressure criteria employed for selection of the patients in a trial. The reproducibility factor is never associated with a systematic clinic minus daytime difference in heart rate, and this further questions its use as a reliable surrogate measure of the true pressor response induced in the patient by the doctor's visit.

▶ In this and another article[1] on a small group of patients, these authors show that the "white-coat effect" is not entirely reflected in the usual criterion for defining "white-coat hypertension" that is, the presence of elevated office readings and normal out-of-the-office readings.

This point, however, is really irrelevant to clinical practice because white-coat or isolated office hypertension should never be based on the first measurement taken in the office, wherein the full "white-coat effect" may occur. Obviously, to make this diagnosis, multiple office readings should be found to be elevated and even more out-of-the-office readings found to be normal.

In making the diagnosis, awake or daytime ambulatory monitoring is preferable,[2] but multiple self-taken home readings are usually adequate, with about a 20% discrepancy between the 2 techniques.[3] A lower level of pressure should be used to define hypertension with either out-of-the-office measure, likely 135/90 or 135/85.[4]

The majority of cross-sectional and follow-up data continue to show that properly defined white-coat hypertension is associated with less current and future target organ damage.[4] Nonetheless, such patients need continued follow-up because they may become persistently hypertensive.

N.M. Kaplan, M.D.

References

1. Parati G, Ulian L, Santucciu C, et al: Difference between clinic and daytime blood pressure is not a measure of the white coat effect. *Hypertension* 31:1185-1189, 1998.
2. Zawadzka A, Bird R, Casadei B, et al: Audit of ambulatory blood pressure monitoring in the diagnosis and management of hypertension in practice. *J Human Hypertens* 12:249-252, 1998.
3. Stergiou GS, Zourbaki AS, Skeva II, et al: White coat effect detected using self-monitoring of blood pressure at home. *Am J Hypertens* 11:820-827, 1998.
4. Hoegholm A, Kristensen KS, Bang LE: White coat hypertension and target organ involvement: the impact of different cut-off levels on albuminuria and left ventricular mass and geometry. *J Human Hypertens* 12:433-439, 1998.

Target-Organ Damage in Stage I Hypertensive Subjects With White Coat and Sustained Hypertension: Results From the HARVEST Study

Palatini P, for the HARVEST Study Investigators (Univ of Padova, Italy)
Hypertension 31:57-63, 1998   1–4

Objective.—Whether white coat hypertension is benign or presages an increased risk of organ damage has not been determined. The relationship

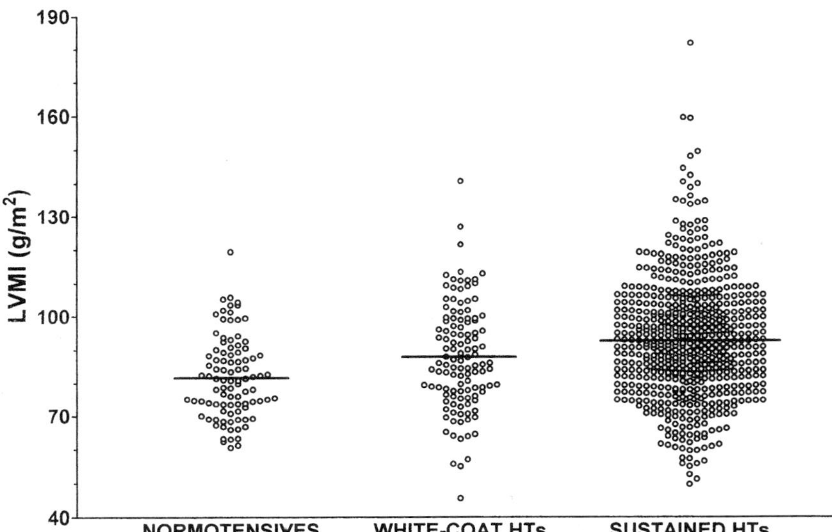

FIGURE 1.—Left ventricular mass indexed by body surface area in the normotensive subjects divided according to whether they had white coat or sustained hypertension according to the 130/80 mm Hg daytime blood pressure partition value. Sustained hypertensive patients (*HTs*): $P < 0.001$ vs. normotensive patients and $P = 0.01$ vs. white-coat hypertensive patients. White-coat hypertensive patients: $P = 0.04$ vs. normotensive patients. (Courtesy of Palatini P, for the HARVEST Study Investigators: Target-organ damage in stage I hypertensive subjects with white coat and sustained hypertension: Results from the HARVEST study. *Hypertension* 31:57-63. Copyright 1998, American Heart Association. Reproduced with permission.)

between white coat hypertension and target-organ damage was investigated in patients enrolled in the multicenter HARVEST study.

Methods.—Early end-organ involvement was assessed by echocardiography, 24-hour ambulatory blood pressure, and dosage of low-level urinary albumin in 722 stage I young hypertensive patients, aged 18 to 45 years, not previously treated for hypertension. Controls consisted of 71 male and 24 female age- and sex-matched normotensive individuals. Individuals were defined as white coat hypertensive patients on the basis of 3 partition values: a mean daytime blood pressure less than 130/80 mm Hg, less than 135/85 mm Hg, or less than 140/90 mm Hg.

Results.—Left ventricular mass index and wall thickness findings from echocardiographic data were higher among sustained hypertensive patients than among white coat hypertensive patients and lowest among normotensive controls (Fig 1). Urinary albumin levels were higher among sustained hypertensive patients than among normotensive patients.

Conclusions.—Whereas white coat hypertensive patients have less target organ complications compared with sustained hypertensive patients, white coat hypertensive patients are at greater risk of organ involvement than their normotensive counterparts.

▶ These data provide the largest and best documented portrayal of the degree of target organ damage found in white coat hypertensives, defined as office readings above 140/90 and 24-hour ambulatory readings below either 130/80 or 135/85 mm Hg. They confirm what has been noted in smaller, less well-defined groups: white coat hypertensives are not as free of cardiovascular involvement as are normotensive individuals, but are much less affected than those with sustained hypertension.

Most of these data are surely cross-sectional. What is needed is more long-term follow-up evidence for the natural history of the white coat phenomenon. The best of these has seen no significant increase in cardiovascular events for up to 8 years in more than 200 white coat patients.[1] Obviously, more such data are needed to confirm the benignity or danger of this condition. For now, careful observation but, in the absence of significant other risk factors or target organ damage, no active drug therapy seems appropriate.

N.M. Kaplan, M.D.

Reference

1. Verdecchia P, Schillaci G, Boldrini F, et al: White coat hypertension. *Lancet* 348:1443-1445, 1996.

Relationship Between Extreme Dippers and Orthostatic Hypertension in Elderly Hypertensive Patients

Kario K, Eguchi K, Nakagawa Y, et al (Jichi Med School, Tochigi, Japan; Madarashima Public Clinic, Saga, Japan)
Hypertension 31:77-82, 1998   1–5

Background.—Hypertensive patients with abnormal patterns of diurnal variation may be at elevated risk of cardiovascular disease. Some elderly hypertensives are "extreme dippers," showing a sharp nocturnal drop in blood pressure (BP); others are "nondippers," with no nocturnal decrease. Both of these groups are at higher risk of cerebrovascular disease than patients with an appropriate nocturnal decrease in BP. There are no data on the relationship between these abnormal patterns of diurnal BP variation and postural BP variation. Relationships among diurnal and postural BP variation patterns were studied in asymptomatic elderly patients with hypertension.

Methods.—Participants were 110 asymptomatic hypertensive elderly patients who underwent ambulatory BP monitoring. Of these, 29 had "white-coat" hypertension. The remaining 81 had sustained hypertension with various patterns of nocturnal BP decline: 14 "extreme dippers," with sleep systolic BP declines of 20% or greater of wake systolic BP; 56 "dippers," with sleep decreases of 0 to less than 20%; and 11 nondippers, with greater sleep BP than wake BP. All patients underwent 70-degree head-up tilt testing for assessment of postural BP variation. The study definition of orthostatic hypertension was a systolic BP increase of 10 mm Hg or greater during tilt; orthostatic hypotension was defined as a systolic BP decrease of 20% or greater during tilt.

Results.—Tilt testing produced mean systolic BP increases of 10 mm Hg in extreme dippers, a 7.5 mm Hg decrease in nondippers, and no change in dippers or white-coat hypertensives. The 4 groups showed similar increases in heart rate during tilt testing. Orthostatic hypertension occurred in 72% of extreme dippers, 11% of dippers, and 9% of nondippers. Orthostatic hypotension occurred in 7% of extreme dippers, 9% of dippers, and 27% of nondippers.

Conclusions.—In elderly patients with hypertension, abnormal patterns of diurnal BP variation are closely linked to abnormal patterns of postural BP variation. Extreme nocturnal dippers have orthostatic hypertension, whereas nondippers show orthostatic hypotension. Being upright in the daytime may thus increase BP in extreme dippers and decrease BP in nondippers. This may be part of the cause of abnormal diurnal variations in BP.

▶ The hodge-podge of the changes in ambulatory BP monitoring (ABPM) noted in these 110 elderly hypertensive subjects is in itself, not surprising. As more elderly hypertensives are put through ABPM, it has become increasingly obvious that their BPs are even more variable than are those in younger hypertensives. They have even more of the "white-coat" effect, with greater differences between their office readings and those taken out of the office,[1] so that, if at all possible, either ABPM or, more practically, home pressures self-recorded with a semiautomatic electronic device should be used both to diagnose their condition and to follow its management. If not, they will be prone to overdiagnosis and overtreatment.

What is surprising from this small study by Kario et al. Is the frequency of orthostatic rises in systolic BP of 10 mm Hg or more in 10 or the 14 patients whose BP naturally dipped the most during sleep, interpreted by the authors as reflecting a greater degree of peripheral vasoconstriction from sympathetic nervous activation. This might be logical if their marked dipping during sleep were related to a greater degree of suppression of such daytime sympathetic overactivity.

Regardless, the more common problem in the elderly with systolic hypertension when seated or supine is postural hypotension, which should always be looked for and managed before the hypertension is treated.

N.M. Kaplan, M.D.

Reference

1. Kaplan NM: Measurement of blood pressure, in *Clinical Hypertension*, ed 7. Baltimore, Md, Williams & Wilkins, 1998, pp 19-39.

Depressor Action of Insulin on Skeletal Muscle Vasculature: A Novel Mechanism for Postprandial Hypotension in the Elderly
Kearney MT, Cowley AJ, Stubbs TA, et al (Univ Med School, Nottingham, England)
J Am Coll Cardiol 31:209-216, 1998   1–6

Objective.—The elderly can have a significant decrease in blood pressure after a meal. One study has suggested that postprandial hypotension may be the result of a failure of insulin-mediated sympathoactivation. The vasodilatory action of insulin and its effect on blood pressure in the elderly was assessed after a high-carbohydrate meal.

Methods.—On 3 occasions at least 1 week apart, after a 6- to 10-hour fast, 10 healthy elderly individuals (8 men), mean age 72.3 years, ate a high-fat meal on 2 occasions and an isoenergetic high-carbohydrate meal on the other occasion. After 1 of the fat meals, an insulin infusion was administered to reproduce the insulin profile recorded during the high-carbohydrate meal. Heart rate and blood pressure were monitored. Cardiac output and superior mesenteric artery blood flow (SMABF) were assessed at baseline and every 20 minutes for 2 hours using Doppler ultrasound, and calf blood flow was measured by venous occlusion plethysmography.

Results.—Cardiac output and heart rate increased significantly after all meals. Although blood pressure did not change after the high-fat meal, it decreased significantly by 8.0 mm Hg after the high-carbohydrate meal and by 9.6 mm Hg after the high-fat meal with insulin (Fig 3). Calf blood

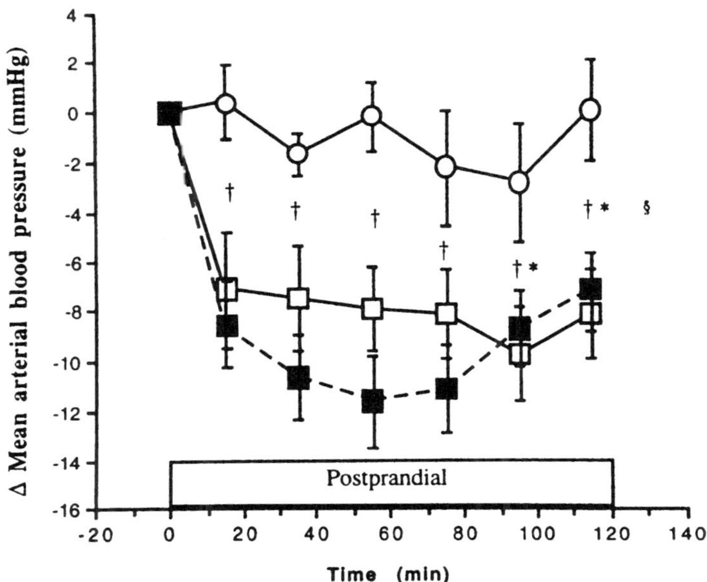

FIGURE 3.—Change (Δ) in mean arterial blood pressure after high-fat meal (*circles*), high-carbohydrate meal (*open squares*), and high-fat meal accompanied by insulin infusion reproducing the insulin profile seen after the high carbohydrate meal (*solid squares*). After both the high-carbohydrate and high-fat meal accompanied by insulin, there was a significant fall in mean arterial blood pressure, which differed significantly from the high fat meal ($P < 0.01$). *Note:* Significant difference between meals: *high-fat meal vs. high-carbohydrate meal; †high-fat meal vs. high-fat meal with insulin. (Reprinted with permission from the American College of Cardiology from Kearney MT, Cowley AJ, Stubbs TA, et al: Depressor action of insulin on skeletal muscle vasculature: A novel mechanism for postprandial hypotension in the elderly. *J Am Coll Cardiol* 31:209-216, 1998.)

flow decreased significantly by 0.8 mL per 100 mL/min after the high-fat meal, but no significant changes were noted after the high-carbohydrate meal and the high-fat meal with insulin. SMABF increased after all meals. Systemic vascular resistance decreased significantly by 2.6 U after the high-fat meal and by 5.3 U and 5.2 U, respectively, after the high-carbohydrate meal and the high-fat meal with insulin.

Conclusion.—Insulin appears to play an important role in the development of postprandial hypotension in the elderly by its vasodepressor action.

▶ As the authors of this study note in their introduction, many elderly people (even if healthy, but more so if hypertensive, diabetic, or frail) have postural and postprandial hypotension. Such hypotension can be debilitating in itself. More commonly, it leads to difficulty in treating the systolic hypertension that is so common in the elderly, even in those who have severe postural hypotension from autonomic failure.[1] Often, the treatment of hypertension must be postponed until the concomitant hypotension is overcome, usually by physical maneuvers (slow rising, isometric exercise before rising, support hose, elevation of the head of the bed, small meals) but occasionally requiring the use of a variety of drugs, which usually are not very successful.

This study documents the role of postprandial rises in insulin from high-carbohydrate food in the usual course of blood pressure: the rise in insulin both stimulates sympathetic nerve activity leading to vasoconstriction and, at the same time, directly dilates the peripheral arteries so that blood pressure normally doesn't change. In these healthy, older subjects, the sympathetic vasoconstriction did not occur, so that the insulin-mediated vasodilatation led to a significant fall in blood pressure.

These were healthy elderly subjects. In hypertensives, the baroreflex sympathetic reflexes may be further blunted; in diabetics, both the reflexes and the peripheral nerves may be inactive so that even greater postprandial hypotension may follow a high carbohydrate meal. Thus, we need to advise the elderly to watch out for high sugar and starch breakfasts if they experience any postural or postprandial symptoms of dizziness or instability.

N.M. Kaplan, M.D.

Reference

1. Shannon J, Jordon J, Costa F, et al: The hypertension of autonomic failure and its treatment. *Hypertension* 30:1062-1067, 1997.

Mechanisms

Evidence for Association and Genetic Linkage of the Angiotensin-Converting Enzyme Locus With Hypertension and Blood Pressure in Men but Not Women in the Framingham Heart Study
O'Donnell CJ, Lindpainter K, Larson MG, et al (Natl Heart, Lung, and Blood Institute's Framingham Heart Study, Mass; Harvard Med School, Boston; Tufts Univ, Boston; et al)
Circulation 97:1766-1772, 1998
1–7

Introduction.—Genetic factors have a significant effect on the occurrence of high blood pressure in the population. The angiotensin-converting enzyme (*ACE*) gene may play an important role in blood pressure regulation though the deletion/insertion (*D/I*) polymorphism in intron 16 of this gene. The relationship of this polymorphism to systemic hypertension and blood pressure was analyzed using data from the Framingham Heart Study.

Methods.—The analysis included data on 3,095 subjects who underwent regular blood pressure measurements through their participation in the Framingham Heart Study. A polymerase chain reaction assay was used to assess *ACE D/I* polymorphism status for each patient. Through association and linkage analyses, the association of *ACE D/I* with blood pressure and hypertension was analyzed.

Results.—Adjusted odds ratios for hypertension using logistic regression analysis were 1.59 for men with the *DD* genotype and 1.18 for men with the *DI* phenotype, compared with those men with the II genotype (Fig 1).

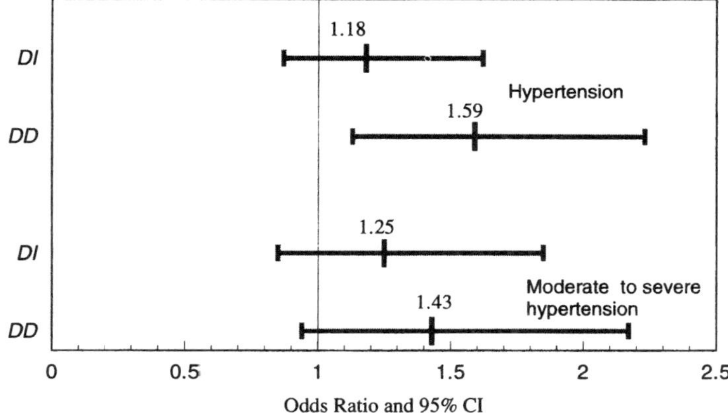

FIGURE 1.—Odds ratios for hypertension according to *ACE* genotype in men. (Courtesy of O'Donnell CJ, Lindpainter K, Larson MG, et al: Evidence for association and genetic linkage of the angiotensin-converting enzyme locus with hypertension and blood pressure in men but not women in the Framingham Heart Study. *Circulation* 97:1766-1772, 1998. Reproduced with permission, *Circulation*. Copyright 1998. American Heart Association.)

For women, these odds ratios were 1.00 and 0.78, respectively. Linear regression analysis showed that the *DD* genotype was associated with elevated diastolic blood pressure in men, but not in women. Linkage analysis suggested that the *ACE* locus affected blood pressure only in men.

Conclusions.—These data suggest that the *ACE* locus is associated with hypertension and increased diastolic blood pressure in men, although not in women. Thus *ACE*, or some gene located near it, may be a sex-specific gene associated with hypertension. This finding must be confirmed in additional population-based studies.

▶ This is one of many studies of the angiotensin-converting enzyme locus as a candidate gene for idiopathic (essential) hypertension. Data on both the *ACE* locus and the angiotensinogen gene have been conflicting, but most support a contribution from both.[1]

Another article in the same issue of *Circulation*[2] provides confirmation of the results reported by O'Donnell et al. In that study of 1,488 young siblings from 583 randomly ascertained 3-generation pedigrees from Rochester, Minnesota, variance components-based linkage analysis found that allelic variation in the region of the *ACE* gene contributed 29% of the interindividual variance in diastolic blood pressure in those with a positive family history of hypertension. As in the Framingham population, genetic variation in the region of the *ACE* gene influenced blood pressure variation only in men.

In an editorial about these 2 studies, Soubrier[3] concludes that these data along with much more evidence "supports the idea that the *ACE* locus might contain a gene for blood pressure." Nonetheless differences in ACE levels are not considered to be critical for the actions of the renin-angiotensin system. As Soubrier notes, the work has just begun in unraveling the genetic mechanisms of hypertension.

N.M. Kaplan, M.D.

References

1. Vasku A, Soucek M, Znojil Z, et al: Angiotensin I-converting enzyme and angiotensinogen gene interaction and prediction of essential hypertension. *Kidney Int* 53:1479-1482, 1998.
2. Fornage M, Amos CI, Kardia S, et al: Variation in the region of the angiotensin-converting enzyme gene influences interindividual differences in blood pressure levels in young white males. *Circulation* 97:1773-1779, 1998.
3. Soubrier F: Blood pressure gene at the angiotensin I-converting enzyme locus. *Circulation* 97:1763-1765, 1998.

Association of Hypertension With T594M Mutation in β Subunit of Epithelial Sodium Channels in Black People Resident in London

Baker EH, Dong YB, Sagnella GA, et al (St George's Hosp Medical School, London; College de France, Paris)
Lancet 351:1388-1392, 1998

1–8

Introduction.—It is well established that Liddle's syndrome is caused by mutations of subunits of the epithelial sodium channel that result in a rise in sodium reabsorption. Sodium-channel activity is increased in the lymphocytes of persons with the threonine 594 methionine (T594M) point mutation. The clinical features of Liddle's syndrome are similar to those of some black patients with hypertension. Almost all mutations in sodium-channel-subunit hypertension have been observed in black people. The frequency of the T594M point mutation in normotensive and hypertensive blacks living in London was assessed.

Methods.—Of 206 blacks with hypertension and a mean age of 48 years, 80 were male and 126 were female. Of 142 blacks who were normotensive and a mean age of 48.7 years, 61 were male and 81 were female. All were screened for T594M mutation. Polymerase chain reaction was used to amplify part of the last exon of the epithelial sodium-channel subunit from genomic DNA. The T594M variant was observed using single-strand conformational polymorphism analysis of PCR products and was confirmed by DNA sequencing.

Results.—Seventeen of 206 (8.3%) hypertensive research subjects had the T594M variant, compared with 3 of 142 (2.1%) who were normotensive. Fifteen of the 17 hypertensive and all 3 normotensive research subjects with the T594M variant were female. Females comprised 61.2% and 57.7% of all hypertensive and normotensive research subjects, respectively. The correlation between the T594M variant and hypertension persisted after adjusting for sex and body-mass index. Plasma renin activity was significantly lower in the 13 research subjects who were hypertensive, compared with 39 untreated persons who were hypertensive and did not have the T594M variant (Fig 2).

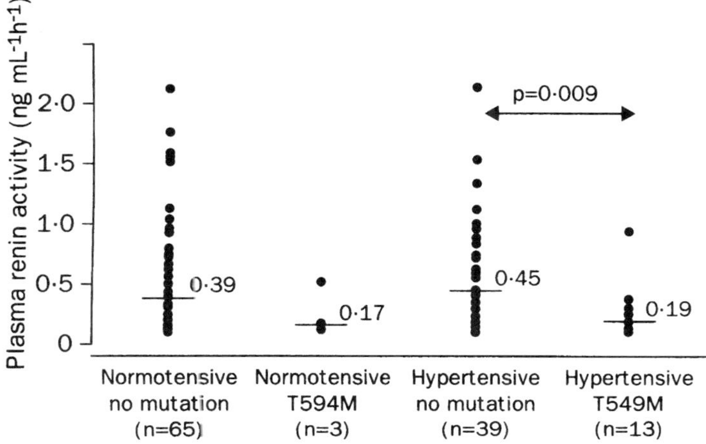

FIGURE 2.—Plasma renin activity in black normotensive and hypertensive individuals with and without T594M mutation. Individual values and median are shown. (Courtesy of Baker EH, Dong YB, Sagnella GA, et al: Association of hypertension with T594M mutation in β subunit of epithelial sodium channels in black people resident in London. *Lancet* 351:1388-1392, 1998. Copyright by The Lancet Ltd., 1998.)

Conclusion.—The T594M sodium-channel-subunit mutation in this series of London residents who were black occurred more frequently in persons with hypertension than in those who were normotensive. It is possible that the T594M variant raises sodium-channel activity and may increase blood pressure in affected persons by increasing renal tubular sodium reabsorption. The T594M variant may be the most frequently occurring secondary cause of essential hypertension in black people.

▶ As more rare monogenic forms of hypertension are recognized, there is a natural desire to identify lesser degrees of dysfunction from various mutations in a larger portion of the hypertensive population. As noted by Baker et al, clinical features of increased renal sodium reabsorption—the known mechanism for Liddle's syndrome involving mutations of subunits of the epithelial sodium channel—are also seen in black hypertensives.

Therefore, this finding of an almost 4 times higher prevalence of a mutation in the beta subunit among black hypertensives than in black normotensives is potentially of great significance. At the same time, no such mutations have been found in nonblack Scandinavian hypertensives.[1] Additional studies particularly in low-renin, volume expanded groups, are obviously needed.

N.M. Kaplan, M.D.

Reference

1. Melander O, Orho M, Fagerudd J, et al: Mutations and variants of the epithelial sodium channel gene in Liddle's syndrome and primary hypertension. *Hypertension* 31:1118-1124, 1998.

Prevention of Renovascular and Cardiac Pathophysiological Changes in Hypertension by Angiotensin II Type 1 Receptor Antisense Gene Therapy

Martens JR, Reaves PY, Lu D, et al (Univ of Florida, Gainesville; Univ of Alabama, Birmingham)
Proc Natl Acad Sci U S A 95:2664-2669, 1998

1–9

Background.—Although drug therapy can normalize elevated blood pressure, whether such normalization reverses the pathophysiologic changes caused by hypertension is less clear. Interruption of the renin-angiotensin system by blockade of angiotensin II type 1 (AT_1) receptors reduces blood pressure. Whether retroviral-mediated delivery of AT_1 receptor antisense (AT_1R-AS) can affect the development of hypertension and prevent other pathophysiologic changes associated with hypertension was studied in a rat model.

Methods.—The animals were 5-day-old spontaneously hypertensive (SH) rats as test subjects and Wistar Kyoto (WYK) rats as controls. The animals were divided into 3 groups. Group 1 received the vehicle alone (controls), group 2 received the retroviral vector alone (LNSV), and group 3 received the retroviral vector containing AT_1R-AS (LNSV-AT_1R-AS). Treatments were injected into the heart, with survival rates of about 95% at 48 hours after injection. Animals were killed 120 days after injection. Smooth muscle cells were isolated and prepared for current recording and analysis. The renal artery was isolated and its tension tested to determine renal vascular reactivity. Total heart and ventricular weights were determined to assess hypertrophy and perivascular fibrosis.

Findings.—At 120 days after injection, LNSV-AT_1R-AS prevented the increase in blood pressure in the SH rats. Blood pressures in groups 1 and 2 SH rats (mean 163.7 mm Hg) were significantly elevated compared with the groups 1 and 2 WYK rats. However, the mean blood pressure in group 3 SH rats (116.3 mm Hg) did not differ from that in normotensive WYK control rats (115.6 mm Hg). Group 3 SH rats had no changes in renal vascular reactivity, whereas the contractile responses to phenylephrine and potassium chloride were increased in the other SH rats. Similarly, the group 3 SH rats had normal vascular relaxation, whereas responses to acetylcholine were decreased in the other SH rats. The Kv current density in vascular smooth muscle cells from interlobar arteries was decreased in groups 1 and 2 SH rats, but not in group 3 SH rats. The SH rats in groups 1 and 2 had increased ventricular weights, multiple focal areas of cardiac fibrosis, and dense perivascular fibrosis in the small coronary arteries. The SH rats in group 3 showed none of these pathophysiologic changes.

Conclusions.—The increase in blood pressure typically seen in SH rats was prevented by LNSV-AT_1R-AS. Furthermore, the use of LNSV-AT_1R-AS prevented the hemodynamic and pathophysiologic changes of hypertension that were seen in other SH rats. Thus retroviral-mediated delivery of AT_1R-AS not only prevented the development of hypertension, it also prevented the pathophysiologic changes that hypertension induces, without increasing plasma levels of angiotensin II.

▶ It may be a long time before the findings reported in this hypertensive rat model are applied to alter the human condition. Nonetheless, these findings are an exciting application of the most advanced concepts of molecular biology, and regardless of their eventual applicability to human disease, they provide additional insights into the workings of the renin-angiotensin system.

All the known functions of the renin-angiotensin system appear to be mediated through the AT_1 receptor. Therefore, the ability to block this receptor over a long period by a single delivery of antisense opens an intriguing prospect for future experiments and possible clinical applications.

The broad effects seen on cardiac, vascular, and renal structures and functions by blockade of the AT_1 receptor document further the primary place of this receptor in both circulatory physiology and hypertensive pathophysiology.

N.M. Kaplan, M.D.

Contribution of Parental Blood Pressures to Association Between Low Birth Weight and Adult High Blood Pressure: Cross Sectional Study
Walker BR, McConnachie A, Noon JP, et al (Univ of Edinburgh, Scotland; Univ of Glasgow, Scotland)
BMJ 316:834-837, 1998   1–10

Introduction.—Recent epidemiologic studies in several countries report a relationship between low birth weight and increased blood pressure later in life. Because both birth weight and blood pressure are influenced by hereditary factors, the assessment of parental background is important. A cross-sectional study was designed to examine the potential contribution of parental blood pressure to the relation between low birth weight and subsequent hypertension.

Methods.—The study cohort was drawn from 603 families who received medical care at a primary care center in Edinburgh, Scotland. Blood pressure had been measured in adults in 1979 and in their young adult offspring in 1986. In 1994, all 603 mothers were asked to report the birth weight of their offspring; case records and replies from 398 mothers provided information for 545 offspring. Analyses were performed on data from 452 offspring, 1 selected at random from each family.

Results.—Blood pressure in young adult offspring was higher in men than in women and showed a positive correlation with current body weight. There was also an association between higher maternal or paternal systolic blood pressure and higher systolic blood pressure in their children and between higher maternal systolic blood pressure and lower birth weight in offspring. When parental blood pressures were not considered, a 1 kg decrease in birth weight was associated with a 2.24-mm Hg increase in systolic blood pressure of offspring. With correction for parental blood pressure, a 1-kg decrease in birth weight was associated with only a 1.71-mm Hg increase in systolic blood pressure.

Conclusion.—Findings suggest that low birth weight is one of the features of the inherited contribution to hypertension. Mothers with elevated blood pressure in later life have babies with lower birth weight, and these offspring also have higher blood pressures as they grow older.

▶ This is a lovely example of clinical research at its best. Using readily available data, a simple hypothesis has been easily documented, providing an original insight into our understanding of the pathogenesis of hypertension. The hypothesis was that both environmental and hereditary factors were responsible for the well-documented association between low birth weight and subsequent hypertension. Most investigators have assumed that the association was related to intra-uterine growth retardation, often from maternal malnutrition during the last trimester of pregnancy.[1]

The data in this paper document an additional contribution from heredity: those mothers with currently higher blood pressure had delivered smaller babies. Unfortunately, the mothers' blood pressure during pregnancy was not ascertained, but the authors quote a recent paper that found higher maternal blood pressure to be associated with lower birth weight.[2]

The data in this paper support a hereditary contribution to the subsequent hypertension in low–birth weight babies of about 25%, the remainder likely coming from intra-uterine growth retardation.

N.M. Kaplan, M.D.

References

1. Barker DJP: Fetal origins of coronary heart disease. *BMJ* 311:171-174, 1995.
2. Churchill D, Perry IJ, Beevers DG: Ambulatory blood pressure in pregnancy and fetal growth. *Lancet* 349:7-10, 1997.

Body Weight, Weight Change, and Risk for Hypertension in Women
Huang Z, Willett WC, Manson JE, et al (Harvard Med School, Boston)
Ann Intern Med 128:81-88, 1998   1–11

Objective.—The association between obesity and hypertension is well known, but the relation between changes in body mass index (BMI) and weight with age and the risk of hypertension have not been investigated.

Methods.—A cohort of 82,473 women, aged 30 to 55 years, without high blood pressure, were examined every 2 years from 1976 to 1992. The follow-up rate was 95%. Incident cases of hypertension were recorded. Age-adjusted and multivariate-adjusted relative risks for hypertension were calculated.

Results.—By 1992, 16,395 women had been diagnosed with hypertension. Higher current BMI and higher BMI at age 18 were strongly and

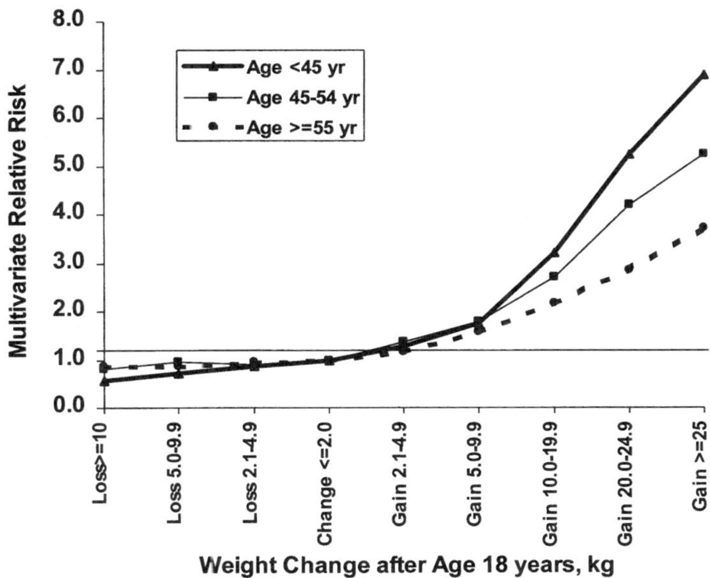

FIGURE 2.—Multivariate relative risk for hypertension according to weight change after age 18 years within strata of age. Adjusted for age, body mass index at age 18 years, height, family history of myocardial infarction, parity, oral contraceptive use, menopausal status, postmenopausal use of hormones, and smoking status. (Courtesy of Huang Z, Willett WC, Manson JE, et al: Body weight, weight change, and risk for hypertension in women. *Ann Intern Med* 128:81-88, 1998.)

independently associated with an increased risk for hypertension. An increase in current BMI of 1 kg/m^2 corresponded to a 12% increase in risk for hypertension, and an increase in BMI at age 18 of 1 kg/m^2 corresponded to an 8% increase in risk for hypertension. When current BMI was held constant, weight change after age 18 increased the relative risk of hypertension by 1.93, but weight loss decreased the risk by 15% for losses of 5.0 to 9.9 kg and by 26% for losses of 20 kg or more. Recent weight loss during midlife significantly lowered the risk of hypertension—24% for a loss of 5.0 to 9.9 kg, and 45% for a loss of 10 kg, or more—particularly when weight loss was maintained for at least 2 years. Weight change and risk for hypertension were related to age (Fig 2). Women with a BMI of less than 21 kg/m^2 in 1976 did not benefit from weight loss, but they increased their risk for hypertension if they gained weight. Women with a BMI of 25 kg/m^2 or more in 1976 dramatically lowered their risk for hypertension if they lost weight.

Conclusion.—Weight gain, even modest increases in midlife, substantially increases the risk for hypertension in women. Weight loss, particularly if sustained for 2 years or longer, dramatically lowers the risk for hypertension.

▶ Because more than half of all Americans are overweight[1] (often defined as a body weight 20 pounds or more above the ideal but more accurately as a BMI between 25 and 29.9), the marked increase in the incidence of hypertension observed with such relatively small amounts of weight gain after age 18 among this large group of women comes as a serious challenge. Once hypertension has been developed, we are currently able to adequately manage it in only 1 of 4 patients,[2] so prevention is obviously critical if we are ever going to be able to handle this most common risk factor for premature cardiovascular disease. But as we get fatter from richer diets and less physical activity, the prospects for meaningful prevention look increasingly dim.

N.M. Kaplan, M.D.

References

1. Flegal KM, Carroll MD, Kuczmarski RJ, et al: Overweight and obesity in the United States: Prevalence and trends, 1960-1994. *Int J Obes Relat Metab Disord* 22:39-47, 1998.
2. The sixth report of the Joint National Committee on detection, evaluation, and treatment of high blood pressure (JNC-VI). *Arch Intern Med* 157:2413-2446, 1997.

Increased Urinary Free Cortisol: A Potential Intermediate Phenotype of Essential Hypertension
Litchfield WR, Hunt SC, Jeunemaitre X, et al (Harvard Med School, Boston; Univ of Utah, Salt Lake City; Hosp Broussais, Paris)
Hypertension 31:569-574, 1998   1–12

Objective.—One of the recently recognized possible indicators of essential hypertension is the abnormal regulation or metabolism of cortisol. Urinary cortisol excretion was evaluated in a hypertensive population as a potential intermediate phenotype of essential hypertension. The influence of sodium intake and any sex-related differences on cortisol excretion were also investigated.

Methods.—Urinary free cortisol (UFC) excretion was measured in 153 white hypertensive patients (68 women) and 18 white controls (7 women) on a high-sodium (200 mmol/day) diet for at least 3 days and then on a low-sodium (10 mmol/day) diet for 7 days. Data were analyzed with respect to age, hypertension status, sex, and interaction of sex and hypertension status.

Results.—The hypertensive group was significantly older than the control group. The UFC was significantly higher in men than in women, and significantly higher for the high-sodium diet than for the low-sodium diet. Levels of UFC were significantly higher in men regardless of diet. Urinary free cortisol levels were higher in hypertensive patients receiving the high-sodium diet and significantly higher for hypertensive patients receiving the low-sodium diet. Levels of UFC were most strongly correlated with sex and blood pressure on the low-sodium diet. Urinary free cortisol levels had a bimodal distribution in hypertensive patients receiving both high- and low-sodium diets. The modal averages for the low-sodium UFC distribution were 127.2 and 224.3 nmol/day, and represented 68.8% and 31.2%, respectively, of hypertensive patients. Bimodality testing was not performed for controls. Change in systolic blood pressure was significantly negatively correlated with age and sex. In the low mode, UFC levels were similar in both groups receiving the low-sodium diet. Blood pressure was least sensitive to sodium level in individuals with the highest UFC.

Conclusions.—A subset of the hypertensive population, which may be as large as 30%, has increased UFC that may be genetic in origin.

▶ The observation that UFC levels are considerably above the normal range in 30% of hypertensive men on a high-sodium diet is provocative and potentially offers a new insight into the pathogenesis of another segment of the hypertensive population. The care taken by these investigators in studying a sizable population of both hypertensive men and women receiving both a low- and high-sodium diet is likely responsible for the uniqueness of the data. Whether this bimodal distribution of UFC connotes a new genetic mechanism or a heightened degree of sympathetic nervous activity as suggested by the authors remains to be seen. At the least, they give us all good warning in the proper collection and interpretation of urine steroid assays increasingly used in the clinical evaluation of Cushing's syndrome.

N.M. Kaplan, M.D.

Direct Evidence for the Importance of Endothelium-derived Nitric Oxide in Vascular Remodeling
Rudic RD, Shesely EG, Maeda N, et al (Yale Univ, New Haven, Conn; Henry Ford Hosp, Detroit; Univ of North Carolina, Chapel Hill)
J Clin Invest 101:731-736, 1998   1–13

Introduction.—Blood vessel architectural changes in response to hemodynamic conditions are mediated by the vascular endothelium. Although various vasoactive molecules and growth factors have been identified, the mechanisms of this effect are unclear. Nitric oxide (NO) has been implicated in this process, but there is no direct evidence to show that NO or any other endothelial-derived mediator is involved in vessel remodeling. The contribution of endothelial-derived NO as a mediator of vascular remodeling was studied in endothelial nitric oxide synthase (eNOS)-knockout mice.

Methods and Findings.—External carotid artery ligation was performed in mice with targeted disruption of the eNOS gene and in control wild-type mice. The wild-type mice showed vascular remodeling of the ipsilateral common carotid arteries, consisting of a decrease in luminal diameter. The eNOS-knockout mice, in contrast, had a paradoxical increase in vessel wall thickness induced by a hyperplastic response. This change occurred only in the vessel sensing a remodeling stimulus.

Conclusions.—In the animal model studied, endothelial-derived NO plays a critical role as a negative regulator of smooth muscle proliferation in response to a remodeling stimulus. Abnormal remodeling may arise from primary defects in the NOS/NO pathway. This abnormal response could lead to pathologic changes in the blood vessel wall, in association with such complex diseases as hypertension and atherosclerosis.

▶ As a long-time student of clinical hypertension, I have almost always avoided data from experimental animals, particularly hypertensive rats. I know that some data are only obtainable from such models, but I've always been leery of applying information from little rodents to big people.

The advent of genetically altered "knockout" mice has opened my mind for the acceptance of useful information that really cannot be obtained in any other way as of now. Smithies and co-workers are among the leaders in the use of this technique to study basic aspects of cardiovascular pathophysiology related to hypertension. This paper is another coup: the proof that vascular remodeling is dependent upon endothelium-derived NO. As the authors note, vascular remodeling is a critical response of the vessel wall to mechanical stress and injury. We will be learning more from these mice models, and the knowledge gained should soon be translated into clinical applications.

N.M. Kaplan, M.D.

Endothelial Dysfunction in Hypertension Is Independent From the Etiology and From Vascular Structure

Rizzoni D, Porteri E, Castellano M, et al (Univ of Brescia, Italy; Univ of Padua, Italy; Univ of Pisa, Italy)
Hypertension 31:335-341, 1998

1–14

Introduction.—Studies assessing the vasodilator response to acetylcholine have found an impairment of endothelial function in the small-resistance arteries among patients with essential and secondary hypertension. This endothelial dysfunction may involve vascular structural changes; animal studies suggest that endothelial dysfunction may be absent in the presence of early vascular structural alterations. Associations between endothelial function, small resistance artery structure, and blood pressure were studied in patients with primary or secondary hypertension.

Methods.—Nine patients with pheochromocytoma, 10 with primary aldosteronism, 17 with renovascular hypertension, 13 patients with essential hypertension, and 11 normotensive controls were studied. All patients had blood pressure measures obtained in the clinic and by 24-hour ambulatory blood pressure monitoring. A subcutaneous fat biopsy specimen was obtained in all individuals, from which small resistance arteries were dissected. These vessels were mounted on a micromyograph for calculation of the media/lumen ratio. The arterial response to acetylcholine was assessed at cumulative concentrations of 10^{-9} to 10^{-5} mol/L.

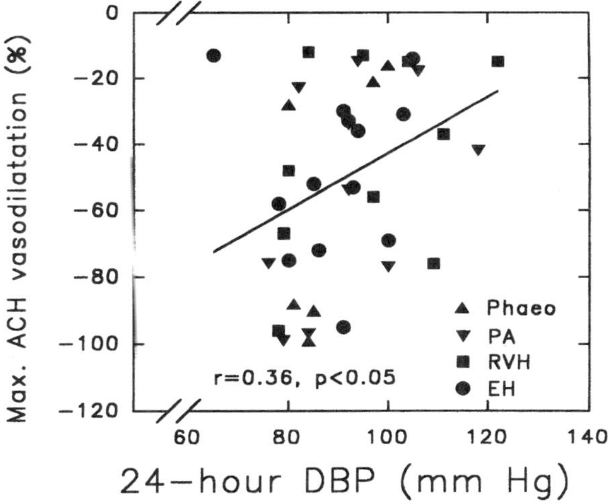

FIGURE 3.—Linear regression between maximum acetylcholine-induced vasodilatation (*Max. ACH vasodilatation*) and 24-hour diastolic blood pressure (*24-hour DBP*) in patients with pheochromocytoma (*filled triangles, up*), with primary aldosteronism (*filled triangles, down*), with renovascular hypertension (*filled squares*) as well as with essential hypertension (*filled circles*). The correlation coefficients in the whole group of hypertensive patients were 0.34 and 0.36, respectively (*P* < 0.05). If the normotensive subjects are included in the computation, the correlation coefficients are 0.47 and 0.48, respectively. (Courtesy of Rizzoni D, Porteri R, Castellano M, et al: Endothelial dysfunction in hypertension is independent from the etiology and from vascular structure. *Hypertension* 31:335-341. Copyright 1998, American Heart Association. Reproduced with permission.)

Results.—All 4 groups of patients with hypertension showed similar impairments of the vasodilator response to acetylcholine, compared with the normotensive controls. Subcutaneous arteries from patients with primary aldosteronism or renovascular hypertension showed a significantly increased media/lumen ratio. For patients with pheochromocytoma, the vascular structural alterations were comparable to those of patients with essential hypertension. The media/lumen ratio and clinical blood pressure measurements were unrelated to maximum acetylcholine-induced vasodilation. The ambulatory blood pressure measurements were significantly correlated with acetylcholine-induced vasodilation, but not very closely (Fig 3).

Conclusions.—The endothelial dysfunction observed in hypertension does not appear to be related to the extent of vascular structural changes or to the cause of hypertension, whether essential or secondary. Hemodynamic loading may have a more important impact on endothelial function in hypertension. More research is needed to determine which aspects of endothelial dysfunction are caused by hypertension, and which contribute to its pathogenesis.

▶ These data provide an interesting insight into the relationship between endothelial dysfunction, defined by the vasodilatory response to acetylcholine, and the presence of hypertension. Since the early 1990s, impaired endothelium-dependent dilation of the peripheral vasculature has been repeatedly found in patients with primary (essential) hypertension, and many have assumed that this impairment is a fundamental defect at least in part responsible for the elevation of blood pressure.

The data in this study involving patients with hypertension secondary to specific causes—excesses of renin, aldosterone, or catecholamines—suggest that the impaired endothelial function may not be primary but rather a secondary reaction to the hemodynamic load placed on the endothelium by the elevated blood pressure.

N.M. Kaplan, M.D.

Magnetic Resonance Evaluation of Ventrolateral Medullary Compression in Essential Hypertension

Colón GP, Quint DJ, Dickinson LD, et al (Univ of Michigan, Ann Arbor)
J Neurosurg 88:226-231, 1998   1–15

Objective.—Several reports have suggested neurovascular compression as a possible cause of hypertension. In particular, neurogenic hypertension may result from neurovascular compression near the ninth and tenth cranial nerve root entry zones and ventrolateral medulla. Magnetic resonance imaging may be a useful screening tool for identifying this patient subpopulation. The role of lateral medullary vascular compression as a cause of neurogenic hypertension was assessed by using MRI.

Methods.—Thin-slice axial brain stem MRI was performed in 30 patients with confirmed essential hypertension, as well as in 45 nonhypertensive patients undergoing MRI scanning for other reasons. The scans were reviewed in blinded fashion by 4 reviewers: 2 neuroradiologists and 2 neurosurgeons. The reviewers noted left vs. right vertebral artery (VA) dominance, medullary compression on the left vs. right side, and brain stem rotation. Medullary compression was defined as vessel contact with and without associated brain stem deformity.

Results.—Hypertensive patients tended to have left VA dominance, compared with the nonhypertensive controls. However, this difference was significant for only 1 of the 4 reviewers. The 2 groups had similar proportions of brain stem compression or rotation.

Conclusions.—In contrast to the results of previous studies using MRI or MR angiography, no significant difference in lateral brain stem vascular compression was demonstrated for patients with essential hypertension vs. those without. This is despite the tendency toward more left VA dominance in patients with hypertension. Neurogenic hypertension may still exist; however, it may not be reliably detected by thin-slice MRI scanning. Current neuroimaging techniques may overestimate the prevalence of neurovascular compression as a cause of hypertension.

▶ Since the Pittsburgh neurosurgeon P. J. Jannetta first proposed a causal connection between microvascular compression of the rostral ventrolateral medulla and hypertension (i.e., neurogenic hypertension), a number of reports have confirmed the anatomical association by MRI, and a number of others have denied the association using similar MRI technology. Better than most, this negative report involves a more carefully selected and larger population whose MRI study was performed in a manner to reduce possible bias.

The authors agree that neurovascular compression could be associated with hypertension but caution against using currently available MRI as an appropriate diagnostic tool. What is obviously essential is a properly controlled trial of decompression for the relief of hypertension. Until those data are available, caution is advised both in making the diagnosis and in operating for relief. Even without such data, medullary decompression is being performed for patients with poorly treated, uncontrolled hypertension,[1] a practice that I believe s premature and unwise.

N.M. Kaplan, M.D.

Reference

1. Geiger H, Naraghi R, Schobel HP, et al: Decrease of blood pressure by ventrolateral medullary decompression in essential hypertension. *Lancet* 352:446-449, 1998.

Complications

Hypertensive Vascular Disease as a Cause of Death in Blacks Versus Whites: Autopsy Findings in 587 Adults
Onwuanyi A, Hodges D, Avancha A, et al (Harlem Hosp Ctr, New York; Columbia Univ, New York)
Hypertension 31:1070-1076, 1998   1–16

Introduction.—For both blacks and whites in the United States, cardiovascular disease remains the leading cause of death, yet substantial differences between blacks and whites in cardiovascular disease mortality have been noted. Specific cardiovascular pathologic findings that underlie the racial differences described in mortality statistics could be found in autopsy; however, few autopsy studies addressing this issue have been conducted. The underlying pathologic causes of death in blacks and whites who died of cardiovascular disease have not been analyzed in existing autopsy studies. The hypothesis that hypertensive vascular disease contributes to cardiovascular mortality to a greater extent among blacks than whites was tested.

Methods.—In a retrospective study, 720 adult cases autopsied in 1991 in New York City in which the coded cause of death was cardiovascular disease were reviewed. The analysis included only 587 bodies (273 white, 314 black); the remainder were excluded for either missing a code for race, missing a code for gender, being extremely obese, or dying of an unusual circumstance. At time of death, black women were younger than white women (mean age, 54.7 vs. 61.5 years). There was no difference in mean age at death among black and white men.

TABLE 3.—Age-Adjusted Odds Ratios* and 95% Confidence Intervals for Black vs. White Autopsy and Clinical Causes of Death

| | Men | | Women | |
Cause of Death	Odds Ratio (95% Cl)	P	Odds Ratio (95% Cl)	P
Autopsy				
Atherosclerotic heart disease	0.4 (0.25-0.55)	<.001	0.4 (0.21-0.81)	<.01
Hypertensive vascular disease	2.2 (1.44-3.38)	<.001	3.1 (1.48-6.46)	<.01
Clinical				
Myocardial infarction	0.5 (0.24-0.88)	<.05	0.2 (0.06-0.91)	<.05
Sudden cardiac death	0.9 (0.56-1.38)	NS	2.1 (0.89-5.01)	NS
Congestive heart failure	1.2 (0.66-2.28)	NS	1.2 (0.34-4.33)	NS

*Age-adjusted odds ratios are derived from logistic regression analysis in which age and specific cause of death are entered simultaneously.

(Courtesy of Onwuanyi A, Hodges D, Avancha A, et al: Hypertensive vascular disease as a cause of death in black versus whites: Autopsy findings in 587 adults. *Hypertension* 31:1070-1076, 1998. Reproduced with permission. *Hypertension* copyright 1998, American Heart Association.)

Results.—In 42% of blacks, hypertensive vascular disease was the autopsy cause of death compared with 23% of whites. The autopsy cause of death in 64% of white subjects was atherosclerotic heart disease, which was found in only 38% of blacks. In both sexes, and after adjustment for age, these patterns were still consistent. For hypertensive vascular disease as the autopsy cause of death, the age-adjusted odds ratio for blacks vs. whites was 2.2 among men and 3.1 among women (Table 3).

Conclusion.—Among blacks in New York City, hypertensive vascular disease was far more common than atherosclerotic heart disease as the cause of death compared with whites. Whites commonly had more atherosclerotic heart disease than blacks. A major factor contributing to increased cardiovascular mortality among urban blacks may be ineffective control of hypertension.

▶ Hypertension clearly causes more morbidity and mortality among blacks than whites in the United States and elsewhere. Much of that increase reflects their lesser access to adequate health care as almost certainly was true in the population served by Harlem Hospital in New York City described in this article.

In addition, hypertension is often more severe in blacks, and their blood pressure often does not go down during the night; that is, they are often nondippers. This, in turn, is associated with more left ventricular hypertrophy and all the excess risk that accompanies LVH.[1]

When socioeconomic factors are comparable, blacks and whites appear to have similar rates of developing hypertension[2] and, in a number of clinical trials, when they are equally treated, they achieve comparable degrees of protection.

N.M. Kaplan, M.D.

References

1. Mayet J, Chapman N, K-C Li, et al: Ethnic differences in the hypertensive heart and 24-hour blood pressure profile. *Hypertension* 31:1190-1194, 1998.
2. He J, Klag MJ, Appel LJ, et al: Seven-year incidence of hypertension in a cohort of middle-aged African Americans and whites. *Hypertension* 31:1130-1135, 1998.

Structural Abnormalities and Not Diastolic Dysfunction Are the Earliest Left Ventricular Changes in Hypertension

Palatini P, and the HARVEST Study Group (Clinica Medica 1, Padova, Italy)
Am J Hypertens 11:147-154, 1998   1–17

Objective.—Although it has been suggested that diastolic dysfunction is the earliest cardiac abnormality in hypertension, few echocardiographic studies have been done in young individuals with borderline to mild hypertension. Left ventricular (LV) filling properties and morphological measurements of hypertensive individuals were compared with those of age-matched controls subjects.

Methods.—Standard EKG, M-mode and 2D echocardiography, blood chemistry, and urinalysis were performed in 722 patients (189 women), aged 18 to 45 years, with stage I hypertension and 95 age- and sex-matched control subjects (24 women). Blood pressure was recorded using 24-hour ambulatory monitoring.

Results.—Left ventricular wall thickness and left ventricular mass index were significantly larger in hypertensive individuals than in controls (1.88 vs. 1.70 cm and 92.2 vs. 81.8 g/m², respectively). Although the maximum velocity at atrial LV diastolic filling (AV_{max}) was higher in hypertensive patients than in control subjects, the ratio of early diastolic filling to atrial filling (E/A) for the hypertensive group was similar to the control group. Compared with the control group, significant changes were noted as follows: LV mass increased 10.4 g/m², LV wall thickness increased 1.8 mm, and relative wall thickness increased 0.032 mm. Atrial filling peak velocity was slightly higher in hypertensive patients than in control subjects. According to multiple regression analysis, 24-hour mean blood pressure was a significant predictor of LV mass index and wall thickness for both men and women with hypertension.

Conclusion.—The earliest cardiac changes in hypertension are an increase in LV wall thickness and mass. LV filling is affected only to a small extent.

▶ Conventional teaching has long held that the earliest cardiac response to an elevated blood pressure is diastolic dysfunction or stiffness—a reduction in filling rates as represented by the peak velocity of early to atrial filling, that is, a lower E/A ratio and prolongation of relaxation times. Structural changes were thought to come later.

The difference between this study and the numerous earlier studies likely reflects the fact that this study involved only young, untreated mild hypertensives rather than older, treated, more severe hypertensives. Therefore, this study is likely correct as to the early changes, particularly because it involved over 700 subjects.

N.M. Kaplan, M.D.

Homogeneously Reduced Versus Regionally Impaired Myocardial Blood Flow in Hypertensive Patients: Two Different Patterns of Myocardial Perfusion Associated With Degree of Hypertrophy
Gimelli A, Schneider-Eicke J, Neglia D, et al (Univ of Pisa, Italy)
J Am Coll Cardiol 31:366-373, 1998   1–18

Purpose.—There is ongoing debate regarding the impact of left ventricular hypertrophy on regional coronary vasodilation among patients with arterial hypertension. Impaired coronary flow reserve is not necessarily related to the existence or extent of left ventricular hypertrophy; however, this correlation has never been quantitatively assessed. The correlation between regional and global myocardial blood flow and left ventricular mass was studied in hypertensive patients free of coronary artery disease.

Methods.—Fifty patients with newly diagnosed, mild-to-moderate arterial hypertension, but without coronary artery disease, were studied. Thirteen normotensive individuals were studied for comparison. Positron emission tomography was performed to measure blood flow at baseline and after administration of dipyridamole, with global and regional measurements obtained by using nitrogen-13 ammonia. These data were used to calculate coronary reserve and resistance. In addition, 2-dimensional echocardiography was performed to measure left ventricular mass.

Results.—There was no difference in baseline flow between hypertensive and control patients. However, flow values in the hypertensive group were reduced after pharmacologic vasodilation. The hypertension-associated impairment in maximal coronary flow was unrelated to left ventricular mass. Some of the hypertensive patients showed a homogeneous distribution of perfusion, which was associated with global reduction of flow. The remaining patients in the hypertensive group showed a heterogeneous flow pattern; this group had abnormal flow only at the site of perfusion defects. Increased left ventricular mass was most likely to be found in patients with regional flow defects.

Conclusions.—No correlation was found between left ventricular mass and global myocardial blood flow among patients with arterial hypertension. However, the presence of ventricular hypertrophy was associated with a heterogeneous flow pattern, characterized by regional flow defects with near-normal flow in unaffected regions. Those hypertensive patients with a homogeneous distribution of perfusion under stress are likely to show a global reduction of myocardial blood flow. The findings may provide insight into the increased incidence of sudden myocardial death and arrhythmias among patients with hypertension and myocardial hypertrophy.

▶ Left ventricular hypertrophy (LVH) is a well-recognized complication of hypertension which, in turn, is associated with the increased risk of sudden death, congestive heart failure, and coronary ischemia. All of these complications may be related to an inability of the hypertrophied myocardium to vasodilate adequately n response to increased demands for cardiac output, i.e., reduced coronary reserve.

These data provide additional evidence of the underlying hemodynamic consequences of LVH. They display both a homogenous and a heterogeneous pattern of reduced perfusion. The failure to show a statistically significant correlation between LV mass and reduced maximal coronary flow may reflect the relatively small number of patients in the study. As noted in the "Discussion" section of the original article by Gimelli et al., most of the published studies on the relation between LVH and coronary reserve have involved few patients, and even fewer provide prognostic follow-up data. Obviously, there is more to be learned about hypertensive LVH.

N.M. Kaplan, M.D.

Prognostic Value of a New Electrocardiographic Method for Diagnosis of Left Ventricular Hypertrophy in Essential Hypertension
Verdecchia P, Schillaci G, Borgioni C, et al (Ospedale R Silvestrini, Perugia, Italy; Ospedale Beato Giacomo Villa, Città della Pieve, Italy)
J Am Coll Cardiol 31:383-390, 1998   1–19

Introduction.—A standard ECG is routinely performed in patients with essential hypertension for the detection of left ventricular hypertrophy (LVH). Various ECG methods for detection of LVH are clinically used. The Perugia score is a new method, based on the sum of the amplitudes of the S wave on lead V_3 and the R wave on lead aVL (greater than 2.4 mV in men or 2.0 mV in women); the presence of left ventricular strain; or a Romhilt-Estes score of 5 points or greater. The Perugia score was compared prospectively with standard methods of diagnosis of LVH in essential hypertension.

Methods.—A total of 1,717 white hypertensive patients from a prospective registry of cardiovascular morbidity and mortality were studied. Fifty-one percent of the patients were men; the mean age was 52 years. The patients were followed for up to 10 years, with a mean follow-up of 3 years. The prognostic value of the Perugia score was compared with that of 5 standard methods: Cornell voltage, the Framingham criterion, the Romhilt-Estes point score, left ventricular strain, and Sokolow-Lyon voltage.

Results.—The baseline prevalence of LVH was 18% by the Perugia score, 9% by Cornell voltage, 4% by the Framingham criterion, 5% by the Romhilt-Estes point score, 6% by left ventricular strain, and 13% by Sokolow-Lyon voltage. The patients had a total of 159 major events of cardiovascular morbidity, 33 of which were fatal. By all methods except the Sokolow-Lyon voltage, the rate of major events was higher for patients

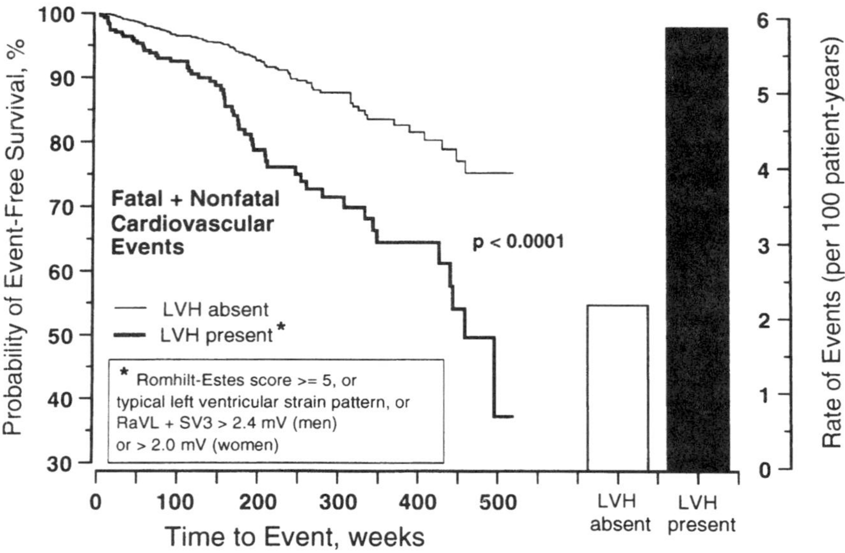

FIGURE 1.—Event-free survival curves for total cardiovascular events (**left**) in the study cohort grouped by the presence or absence of left ventricular hypertrophy (*LVH*) according to the Perugia score. The rate of major cardiovascular morbid events (**right**) was significantly higher in the subset with LVH. (Courtesy of Verdecchia P, Schillaci G, Borgioni C, et al: Prognostic value of a new electrocardiographic method for diagnosis of left ventricular hypertrophy in essential hypertension. *J Am Coll Cardiol* 31:383-390, 1998. Reprinted with permission from the American College of Cardiology.)

with vs. without LVH (Fig 1). On multivariate analysis, hazard ratios for cardiovascular disease risk were 2.04 for the Perugia score, 1.91 for the Framingham criterion, 2.63 for the Romhilt-Estes point score, and 2.11 for the left ventricular strain method. Population-attributable risk for cardiovascular events was 16% with the Perugia score, compared with 3% for the Framingham criterion, 7% for the Romhilt-Estes point score, and 7% for the left ventricular strain method. Hazard ratio for cardiovascular mortality among patients with LVH diagnosed by the Perugia score was 4.21, with a population-attributable risk of 37%.

Conclusions.—In patients with essential hypertension, the Perugia score for diagnosis of LVH is associated with a higher population-attributable risk for cardiovascular morbidity and mortality than standard diagnostic methods. Traditional interpretations of the standard ECG continue to play an important role in cardiovascular risk stratification for patients with essential hypertension. Prognostic validation will be needed to determine the role of sophisticated new computer-assisted ECG analysis techniques.

▶ After all of these years, the discovery of a better way to recognize clinically significant LVH by ECG comes as a surprise to this noncardiologist. I guess it proves that even well-established procedures can be improved upon, so that fresh looks at old precepts are often productive.

The considerably greater sensitivity in detecting LVH and the greater prognostic value of the Perugia score have been derived from a large database and a long follow-up. Therefore, all who use and interpret ECGs should be aware of these data. As the authors note, they were obtained in an all-white population so they may not apply to other racial groups. Moreover, computer-assisted calculations of the 12-lead voltage duration product[1] may prove to be even more accurate in detecting LVH, but that technique needs prognostic validation.

N.M. Kaplan, M.D.

Reference

1. Okin PM, Romar MJ, Devereaux RB, et al: Time-voltage area of the QRS for the identification of left ventricular hypertrophy. *Hypertension* 26:251-258, 1996.

Prognostic Significance of Serial Changes in Left Ventricular Mass in Essential Hypertension
Verdecchia P, Schillaci G, Borgioni C, et al (Ospedale Generale Regionale R Silvestrini, Perugia, Ita y; Ospedale Beato G Villa, Città della Pieve, Italy; DIMISEM Università di Perugia, Italy)
Circulation 97:48-54, 1998   1–20

Objective.—In patients with hypertension, increasing left ventricular (LV) mass increases the risk for cardiovascular disease. Whether the reverse is true has not been studied. The prognostic significance of serial changes in LV mass in patients being treated for hypertension was evaluated prospectively.

Methods.—Blood pressure (24-hour ambulatory BP) was measured and echocardiography and ECG were performed in 430 hypertensive patients (54% men), whose average age was 48 years, before therapy and at subsequent follow-up visits. The average follow-up was 2.8 years. Cardiovascular morbid events were recorded. The relationship between cardiovascular events and LV mass was compared statistically.

Results.—The LV mass index was more strongly correlated with average 24-hour ambulatory BP than with clinic BP. During the follow-up period, BP and LV mass were significantly reduced, whereas body weight, body mass index, total and high-density lipoprotein cholesterol, and serum creatinine were slightly but significantly increased. There were 31 nonfatal cardiovascular events during the 1,367 person-years of observation, 15 (1.78/100 person-years) in the group with decreased LV mass, and 16 (3.03/100 person-years) in the group with increased LV mass. In the Cox regression model, the former group had a significantly lower risk (odds ratio, 0.46) of a cardiovascular event even after adjustment for age. Multivariate analysis showed that patients with a LV mass of greater than 125 g/m² at baseline whose LV mass declined during follow-up had a significantly lower cardiovascular event rate than those whose LV mass did not decline (1.58 vs. 6.27 events per 100 person-years) (Fig 3).

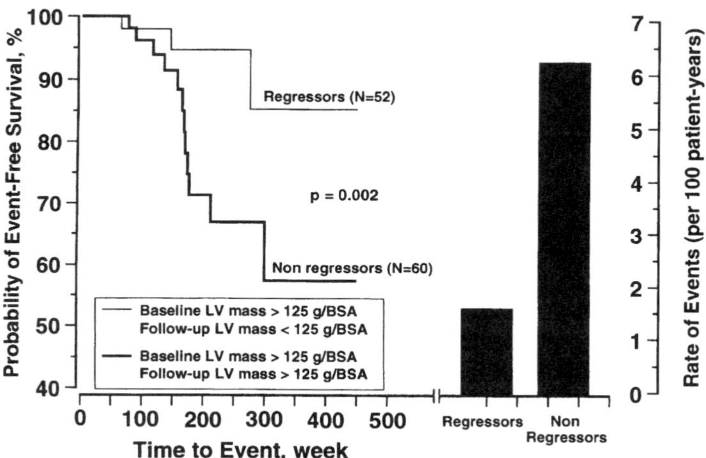

FIGURE 3.—Event rate in subset with echocardiographic left ventricular hypertrophy (LVH) at baseline visit. *Survival curves* differed between those with regression (*thin line*) or persistence (*thick line*) of LVH at follow-up visit. *Abbreviation: BSA*, body surface area. (Courtesy of Verdecchia P, Schillaci G, Borgioni C, et al: Prognostic significance of serial changes in left ventricular mass in essential hypertension. *Circulation* 97:48-54. Copyright 1998, American Heart Association. Reproduced with permission.)

Conclusions.—Hypertensive patients whose LV mass declines during treatment have a better cardiovascular risk profile than patients whose LV mass does not decrease. The relationship holds regardless of baseline LV mass, clinic and ambulatory BP, and reduction in BP.

▶ This is the largest follow-up of the prognostic significance of changes in LV mass as determined by echocardiography. A prior publication from Framingham showed an improved prognosis for cardiovascular disease with decreases in LV mass by ECG[1] but, as reconfirmed in this paper by Verdecchia et al., ECG is a much less sensitive indicator for increased LV mass as is commonly noted by echocardiography in hypertensives.

These data are only among the earliest to be presented. Many large-scale, long-term studies are evaluating the value of echo-determined regression of LV hypertrophy so that clinical judgments as to its overall value will become increasingly easier. For now, most expert groups[2] do not recommend echocardiography, even the less-expensive, limited procedure that some utilize, for routine evaluation and follow-up of hypertensive patients. With more such data as in this paper, our position may change and echocardiography may replace ECG as a routine part of the hypertensive evaluation and follow-up.

N.M. Kaplan, M.D.

References

1. Levy D, Salomon M, D'Agostino RB, et al: Prognostic implications of baseline electrocardiographic features and their serial changes in subjects with left ventricular hypertrophy. *Circulation* 90:1786-1793, 1994.

2. Joint National Committee: The sixth report of the Joint National Committee on Detection, Evaluation and Treatment of High Blood Pressure (JNC-VI). *Arch Intern Med* 157:2413-2446, 1997.

Heterogeneous Vasomotor Responses of Coronary Conduit and Resistance Vessels in Hypertension

Houghton JL, Davison CA, Kuhner PA, et al (State Univ of New York, Albany; Augusta Preventive Cardiology, Ga)
J Am Coll Cardiol 31:374-382, 1998   1–21

Objective.—Little information is available about the relation between conduit and resistance vasomotor function in contiguous human coronary vessels. The relation between conductance and resistance coronary vasomotor responses to the endothelium-dependent agonist, acetylcholine (ACh), in hypertensive patients with and without left ventricular hypertrophy (LVH) and in normotensive controls was investigated.

Methods.—Left ventricular mass, coronary flow, and endothelium-independent coronary vascular relaxation were measured in 98 individuals (46 men) without evidence of coronary artery disease. Invasive coronary angiography was performed under baseline conditions and at the end of each graded infusion of ACh. Quantitative coronary angiography was performed, and coronary artery blood flow was calculated.

Results.—There were 31 normotensive individuals, 28 with hypertension but no LVH, and 39 with hypertension and LVH. Patients with hypertrophy were more likely to be female, obese, and older. The increase in coronary blood flow in response to adenosine was significantly depressed in hypertensive individuals with LVH compared with normotensive individuals and hypertensive individuals without LVH (169% vs. 234% vs. 232%, respectively). Whereas the increase in coronary blood flow in response to ACh was similar for normotensive individuals and for individuals with hypertension without LVH, blood flow was significantly constricted in hypertensive individuals with LVH (Fig 1). The correlation coefficients for conduit and resistance artery responses to ACh were $r = 0.73$ for the 31 normotensive individuals, $r = 0.5$ for 28 hypertensive individuals without LVH, and $r = 0.38$ for 39 hypertensive individuals with LVH.

Conclusions.—Although normotensive individuals and hypertensive individuals had no evidence of coronary artery disease, they demonstrated heterogeneous vasomotor responses in both conduit and resistance coronary vessels. The response to ACh was a significantly constricted blood flow for hypertensive patients with LVH.

▶ The general applicability of these findings in 98 patients who had cardiac catheterization for chest pain to the larger population of hypertensives is obviously uncertain. Nonetheless, these patients were found to have normal-looking coronary arteries, presumably representing the "cardiac syn-

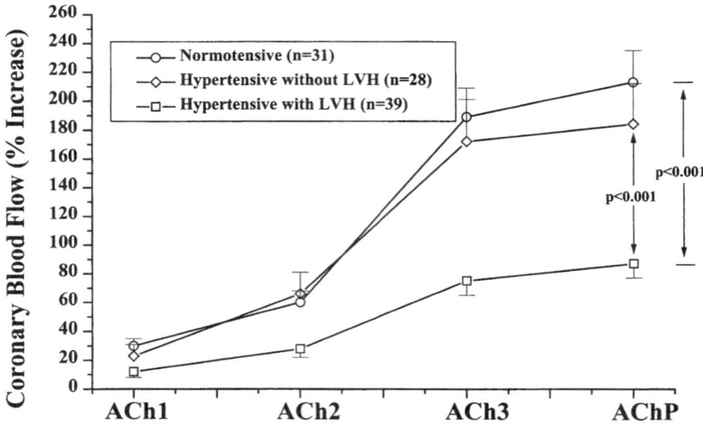

FIGURE 1.—Percent increase in coronary blood flow above baseline in response to graded intracoronary infusion of the endothelium-dependent agent acetylcholine (*ACh*) in 31 normotensive patients, 28 hypertensive patients without left ventricular hypertrophy (*LVH*) and 39 hypertensive patients with LVH. Data are expressed as mean value ± SE. *ACh1*, acetylcholine infusion rate of 0.15 µg/min; *ACh2*, 1.5 µg/min; *ACh3*, 15 µg/min; *AChP*, peak response to ACh infusion rates of 15 or 30 µg/min. (Courtesy of Houghton JL, Davison CA, Kuhner PA, et al: Heterogeneous vasomotor responses of coronary conduit and resistance vessels in hypertension. *J Am Coll Cardiol* 31:374-382, 1998. Reprinted with permission from the American College of Cardiology.)

drome X" in many of them, a syndrome previously shown to involve abnormal coronary vascular reserve or vasodilatory capacity.

The major finding is reflected in Figure 1: a marked attenuation of the ACh-provoked increase in coronary blood flow in those hypertensives with LVH compared with both normotensive and hypertensive patients without LVH.

N.M. Kaplan, M.D.

Hypertension Is Related to Cognitive Impairment: A 20-Year Follow-up of 999 Men

Kilander L, Nyman H, Boberg M, et al (Karolinska Hosp, Stockholm)
Hypertension 31:780-786, 1998   1–22

Background.—The significance of cognitive deterioration with aging—whether it is an inevitable part of the aging process or an early stage of dementia—is a topic of ongoing debate. Recent studies have shown an association between hypertension and later onset of dementia. These findings have focused attention on the possibility of cerebral target-organ damage in hypertension, and the concept of "preventable senility." The effects of hypertension, circadian blood pressure (BP) profile, and disturbances of glucose and lipid metabolism on cognitive function in elderly men were studied.

Methods.—The population-based cohort study included 999 men, aged 70 years, who had been followed up for cardiovascular risk factors since

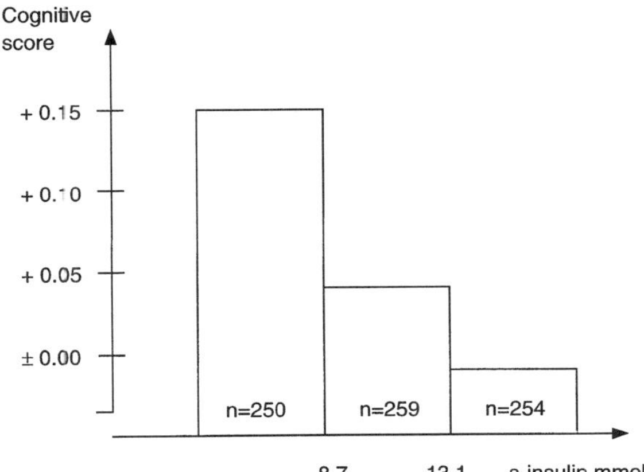

FIGURE 1.—Tertiles of serum insulin at age 50 years relative to cognitive score 20 years later. Cognitive score in tertile 1 vs. tertile 3, analysis of covariance (ANCOVA): P^1 (adjusted for age, education, occupation) = 0.031; P^2 (as P^1 + diastolic blood pressure at age 50) = 0.145. (Courtesy of Kilander L, Nyman H, Boberg M, et al: Hypertension is related to cognitive impairment: A 20-year follow-up of 999 men. *Hypertension* 31:780-786. Copyright 1998, American Heart Association. Reproduced with permission.)

age 50 years. All patients underwent 20-hour ambulatory BP monitoring. Also measured were insulin sensitivity, glucose tolerance, serum lipids, and lipoproteins. The effects of these variables on cognitive function—as assessed by the Mini-Mental State Examination and Trail-Making Test—were analyzed.

Results.—Diastolic blood pressure (DBP) at baseline was inversely related to cognitive performance at follow-up. Men with a baseline DBP of 70 mm Hg or lower had the best cognitive function at age 70 years, whereas those with a baseline DBP of 105 mm Hg or greater had the poorest cognitive results at follow-up (Fig 1). Cross-sectional factors related to low cognitive function were high 24-hour BP, a "nondipping" BP profile, insulin resistance, and diabetes. Men not receiving antihypertensive therapy showed the strongest relationship between high BP and cognitive impairment.

Conclusions.—The findings of this longitudinal, population-based study strengthen the hypothesis that cerebral target-organ damage caused by high BP plays a role in cognitive deterioration with aging. The next step is to determine whether more aggressive treatment of vascular risk factors can prevent further cognitive decline. Antihypertensive drug treatments that preserve the normal 24-hour BP profile and do not have metabolic side effects should be preferred for use in elderly patients.

▶ The beauty of this study is the careful 20-year follow-up of almost 1,000 men, providing the best evidence now available for an association between cognitive impairment and a variety of possible contributing factors.

Not surprisingly, the level of DBP showed the strongest correlation but, surprisingly, isolated systolic hypertension was not related to impaired cognition at 70 years of age. The need to look for and to control insulin resistance and resultant hyperinsulinemia is documented by the relationship shown in Figure 1.

Obviously, everything possible to prevent age-related impairment of cognitive function should be provided to the rapidly growing elderly population. Control of hypertension must be at the top of the list, particularly because it has been shown to prevent dementia.[1]

N.M. Kaplan, M.D.

Reference

1. Forette FA, Seux ML, Thijs L, et al: Antihypertensive treatment and prevention of dementia in older patients with isolated systolic hypertension: The SYST-Eur results. *J Hypertens* 16:22S, 1998.

Nondrug Therapy

Sodium Reduction and Weight Loss in the Treatment of Hypertension in Older Persons: A Randomized Controlled Trial on Nonpharmacologic Interventions in the Elderly (TONE)
Whelton PK, for the TONE Collaborative Research Group (Tulane Univ, New Orleans, La; Johns Hopkins Univ, Baltimore, Md; Wake Forest Univ, Winston-Salem, NC; et al)
JAMA 279:839-846, 1998

1–23

Background.—Nonpharmacologic treatments are often recommended to treat hypertension in the elderly. However, there is little evidence from randomized controlled trials to support this recommendation. The current study assessed the efficacy of weight loss or decreased sodium intake in elderly persons with hypertension.

Methods.—Nine hundred seventy-five men and women, aged 60 to 80, were enrolled in the study. All had systolic blood pressure lower than 145 mm Hg and a diastolic pressure lower than 85 mm Hg while taking a single antihypertensive medication. Five hundred eighty-five obese persons were randomly assigned to reduced sodium intake, weight loss, both, or usual care. The 390 nonobese participants were randomly assigned to decreased sodium intake or usual care. After 3 months, antihypertensive medication withdrawal was attempted. Main outcome measures were diagnosis of high blood pressure at 1 or more follow-up visits, treatment with antihypertensive agents, or a cardiovascular event during the 15- to 36-month follow-up.

Findings.—The combined outcome measure occurred less frequently among participants assigned to decreased sodium intake compared with those not assigned to this intervention, as well as in obese patients assigned to weight loss compared with obese patients not assigned to weight loss. Compared with usual care, reduced sodium intake alone was associated with a 0.60 hazard ratio among obese subjects; weight loss alone, 0.64; and decreased sodium intake and weight loss combined, 0.47. The frequency of cardiovascular events during follow-up was comparable in all intervention groups.

Conclusions.—Decreased sodium intake and weight loss is a safe, effective nonpharmacologic treatment for hypertension in the elderly. These findings are consistent with a large body of observational evidence.

▶ This is truly a landmark study. First, it involved a large group of older hypertensive patients, the largest population of patients who must be treated. Second, it chose a clear experimental design: return of hypertension or development of cardiovascular events after cessation of minimal but successful antihypertensive drug therapy. Third, it used the two lifestyle changes—dietary sodium restriction and weight reduction—that are most likely to be needed and to succeed. Fourth, it followed the subjects for a meaningful 30 months.

The results are striking. Despite only relatively small decreases in sodium intake and weight, there was almost a 3-fold increase in the percentage of patients who remained free of hypertension or cardiovascular events among those who followed both lifestyle changes compared to those who did nothing (usual care).

Let those who ascribe putative dangers to moderate sodium restriction or who deny the potential benefit from even small changes in lifestyle pay attention. The efforts are well worth the trouble.

N.M. Kaplan, M.D.

Dietary Sodium Intake and Mortality: The National Health and Nutrition Examination Survey (NHANES I)
Alderman MH, Cohen H, Madhavan S (Albert Einstein College of Med, Bronx, NY)
Lancet 351:781-785, 1998   1–24

Purpose.—A large body of data suggests that reducing the amount of sodium in the diet can reduce blood pressure. However, there is little evidence to show that restriction of dietary sodium reduces morbidity or mortality. The effects of dietary sodium on mortality were assessed in a general population sample.

Methods.—The study was based on a representative sample of 20,729 U.S. adults, aged 25 to 75 years, from the first National Health and Nutrition Examination Survey. Baseline data were collected on these individuals between 1971 and 1975. A total of 11,348 individuals underwent medical examination and nutritional investigation, based on 24-hour recall. Information on sodium intake was available for all individuals but 2. The individuals were followed up for vital status through 1992. The mortality effects of sodium intake, caloric intake, and sodium/calorie ratio were assessed in sex-specific quartiles.

Results.—At follow-up, 3,923 individuals had died, 1,970 of cardiovascular disease (CVD). Age- and sex-adjusted all-cause mortality was inversely related to sodium intake, decreasing from 23/1,000 person-years in the lowest quartile of sodium intake to 19/1,000 in the highest quartile. Mortality was also inversely related to total calorie intake, decreasing from 25/1,000 to 18/1,000 from the lowest to the highest quartile. There was also a weak positive association between all-cause mortality and sodium/calorie ratio, from 20/1,000 to 22/1,000. A similar pattern was noted for CVD mortality, which decreased from 12/1,000 to 10/1,000 from the lowest to highest quartile of sodium intake and from 13/1,000 to 9/1,000 from the lowest to highest quartile of caloric intake, while increasing from 10/1,000 to 11/1,000 from the lowest to highest quartile of sodium/calorie ratio.

On multiple regression analysis, an inverse association was noted between sodium intake and all-cause and CVD mortality. There was also a direct relationship between sodium/calorie ratio and all-cause and CVD mortality. Caloric intake was not independently related to mortality, after adjustment for sodium intake and sodium/calorie ratio. Similar conclusions were reached when the analysis was restricted to individuals with no baseline history of CVD.

Conclusions.—Dietary sodium intake is inversely associated with all-cause and CVD mortality, and dietary sodium/calorie ratio is directly associated with both mortality rates. Although small, these associations are significant and independent. The findings do not support current recommendations to reduce dietary sodium, nor any other dietary recommendation. If there is a relationship between sodium intake and survival, it is not a simple one, and it must be considered in context of the total diet.

▶ A great deal of controversy arose in the lay press when this paper was published because it was used as a direct attack on the virtually universal recommendation to restrict sodium intake moderately both to treat established hypertension and, even more importantly, to prevent its development. The evidence is exceedingly strong that the current level of sodium intake is excessive, well beyond any physiologic need, and almost certainly a necessary component of the pathogenesis of hypertension. Moreover, moderate sodium restriction lowers blood pressure and, as beautifully shown in the TONE study (Abstract 1–23), reduces the onset of cardiovascular events. Therefore, the findings reported by Alderman et al. must be carefully considered before accepting them at face value.

First, there are multiple methodological problems: the estimate of sodium and caloric intake was a single-day dietary recall, of questionable accuracy because the body weight was identical in those men who supposedly consumed 1,473 calories per day (lowest quintile) as those who consumed 2,937 calories per day (highest quintile); the blood pressure was recorded 1 time; and those in the lowest quintile of dietary sodium intake (estimated as only 678 mg/day in women and only 1,041 mg/day in men) were older, more likely to be black, hypertensive, and to have preexisting CVD—all features that would lead to higher all-cause and cardiovascular mortality.

Second, the inverse association between mortality and daily caloric intake was even more statistically significant than was the association with sodium intake, which goes against a great deal of evidence that longevity is prolonged by lower caloric intake. Lastly, when sodium per calorie, likely the most meaningful index of intake, was examined, there was a progressive direct increase in mortality the higher the sodium per calorie, not the reverse seen with sodium or calories alone. Alderman and co-workers are to be congratulated for examining an important issue that certainly has not received enough attention. But, the overwhelming epidemiologic, experimental, and clinical evidence now available favors moderate sodium restriction.

N.M. Kaplan, M.D.

Effects of Sodium Restriction on Blood Pressure, Renin, Aldosterone, Catecholamines, Cholesterols, and Triglyceride: A Meta-analysis
Graudal NA, Galløe AM, Garred P (Univ of Copenhagen)
JAMA 279:1383-1391, 1998   1–25

Purpose.—There is a long history of debate regarding the effects of sodium intake on blood pressure. One issue of contention is whether a reduction in sodium intake in the population can reduce blood pressure and thus reduce the number of strokes and myocardial infarctions. Recent studies have suggested that sodium restriction may even have adverse effects. In this meta-analysis, the effects of sodium restriction on blood pressure and other variables were evaluated, as well as the apparent stability of the effect size of reduced sodium intake on blood pressure.

Methods.—A total of 58 trials in which hypertensive patients were randomly assigned to high- and low-sodium diets were analyzed. The studies had a median duration of 28 days. Also included were 56 trials of normotensive individuals, with a median duration of 8 days. Each trial evaluated at least 1 of the following outcome measures: systolic and diastolic blood pressure, body weight, or plasma or serum levels of renin, aldosterone, catecholamines, cholesterols, and triglyceride.

Results.—In the studies of hypertensive patients, mean urinary sodium excretion on the low-sodium diets was 118 mmol per 24 hours. Reduction in sodium intake reduces systolic blood pressure by a mean of 3.9 mm Hg and diastolic blood pressure by 1.9 mm Hg. In the studies of normotensive individuals, mean urinary sodium excretion on the low-sodium diets was 160 mmol per 24 hours; systolic blood pressure was reduced by 1.2 mm Hg and diastolic blood pressure by 0.26 mm Hg. On cumulative meta-analysis, the size of this effect had remained stable since 1985. Sodium restriction was associated with a 3.6-fold increase in plasma renin level and a 3.2-fold increase in plasma aldosterone level; these decreases occurred in proportion to the degree of sodium reduction. Sodium restriction was also associated with a significant reduction in body weight, and significant increases in noradrenaline, cholesterol, and low-density lipoprotein cholesterol. Adrenaline, triglyceride, and high-density lipoprotein cholesterol levels were unaffected.

Conclusions.—Meta-analysis of the effects of low-sodium diets on blood pressure and other parameters does not support general recommendations for reduced sodium intake. Sodium restriction may be a useful part of treatment for hypertension; however, the effect of reduced sodium intake on blood pressure in randomized trials has been consistent since 1985. Sodium restriction also has short-term effects on hormones and lipid profile, the persistence and clinical significance of which are unknown. Long-term trials assessing such end points as stroke, acute myocardial infarction, and survival are needed to settle the debate regarding the influence of sodium on blood pressure.

▶ This paper was authored by immunologists who obviously do not understand clinical medicine. They focus on short (as little as 4-day) studies that examined the effects of very rigid (as little as 10 mmol/day) sodium restriction on blood pressure and various hormones and lipids. To infer that the effects of moderate sodium restriction over many months are in any way comparable to these explosive short-term aberrations is pure nonsense.

The danger, of course, is that patients and the general public and unknowing physicians will accept these abrupt aberrations and deny the benefits of moderate sodium restriction. Along with the flawed data of Alderman et al.,[1] who reported an increase in coronary events with either a lower sodium or caloric intake, based on a highly inaccurate 1-day dietary recall (Abstract 1–24) such reports tend to get a lot of publicity fueled by press releases from the Salt Institute lobby.

There is absolutely no question that moderate sodium restriction is both safe and effective (Abstract 1–23) in lowering elevated blood pressure.[2] We do not know whether such moderation will prevent hypertension, but there is no reason not to try.

N.M. Kaplan, M.D.

References

1. Alderman MH, Cohen H, Madhavan S: Dietary sodium intake and mortality: The National Health and Nutrition Examination Survey (NHANES I). *Lancet* 351:781-785, 1998.
2. Whelton PK, Appel LJ, Espeland MA, et al: Sodium reduction and weight loss in the treatment of hypertension in older persons. *JAMA* 279: 839-846, 1998.

Salt Sensitivity Is Associated With Insulin Resistance in Essential Hypertension
Fuenmayor N, Moreira E, Cubeddu LX (Central Univ of Venezuela, Caracas)
Am J Hypertens 11:397-402, 1998   1–26

Introduction.—Insulin resistance has been linked to abnormal responses to dietary salt. Depending on their response to salt, patients with essential hypertension may be classified as salt sensitive or salt resistant. The evidence suggests a possible relationship between insulin resistance and salt-sensitive hypertension. This relationship was assessed in patients with untreated essential hypertension.

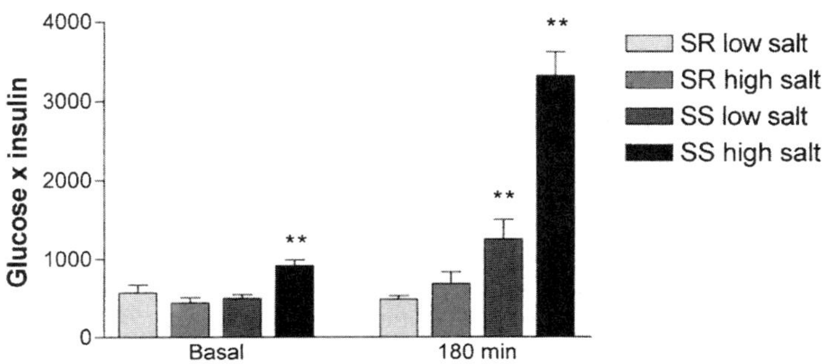

FIGURE 3.—Differences in the product glucose times insulin concentrations during the insulin suppression test, in salt sensitive (SS) and salt resistant (SR) hypertensive patients under low and high salt intake. Shown are mean values ± SEM of the product glucose times insulin concentrations at 180 minutes (steady state) during the insulin suppression test. SS high salt values were significantly different from other basal values at $P < 0.01$. *SS low salt and SS high salt were significantly different from their respective basal values and from other steady state values at $P < 0.01$. (Reprinted by permission of Elsevier Science Inc. from Fuenmayor N, Moreira E, Cubeddu LX: Salt sensitivity is associated with insulin resistance in essential hypertension. *Am J Hypertens* 11:397-402. Copyright 1998 by American Journal of Hypertension Ltd.)

Methods.—The study included 16 patients with mild to moderate, untreated, uncomplicated essential hypertension. All patients were nonobese, that is, body mass index of no higher than 28, and nondiabetic. Eight patients were classified as salt sensitive and 8 as salt resistant based on their blood pressure response to low- and high-salt intake (40-60 and 240 mEq/day, respectively). Each patient underwent an insulin suppression test to measure insulin-mediated glucose suppression.

Results.—The 2 groups were similar in their fasting serum glucose levels. In the salt-sensitive group, a high-salt intake was associated with a rise in fasting serum insulin levels. The insulin suppression test showed markedly higher steady-state glucose values in salt-sensitive patients than in salt-resistant patients. In the salt-sensitive group, the product of glucose times insulin at steady state was 2.5 times higher during low-salt intake and 5 times higher during high-salt intake, compared with the salt-resistant group (Fig 3). Salt-sensitive patients had impaired insulin-mediated glucose disposal during both low- and high-salt intake, although it was worse during high-salt intake.

Conclusions.—Hypertension in salt-sensitive patients is associated with insulin resistance causing impairment of insulin-mediated glucose disposal. In salt-sensitive patients, but not salt-resistant patients, high-salt intake leads to increased blood pressure, induced hyperinsulinemia, and worsening of insulin-mediated glucose disposal. Thus, salt sensitivity apparently makes a separate contribution to insulin resistance and acts as an additional cardiovascular disease risk factor.

▶ Insulin resistance with resultant hyperinsulinemia is commonly seen in hypertensives, in virtually all who are obese, and in about one third of those who are not obese. The association is largely related to excessive body fat, particularly when predominately visceral or abdominal in location, but goes beyond that alone.[1] Among patients with impaired glucose tolerance, hyperinsulinemia preceded the onset of hypertension,[2] suggesting a causal connection. This is further supported by the finding of insulin resistance in still normotensive children of hypertensive parents.[3]

The results of the study by Fuenmayor et al suggest yet another connection: insulin resistance was only found in the nonobese hypertensives who were also salt sensitive, that is, those subjects whose blood pressure went up on a high sodium intake. As the authors note: "Salt sensitivity and insulin resistance may be genetically determined and may cosegregate in genetically hypertensive-susceptible men" (and women). At least the data support the idea that the lowering of blood pressure by moderate sodium restriction may involve an improvement in insulin sensitivity.

N.M. Kaplan, M.D.

References

1. Donahue RP, Prineas RJ, Bean JA, et al. The relation of fasting insulin to blood pressure in a multiethnic population: The Miami community health study. *Ann Epidemiol* 8:236-244, 1998.
2. Qiao Q, Rajala U, Keinanen-Kiukaanniemi S: Hypertension, hyperinsulinaemia and obesity in middle-aged Finns with impaired glucose tolerance. *J Human Hypertens* 12:265-269, 1998.
3. Mattiasson I, Endre T, Berglund G, et al: Insulin sensitivity, sodium-lithium countertransport and platelet free calcium concentrations in normotensive men with a family history of hypertension. *J Human Hypertens* 12:259-264, 1998.

Ethanol Suppresses Smooth Muscle Cell Proliferation in the Postprandial State: A New Antiatherosclerotic Mechanism of Ethanol?

Locher R, Suter PM, Vetter W (Univ Hosp, Zürich, Switzerland)
Am J Clin Nutr 67:338-341, 1998   1–27

Objective.—Drinking alcohol in moderation may reduce cardiovascular risk, recent epidemiologic studies have suggested. However, the mechanism of this effect is unclear—it may involve increased high-density lipoprotein (HDL) cholesterol or changes in fibrinolytic activity. The effects of ethanol in postprandial plasma on smooth muscle cell (SMC) proliferation were studied in vitro.

Methods.—Healthy young men were given identical test meals containing 1 g/kg of fat, either with or without 38 g of ethanol—equivalent to about 2 glasses of wine or 3 cans of beer. During the 8 hours after this meal, hourly blood samples were obtained. The plasma from these samples was then separated and added to rat SMC cultures, 0.3% by volume. The SMC proliferative response to plasma was measured via incorporation of [methyl-^{3}H]thymidine.

Results.—The volunteers' blood ethanol concentration peaked at 11.5 mmol/L within the first hour after the test meal. Postprandial plasma from the ethanol group showed a 20% reduction in its capacity to induce thymidine incorporation into SMCs, compared with plasma from the nonethanol group.

Conclusions.—Drinking alcohol with meals reduces the stimulatory effect of postprandial plasma on SMC proliferation. Thus, the benefits of ethanol in reducing cardiovascular risk may arise from modulation of postprandial vascular muscle cell growth. Given the time spent in the postprandial state during a lifetime, these findings have important implications for the pathogenesis of atherosclerosis.

▶ These data provide another explanation for what has repeatedly been shown: a cardioprotective effect of small amounts of ethanol consumed on a regular repetitive basis. The recent paper by Thun et al. is perhaps the strongest of all because the size of the population was more than 500,000 and the duration of follow-up was long.[1]

In addition to the findings reported there, the manner by which small amounts of ethanol protect against coronary disease almost certainly involves increases n HDL-cholesterol.[2] Regardless of how it happens, it's a happy consequence of a pleasant habit. Women need drink as little as one half the usual portion per day to gain full cardioprotection with no significant increase in the incidence of breast cancer.[3] Of course, those who drink too much, more than 2 portions per day, may have more hypertension and develop even more left ventricular hypertrophy than those who drink in moderation.[4]

N.M. Kaplan, M.D.

References

1. Thun MJ, Peto R, Lopez AD, et al: Alcohol consumption and mortality among middle-aged and elderly U.S. adults. *N Engl J Med* 337:1705-1714, 1997.
2. McConnell MV, Vavouranakis I, Wu LL, et al: Effects of a single, daily alcohol beverage on lipid and hemostatic markers of cardiovascular risk. *Am J Cardiol* 80:1226-1228, 1997.
3. Smith-Warner S, Spiegelman D, Yaun S-S, et al: Alcohol and breast cancer in women. *JAMA* 279:535-539, 1998.
4. Ishimitsu T, Yoshida K, Nakamura M, et al: Effects of alcohol intake on organ injuries in normotensive and hypertensive human subjects. *Clin Sci* 93:541-547, 1997.

Effect on Blood Pressure of Potassium, Calcium, and Magnesium in Women With Low Habitual Intake

Sacks FM, Willett WC, Smith A, et al (Harvard Med School, Boston)
Hypertension 31:131-138, 1998   1–28

Objective.—Whereas potassium, calcium, and magnesium are associated with lower blood pressure, studies have failed to confirm their blood pressure–lowering potential in normotensive individuals. The hypothesis that normotensive individuals with low intake of these minerals have an enhanced response to mineral supplements was tested by giving supplements to participants in the Nurses Health Study II who habitually had low intakes of these minerals.

Methods.—Daily supplements of either 40 mmol of potassium, 30 mmol of calcium, 14 mmol of magnesium, all 3, or placebo were administered to a randomized, parallel group of 321 normotensive women for 16 weeks. Baseline and 16-week 24-hour ambulatory blood pressures and dietary mineral intakes were measured and compared between groups.

Results.—Three hundred women, with an average age of 39 years, completed the study. Potassium, magnesium, and calcium intakes rose from the 10th, 17th, and 10th percentiles, respectively, at baseline to the 90th, 95th, and greater than the 95th percentile at the end of the study. Baseline average 24-hour systolic and diastolic blood pressures were 116 and 73 mm Hg, respectively. The potassium group had a significant decrease of 2 mm Hg in systolic blood pressure compared with the placebo group. There were no significant changes in the calcium or magnesium groups.

Conclusions.—Potassium supplementation has a small but significant blood pressure–lowering effect in normotensive women with low dietary mineral intake.

▶ These data add to an already impressive and convincing number of carefully controlled observations that make these points: potassium supplements will usually lower the blood pressure, but neither calcium nor magnesium supplements will have an effect. These data suggest that the latter supplements are ineffective, even in individuals who are ingesting relatively small amounts of them in their natural diet.

Potassium supplements are too expensive to be used for either prevention or treatment of hypertension. Fortunately, consumption of natural foods— virtually all high in potassium and low in sodium—rather than artificially processed foods—virtually all altered by the addition of sodium and the removal of potassium—will provide the extra benefit of potassium supplements.[1]

There may be a benefit to calcium supplements in preventing preeclampsia in women who have a very low calcium intake as has been reported from developing countries.[2] No such benefit has been seen among women in the United States.[3]

N.M. Kaplan, M.D.

References

1. Appel LJ, for the DASH Collaborative Research Group: A clinical trial of the effects of dietary patterns on blood pressure. *N Engl J Med* 336:1117-1124, 1997.
2. Bucher HC, Guyatt GH, Cook RJ, et al: Effect of calcium supplementation on pregnancy-induced hypertension and pre-eclampsia. *JAMA* 275:1113-1117, 1996.
3. Levine RJ, Hauth JC, Curet LB, et al: Trial of calcium to prevent preeclampsia. *N Engl J Med* 337:69-76, 1997.

Vitamin C Improves Endothelium-Dependent Vasodilation by Restoring Nitric Oxide Activity in Essential Hypertension

Taddei S, Virdis A, Ghiadoni L, et al (Univ of Pisa, Italy)
Circulation 97:2222-2229, 1998

1–29

Background.—Patients with essential hypertension may demonstrate impairment of endothelium-dependent vasodilation. Experimental models of hypertension suggest that this endothelial dysfunction involves oxygen free-radical inactivation of endothelium-derived nitric oxide (NO). The effects of treatment with vitamin C, an antioxidant, on endothelial responses were assessed in patients with essential hypertension.

Methods.—The study included 14 patients with essential hypertension aged a mean of 47 years, with mean blood pressure 154/102 mm Hg and 14 healthy control subjects. All patients underwent forearm blood flow measurements using strain-gauge plethysmography to assess responses to acetylcholine or sodium nitroprusside, which are endothelium-dependent and endothelium-independent vasodilators, respectively. Both vasodilators were administered intrabrachially in a range of doses. Measurements were performed once under control conditions and once during intrabrachial infusion of vitamin C, 2.4 mg per 100 mL of forearm tissue per minute. Additional hypertensive patients were studied to assess responses to the NO synthase inhibitor N^G-monomethyl-L-arginine and the cyclooxygenase inhibitor indomethacin.

Results.—In the patients with essential hypertension, the vasodilatory impairment in response to acetylcholine was impaired during vitamin C infusion, while the response to sodium nitroprusside was unaffected. This change was not observed in the control subjects. N^G-monomethyl-L-arginine reversed the effect of vitamin C on the vasodilatory response to acetylcholine, consistent with superoxide anion impairment of endothelium-dependent vasodilation via NO breakdown. Indomethacin prevented the potentiating effect of vitamin C on vasodilation to acetylcholine, suggesting that the cyclooxygenase pathway could be an important source of superoxide anions in patients with hypertension.

Conclusions.—Vitamin C can improve the impaired endothelial vasodilation function observed in patients with essential hypertension. This effect is reversed by treatment with N^G-monomethyl-L-arginine, a NO synthase inhibitor. In patients with essential hypertension, endothelial dysfunction may be related to NO inactivation by oxygen-free radicals.

▶ It would be lovely if not even megadoses of vitamin C could improve endothelial function in "real life." Obviously, these short-term findings, as impressive as they are, do not document any clinical benefits of vitamin C or any other antioxidant. As the authors note, large scale randomized controlled trials are in progress (including another involving physicians in which the author is enrolled). For now, extra vitamin E seems to be worthwhile because it is hard to get from foods. And its likely that a little folic acid will reduce elevated homocysteine levels, but as to vitamin C—let's wait for the evidence.

N.M. Kaplan, M.D.

Drug Therapy

Mortality Rates in Treated Hypertensive Men With Additional Risk Factors Are High But Can Be Reduced: A Randomized Intervention Study
Fagerberg B, for the Risk Factor Intervention Study Group (Göteborg Univ, Gothenburg, Sweden; Lund Univ, Malmö, Sweden)
Am J Hypertens 11:14-22, 1998   1–30

Purpose.—For patients with hypertension, the presence of concomitant risk factors—i.e., hypercholesterolemia, diabetes mellitus, and smoking—substantially increases cardiovascular disease risk. Thus, multifactorial risk factor intervention programs have been proposed. Previous studies of these interventions have not clearly shown that they can reduce risk factors while improving prognosis. The effects of a multifactorial risk factor intervention program for hypertensive patients at high cardiovascular risk were examined.

Methods.—Participants were 508 men, aged 50 to 72 years, receiving treatment for hypertension. All patients had at least 1 additional risk factor: serum cholesterol concentration of 7.5 mmol/L or greater, diabetes mellitus, or smoking. They were randomly assigned to receive either the multifactorial risk factor intervention or usual care. Patients in the intervention group attended group meetings directed at encouraging a lipid-lowering diet and smoking cessation. For patients in whom nonpharmacologic measures were insufficient, drug therapy with cholestyramine, nicotinic acid, fibrates, and/or statin drugs was given according to agreed-on guidelines. Diabetic patients were taught glucose self-monitoring. The patients were followed up for a median of 6.6 years.

Results.—At follow-up, 25% of patients in the usual care group vs. 16% of those in the intervention group had died (Fig 2). The study intervention was associated with a 44% reduction in the risk of cardiovascular death (95% confidence interval, relative risk 0.42-0.92). Overall risk of fatal and nonfatal cardiovascular events was reduced by 29% in the intervention group. Compared with the usual care group, serum total cholesterol was 6.3% lower in the intervention group; low-density lipoprotein cholesterol was 9.1% lower, and blood glucose level was 0.2 mmol/L lower. Three-year smoking cessation rate, adjusted for serum cotinine, was 28% in the intervention group vs. 11% in the usual care group.

Conclusions.—Even with good blood pressure control, cardiovascular risk remains high for hypertensive patients with concomitant risk factors. However, a multifactorial intervention approach can improve the prognosis for this group of patients. The authors believe their good results can be attributed to the entire multiple risk approach, emphasizing education in a healthier lifestyle.

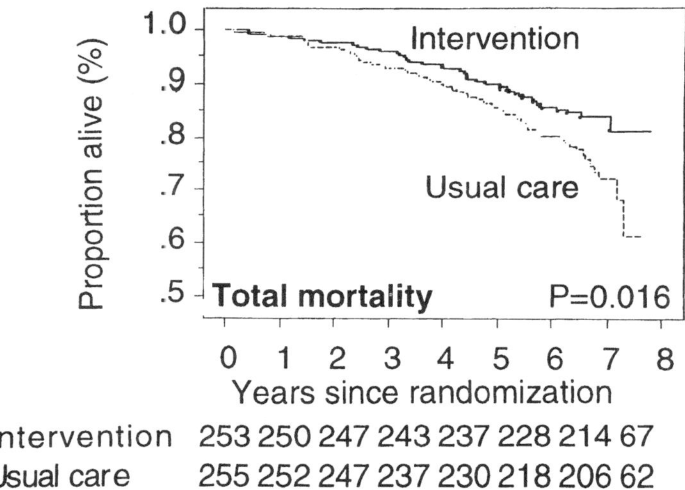

FIGURE 2.—Kaplan-Meier curve for total mortality. Number of patients at risk at the beginning of each year is given for the intervention and usual care groups, respectively. (Courtesy of Fagerberg B, for the Risk Factor Intervention Study Group: Mortality rates in treated hypertensive men with additional risk factors are high but can be reduced: A randomized intervention study. *Am J Hypertens* 11:14-22. Copyright 1998, by American Journal of Hypertension, Inc. Reprinted by permission of Elsevier Science Inc.)

► These results may not seem so surprising, but they are among the best to document the ability to keep high-risk patients alive by a multifactorial but practical intervention program. In view of the striking benefits recently reported for statin therapy in multiple large populations, the greater use of these and other lipid-lowering agents may explain most of the protection, and the greater rate of smoking cessation likely contributed.

It should also be noted that most of these hypertensives continued to receive diuretics and β-blockers to control their blood pressure. Whatever metabolic mischief that might have been stirred up by those drugs was obviously overcome by the multiple interventions that are appropriate for a modern risk-reduction program.

N.M. Kaplan, M.D.

Effects of Intensive Blood-Pressure Lowering and Low-Dose Aspirin in Patients With Hypertension: Prinicipal Results of the Hypertension Optimal Treatment (HOT) Randomised Trial

Hansson L, for the HOT Study Group (Univ of Uppsala, Sweden; Università di Milano, Italy; Univ of Western Ontario, London; et al)
Lancet 351:1755-1762. 1998   1–31

Objective.—Even with treatment, patients with hypertension are at elevated risk of cardiovascular complications, compared with normotensive individuals. One probable reason is inadequate blood pressure reduction; however, the optimal target blood pressure is unknown. There are no data on the possible health benefits of aspirin for patients with hypertension. The Hypertension Optimal Treatment (HOT) Study sought to determine the optimal target blood pressure for patients with hypertension, and to assess the benefits of low-dose aspirin for these patients.

Methods.—A toal of 18,790 hypertensive patients from 26 countries were studied. Mean age was 61.5 years; diastolic blood pressure was between 100 and 115 mm Hg. The patients were randomly assigned to a target diastolic pressure of 90 mm Hg or less, 85 mm Hg or less, or 80 mm Hg or less. Antihypertensive therapy started with the long-acting calcium antagonist felodipine, with other agents added as needed, according to a 5-step protocol. The patients were also randomly assigned to receive aspirin, 75 mg/day, or placebo.

Results.—The lower the target blood pressure, the greater the blood pressure reduction achieved: 20.3 mm Hg in the 90 mm Hg or less group, 22.3 mm Hg in the 85 mm Hg or less group, and 24.3 mm Hg in the 80 mm Hg or less group. The mean diastolic blood pressure associated with the lowest major cardiac event rate was 82.6 mm Hg; the blood pressure with the lowest rate of cardiovascular mortality was 86.5 mm Hg. Blood pressure could be reduced even further without adverse effects. For patients with diabetes mellitus, the major cardiovascular event rate was more than 50% lower in the 80 mm Hg or less group than in the 90 mm Hg or less group.

Patients receiving aspirin had a 15% reduction in the rate of major cardiovascular events, and a 36% reduction in myocardial infarction rate. The risk of stroke was unaffected. The risk of fatal bleeding episodes was similar in the aspirin and placebo groups. However, the aspirin group had more than double the rate of nonfatal major bleeding episodes.

Conclusions.—Intensive blood pressure reduction lowers the risk of cardiovascular events and cardiovascular death among patients with hypertension. The results demonstrate the benefits of reducing diastolic blood pressure to 82.6 mm Hg or lower. Blood pressure reduction has especially important benefits for diabetic patients. Low-dose aspirin treatment for hypertensive patients also reduces the risk of major cardiovascular events, particularly myocardial infarction. As long as blood pressure is well controlled and the associated risk of bleeding is assessed, aspirin therapy is recommended for patients receiving antihypertensive treatment.

▶ As I noted in an editorial that accompanied this paper, the results of the HOT Study are both a triumph and a disappointment. The disappointment comes from the failure to answer the primary goal of the study: the existence of a J-curve, the increase in mortality from coronary ischemia as pressure is reduced below some critical level needed to maintain myocardial perfusion. This failure is a consequence of the minimal differences in blood pressure achieved in the 3 groups, differences less than half of those intended. Nonetheless, the HOT results show no rise in morbidity or mortality below the "best" blood pressure—138/83 mm Hg. On the other hand, no further decrease in events was noted in those with blood pressure below

138/83, so that there seems no justification for more aggressive therapy in most patients because both costs and side effects would increase if more therapy was given.

Some patients likely need more therapy to reach lower goals. As recommended in the sixth report of the Joint National Committee and documented in the HOT data, diabetic hypertensives need even greater reductions of blood pressure, certainly well below 140/90 to be maximally protected. Patients with renal insufficiency or heart failure similarly need more aggressive therapy.

The triumph of the HOT study was the ability to lower diastolic blood pressure by more than 20 mm Hg in most of the patients, considerably more than achieved in previous trials. The lower rates of cardiovascular events certainly must reflect the greater degree of blood pressure reduction.

Although no breakdown of events by the type of drug is given in this first report of the HOT data, the fact that 78% of the patients continued to receive the primary drug felodipine, a dihydropyridine calcium antagonist (CA), should put the final nail in the coffin of those who have preached about multiple dangers of such drugs. In particular, the remarkable protection noted among the 1,500 diabetics in the HOT trial with a dihydropyridine CA should allay any concerns about the use of these drugs in diabetic hypertensives as raised in the ABCD[1] and FACET[2] studies. The final line about diabetic hypertensives is: ACE inhibitors are best but CAs are safe and, if needed to lower the blood pressure, definitely indicated.

Lastly, the protection against myocardial infarction by 75 mg of aspirin supports the use of this agent in well-controlled hypertensives. Caution is still needed in those who remain poorly controlled.

N.M. Kaplan, M.D.

References

1. Estacio RO, Jeffers BW, Hiran WR, et al: The effect of nisoldipine as compared with enalapril on cardiovascular outcomes in patients with non-insulin dependent diabetes and hypertension. *N Engl J Med* 338:645-652, 1998.
2. Tatti P, Pahor M, Byington RP, et al: Outcome results of the fosinopril versus amlodpine cardiovascular events randomised trial (FACET) in patients with hypertension and NIDDM. *Diabetes Care* 21:597-560, 1998.

Effect of Treatment of Isolated Systolic Hypertension on Left Ventricular Mass
Ofili EO, Cohen JD, St Vrain JA, et al (Morehouse School of Medicine, Atlanta, Ga; St Louis Univ; Ohio State Univ, Columbus)
JAMA 279:778-780, 1998   1–32

Objective.—Whereas there is a high prevalence of left ventricular (LV) hypertrophy in elderly individuals with isolated systolic hypertension (ISH), the effect of treatment on LV mass in such patients is unknown. The long-term effects of treatment with antihypertensive drugs on echocardiographic LV mass in an elderly cohort were reported.

Methods.—Either placebo or chlorthalidone (12.5-25 mg/day) was administered to 104 hypertensive patients, aged 60 years or older, in the Systolic Hypertension in the Elderly Program (SHEP). Atenolol (25-50 mg/day) was administered to patients in the treatment group who were unable to attain the target systolic blood pressure of 140 to 159 mm Hg. Echocardiography was used to monitor changes in LV mass during the minimum 3-year follow-up period.

Results.—There were 47 patients in the treatment group and 47 in the placebo group available for follow-up at 3 years. At 1 and 3 years, 91% and 80%, respectively, of patients in the treatment group were receiving chlorthalidone. Compared with the placebo group, treatment group systolic (144 vs. 163 mm Hg) and diastolic (62 vs. 75 mm Hg) blood pressures were significantly reduced throughout the study period. Left ventricular mass index and ventricular septal thickness were significantly lower in the treatment group compared with measurements in the placebo group (93 vs. 110 g/m^2 and 1.02 vs. 1.17 cm, respectively). In the treatment group, LV mass index decreased significantly by 13% and ventricular septal thickness was lower than baseline values, whereas in the placebo group, LV mass index increased by 6% and septal wall thickness increased compared with baseline values.

Conclusions.—Antihypertensive treatment with chlorthalidone significantly lowers systolic blood pressure and LV mass in elderly patients with ISH.

► Left ventricular hypertrophy (LVH) has long been recognized as a strong and independent risk factor for cardiovascular disease. Regression of LVH is increasingly being considered as a useful though surrogate end point for successful antihypertensive therapy. Although reduction of blood pressure clearly remains the best index of success, a concomitant regression of LVH is an attractive extra attraction.

The ability of diuretics to achieve equal degrees of LVH regression as other drugs has been questioned. In one of the better meta-analyses, the overall impact of angiotensin-converting enzyme (ACE) inhibitors and calcium antagonists was portrayed as superior to diuretics.[1] On the other hand, the only currently available head-to-head comparison between all 5 major classes of drugs, the Treatment of Mild Hypertension Study (TOMHS), found equal regression with all 5.[2] However, the degree of initial LVH among the TOMHS participants was so minimal that the degree of regression with all agents was quite small.

The results reported among the SHEP patients are more impressive, documenting an almost 20% difference between placebo and a low dose of diuretic. Once again, diuretics look terrific.

N.M. Kaplan, M.D.

References

1. Gottdiener JS, Reda DJ, Massie BM, et al: Effect of single-drug therapy on reduction of left ventricular mass in mild to moderate hypertension. *Circulation* 95:2007-2014, 1997.
2. Liebson PR, Grandits GA, Dianzumba S, et al: Comparison of 5 antihypertensive monotherapies and placebo for change in left ventricular mass in patients receiving nutritional-hygienic therapy in the Treatment of Mild Hypertension Study (TOMHS). *Circulation* 91:698-706, 1995.

Treatment of Diastolic Dysfunction in Hypertensive Patients Without Left Ventricular Hypertrophy

Molinero E, Murga N, Sagastagoitia JD (Basurto Hosp, Bilbao)
J Hum Hypertens 12:21-27, 1998   1–33

Objective.—In patients with hypertension, diastolic dysfunction develops before left ventricular hypertrophy (LVH). A number of different treatments have been used in an attempt to correct these diastolic abnormalities, on the belief that restoring normal physiologic heart conditions will be of benefit to the patient. Verapamil and the combination of amiloride and hydrochlorothiazide were compared for their effects on diastolic dysfunction in patients with hypertension who have not yet developed LVH.

Methods.—The study included 26 patients with hypertension who had diastolic dysfunction but normal systolic function and no LVH. After a 2-week washout period, the patients were randomized to receive 6 months of treatment with verapamil SR, 240 mg/day; or a combination of amiloride, 5 mg/day. plus hydrochlorothiazide, 50 mg/day. Follow-up Doppler echocardiograms were performed at 4, 12, and 24 weeks to assess left ventricular volumes and systolic and diastolic function.

Results.—Both treatments provided good control of blood pressure. Patients receiving verapamil had significant improvement in diastolic function. This group showed a tendency toward reduction in peak A and toward an increased peak E/A ratio, with a significantly reduced deceleration time. Diastolic function was unchanged in patients receiving amiloride plus hydrochlorothiazide. By the 24-week follow-up, left ventricular wall thickness was significantly reduced in the verapamil group, compared with the combination therapy group.

Conclusions.—In hypertensive patients, treatment with verapamil can improve ventricular diastolic function, whereas the combination of amiloride and hydrochlorothiazide does not. Verapamil treatment leads to a reduction in left ventricular wall thickness, even in patients without LVH. Larger studies are needed to confirm these findings.

▶ As noted in Abstract 1–17 (Palatini), diastolic dysfunction occurs before LVH and in these 26 patients with established hypertension, dysfunction was present without LVH. Whereas most studies have analyzed the effects of various antihypertensive drugs on LVH, this study compared the effects of 2 agents—a calcium antagonist or a diuretic—on indices of diastolic function. The fact that the calcium antagonist came out ahead is not surprising, adding to the already considerable evidence of their value with diastolic dysfunction from LVH.

The mechanisms that lead to diastolic dysfunction likely include plasma aldosterone which appears to stimulate myocardial fibrosis.[1] With atrial involvement, increased production of atrial natriuretic factor may oppose some of the effects of aldosterone.

N.M. Kaplan, M.D.

Reference

1. Fagard RH, Lijnen PJ, Petrov VV: Opposite associations of circulating aldosterone and atrial natriuretic peptide with left ventricular diastolic function in essential hypertension. *J Human Hypertens* 12:195-202, 1998.

Tight Blood Pressure Control and Risk of Macrovascular and Microvascular Complications in Type 2 Diabetes: UKPDS 38

Turner R, for the UK Prospective Diabetes Study Group (Radcliffe Infirmary, Oxford, England)
BMJ 317:703-713, 1998   1–34

Introduction.—Type 2 diabetes and hypertension are commonly associated conditions, and they both carry an increased risk of renal and cardiovascular disease. The incidence of stroke and myocardial infarction in the general population is reduced by treatment to lower blood pressure. It is unknown whether treating hypertension in type 2 diabetes patients reduces the risk of end-stage renal disease. Whether tight blood pressure control could reduce morbidity and mortality in hypertensive patients with type 2 diabetes was analyzed. Tight blood pressure control was defined as aiming for a blood pressure of less than 150/85 mm Hg.

Methods.—The study included 1,148 hypertensive patients with type 2 diabetes aged a mean of 56 years with a mean blood pressure of 160/94 mm Hg. Seven hundred fifty-eight patients were allocated to tight control of blood pressure (<150/85 mm Hg) and 390 to less tight control (<180/105 mm Hg). They were controlled with an angiotensin-converting enzyme inhibitor captopril or a β-blocker atenolol.

Results.—In the group assigned tight blood pressure control, the mean blood pressure was significantly reduced (144/82 mm Hg) compared with the group assigned to less tight control (154/87 mm Hg). There was a 24% reduction in risk in diabetes-related end points, 32% reduction in deaths related to diabetes, 44% reduction in strokes, and 37% reduction in microvascular end points in the group assigned to tight control compared with that assigned to less tight control. In mortality from all causes, there was a nonsignificant reduction. The group assigned to tight blood pressure control had a 34% reduction in risk in the proportion of patients with deterioration of retinopathy and 47% reduced risk of deterioration in visual acuity, after 9 years of follow-up. There were 29% of patients in the tight control group that required 3 or more treatments to lower blood pressure to achieve target blood pressures after 9 years of follow-up.

Conclusion.—A clinically important reduction in the risk of deaths related to diabetes, complications related to diabetes, progression of diabetic retinopathy, and deterioration in visual acuity occurred in patients with hypertension and type 2 diabetes who were treated with tight blood pressure control.

▶ This large and long trial of the treatment of type 2 diabetics examined 2 major issues: whether tight control of hyperglycemia with various agents reduced the incidence of diabetic complications and whether tighter control of hypertension was beneficial. The results of the effects of tighter glycemic control were published simultaneously[1] to these on tighter blood pressure control.[2] It should be noted that tighter blood pressure control provided more than twice the benefit than did tighter glycemic control.

This study was formulated over 10 years ago at a time when there was real uncertainty about the value of tighter control of both glycemia and blood pressure. Therefore, the relatively high levels of blood pressure, less than 150/85 mm Hg, that were used as the criterion for tighter control might now be considered too high to document the real value of tighter control. Nonetheless, the 10/5 mm Hg difference achieved between the 2 groups was enough to show a significant benefit of tighter blood pressure control.

The study was designed to compare 2 principal types of antihypertensive drug: the beta-blocker atenolol and the angiotensin-converting enzyme (ACE) inhibitor captopril. As noted in an article following this one,[2] the overall results with the 2 were virtually identical, in both the degree of blood pressure control and the rates of nonfatal and fatal diabetic complications. The authors concluded that "The suggestion that angiotensin converting enzyme inhibitors have a specific renal protective effect in the treatment of type 2 diabetes is not supported."

This comes as a bit of a surprise because everyone has jumped on the ACE inhibitor bandwagon for protection against diabetic nephropathy. The UKPDSG investigators suggest that these benefits may simply reflect lower blood pressure and not a specific additional effect of the ACE inhibitor.

N.M. Kaplan, M.D.

References

1. United Kingdom Prospective Diabetes Study Group. UK prospective diabetes study: 33 intensive blood glucose control with sulphonylureas or insulin compared with conventional treatment and risk of complications in patients with type 2 diabetes. *Lancet* 352:837-853, 1998.
2. UK Prospective Diabetes Study Group: Efficacy of atenolol and captopril in reducing risk of macrovascular and microvascular complications in type 2 diabetes: UKPDS 39. *BMJ* 317:713-720, 1998.

Are β-Blockers Efficacious as First-line Therapy for Hypertension in the Elderly? A Systematic Review

Messerli FH, Grossman E, Goldbourt U (Alton Ochsner Med Found, New Orleans, La; Chaim Sheba Med Ctr, Tel Hashomer, Israel)
JAMA 279:1903-1907, 1998

1–35

Background.—In addition to reducing blood pressure, the goal of antihypertensive therapy is to reduce cardiovascular morbidity and mortality. The safety and efficacy of diuretics are well established, but the case for β-blocker treatment in elderly patients has not been as well confirmed. This meta-analysis assessed the effects of diuretics and β-blockers in elderly patients with hypertension with respect to cardiovascular morbidity and mortality and mortality from all causes.

Methods.—A review of the literature identified 10 randomized trials of diuretic or β-blocker therapy in hypertensive elderly patients, aged 60 years or more. All studies lasted 1 year or longer and provided information on morbidity and mortality. The trials included a total of 16,164 patients. In 8 trials, a diuretic was used as first-line therapy; in 2, a β-blocker.

Results.—Although two thirds of patients had their blood pressure well controlled with diuretic monotherapy, this result was true for less than one third of patients receiving β-blocker monotherapy. In all outcomes assessed, the analysis demonstrated the superiority of diuretics over β-blockers. This superiority was evident for prevention of cerebrovascular events, odds ratio (OR) 0.61; of fatal stroke, OR 0.67; of coronary heart disease, OR 0.74; and of cardiovascular mortality, OR 0.75. Diuretic therapy also reduced mortality from all causes, OR 0.86. β-Blocker therapy significantly reduced the likelihood of cerebrovascular events (OR 0.75) but had no effect on risk of coronary heart disease, cardiovascular mortality, or mortality from all causes.

Conclusions.—The available data suggest that β-blockers are not appropriate as first-line therapy for uncomplicated hypertension in elderly patients. The findings are consistent with the recommendations of the sixth Joint National Committee. Diuretics should continue to be the standard first-line therapy for hypertension in the elderly.

▶ Because the members of the sixth Joint National Committee (JNC-6) were aware of these data, the report gives preference to diuretics and then to long-acting dihydropyridine calcium antagonists for the treatment of systolic hypertension in the elderly. The report states that if beta-blockers are used , they should be given with a diuretic.

The value of this paper by Messerli et al is that it documents better than any other the lack of both cardioprotection and antihypertensive efficacy of beta-blockers in the elderly. Beta-blockers should be used for the known secondary protection they provide in survivors of myocardial infarction, and they may be useful for treatment of angina and heart failure. But heed should be given to these data suggesting that by themselves they are not as useful for treatment of hypertension in the elderly as are diuretics and long-acting DHP calcium antagonists.

N.M. Kaplan, M.D.

Influence of Race and Dietary Salt on the Antihypertensive Efficacy of an Angiotensin-Converting Enzyme Inhibitor or a Calcium Channel Antagonist in Salt-Sensitive Hypertensives
Weir MR, Chrysant SG, McCarron DA, et al (Univ of Maryland, Baltimore; Oklahoma Cardiovascular and Hypertension Ctr, Oklahoma City; Oregon Health Sciences Univ, Portland; et al)
Hypertension 31:1088-1096, 1998   1–36

Introduction.—Racial differences may have an effect on the response to antihypertensive drugs. Critical physiologic factors that may also explain the difference are dietary salt sensitivity and low plasma renin activity. Debate still exists as to whether race affects the relationship between blood pressure and dietary salt intake. Hypertensive black, white, and Hispanic patients on low- and high-salt diets who had been previously profiled as being salt sensitive were assessed to determine possible racial differences in response to the full dosing range of isradipine and enalapril.

Methods.—The study included 96 blacks, 63 Hispanics, and 232 whites who were preselected for stage I to III hypertension and further selected for salt sensitivity, which was defined as an increase of 5 mm Hg or more in diastolic blood pressure after 3 weeks of a low-salt ($\leq$88 mmol/day Na$^+$) and high-salt (>190 mmol/day Na$^+$) diet. In this multicenter, randomized, double-blind, placebo-controlled, parallel-group clinical trial, the antihypertensive effect of an angiotensin-converting enzyme inhibitor (enalapril 5 or 20 mg BID) was compared to a calcium channel antagonist (isradipine 5 or 10 mg BID) during alternating periods of high- and low-salt intake. Blood pressure change and absolute blood pressure level achieved with therapy were the main outcome measures.

Results.—With both enalapril and isradipine, there was a greater mean decrease in blood pressure during the high-salt diet (314.7 mmol/day urinary Na$^+$) compared with the low-salt diet (90.1 mmol/day Na$^+$). However, for both agents, the absolute blood pressure achieved in all races was consistently lower on a low-salt diet. Isradipine-treated salt-sensitive hypertensives showed a smaller difference between high- and low-salt diets with respect to race (black, −3.6 vs. −1.6 mm Hg; white, −6.2 vs. −3.9 mm Hg; Hispanic, −8.1 vs. −5.3 mm Hg) than was seen in enalapril-treated salt-sensitive hypertensives (black, −9.0 vs. −5.3 mm Hg; white, −11.8 vs. −7.0 mm Hg; Hispanic, −11.1 vs. −5.6 mm Hg). With both drugs, blood pressure control was similar with respect to race on the low-salt diet. Blacks had better blood pressure control with isradipine than with enalapril on the high-salt diet, whereas no difference in the blood pressure control was seen in whites and Hispanics treated with either drug.

Conclusion.—In salt-sensitive hypertensive blacks, whites, and Hispanics treated with enalapril or isradipine, dietary salt reduction helps reduce blood pressure. Race-related differences in antihypertensive activity are diminished by controlling for salt sensitivity.

▶ These data could help explain 2 previously reported differences in the efficacy of various antihypertensive drugs: first, the relatively lesser responsiveness of blacks to angiotensin-converting enzyme (ACE) inhibitors compared with whites; second, the lesser impact of a low-sodium diet on the efficacy of calcium antagonists. The second point seems to be unrelated to sodium sensitivity because fewer changes were noted with the 2 extremes of sodium intake with the CA than with the ACE inhibitor in these patients who were all preselected to be sodium sensitive.

What is most apparent is the improved efficacy of both the ACE inhibitor and the calcium antagonists in all 3 ethnic groups when on a lower-sodium (90 mmol/day) diet than on a high-sodium diet. This fits very well with the recommendation by JNC-6 to reduce sodium to 100 mmol/day in all hypertensives.[1] In addition, the data suggest that a lower sodium intake will restore the full effectiveness of ACE inhibitors in blacks, who are more likely to be sodium sensitive than are whites.

N.M. Kaplan, M.D.

Reference

1. The sixth report of the Joint National Committee on prevention, detection, evaluation and treatment of high blood pressure. *Arch Intern Med* 157:2413-2446, 1997.

Effects of Combination Therapy With an Angiotensin Converting Enzyme Inhibitor and Thiazide Diuretic on Insulin Action in Essential Hypertension
Hunter SJ, Harper R, Ennis CN, et al (Royal Victoria Hosp, Belfast, N Ireland; Greenisland Health Centre, Ireland; Queen's Univ of Belfast, N Ireland)
J Hypertens 16:103-109, 1998   1–37

Objective.—Whether the use of high doses of thiazides reduce the potential benefits of angiotensin-converting enzyme (ACE) inhibitors on insulin sensitivity in patients with essential hypertension has not been studied. The effects of 50 mg of captopril twice daily used alone or in combination with 5 mg of bendrofluazide on insulin action in nondiabetic hypertensive patients was assessed in a double-blind, randomized, crossover study.

Methods.—After a 6-week washout period, 15 patients (7 males), aged less than 65 years, were titrated up to 50 mg of captopril twice daily in the first week. Then patients received bendrofluazide or placebo concurrently with captopril for 12 weeks, were given captopril and placebo for an additional 6 weeks, and were crossed over to the alternative regimen for the final 12 weeks. Systolic and diastolic blood pressures were measured, and insulin action was assessed using the euglycemic glucose clamp technique at the end of each period.

Results.—Two patients did not complete the study. Combination therapy lowered both systolic and diastolic blood pressures significantly compared with captopril alone (139 vs. 160 mm Hg and 89 vs. 97 mm Hg, respectively). The combination significantly increased fasting serum insulin levels compared with captopril alone (7.9 vs. 6.2 mU/L), significantly lowered potassium levels (3.8 vs. 4.2 mmol/L), and significantly increased postabsorptive endogenous glucose production (10.8 vs. 10.0 μmol/kg/min). Total cholesterol, low-density lipoprotein cholesterol, high-density lipoprotein cholesterol, total triglyceride, glucose, and urate levels were unchanged. Both captopril and combination therapy lowered glucose production similarly.

Conclusions.—Compared with captopril alone, the combination of captopril and bendrofluazide significantly reduced blood pressure and significantly increased insulin production, indicating increased hepatic resistance to insulin, and a tendency toward decreased potassium levels. Thus if both ACE inhibitors and diuretics are prescribed, the lowest dose of diuretic should be used.

▶ These results are a bit disturbing, denying both a favorable effect of the ACE inhibitor captopril on insulin resistance and the ability to ameliorate the adverse effect of diuretics with an ACE inhibitor.

As these authors have previously shown, low doses of diuretic do not significantly worsen insulin sensitivity, so the major message is to only use low doses rather than depending on other drugs to soften the impact of high doses, not only on insulin resistance but also on other metabolic and hormonal changes.

We still do not know the role of insulin resistance as found in virtually all obese hypertensives and about one third of nonobese hypertensives. High insulin levels arising as a consequence of insulin resistance are associated with increased cardiovascular risk, so it is likely that ameliorating insulin resistance is worth the effort.

N.M. Kaplan, M.D.

Influence of a History of Arterial Hypertension and Pretreatment Blood Pressure on the Effect of Angiotensin Converting Enzyme Inhibition After Acute Myocardial Infarction

Gustafsson F, for the Trandolapril Cardiac Evaluation Study (Frederiksberg Univ Hosp, Denmark; Gentofte Univ, Denmark)
J Hypertens 16:65S-70S, 1998   1–38

Background.—Angiotensin-converting enzyme (ACE) inhibitor therapy reduces mortality in patients with acute myocardial infarction (AMI) and impaired left ventricular systolic function. About one third of AMI survivors have a history of arterial hypertension, and these patients appear to have a worse prognosis than nonhypertensive patients. The effects of ACE inhibition after AMI in patients with arterial hypertension are unclear. The impact of treatment with the ACE inhibitor trandolapril on morbidity and mortality in patients with AMI and left ventricular dysfunction was investigated retrospectively.

Methods.—Data from the randomized, controlled Trandolapril Cardiac Event study were used. In this study, 1,749 patients with enzyme-confirmed AMI and echocardiographically confirmed left ventricular dysfunction were randomly assigned to receive either trandolapril or placebo. The patients were followed up for a mean of 26 months. The effects of arterial hypertension and of pretreatment blood pressure on the treatment results were examined.

Results.—A history of arterial hypertension was noted for 400 patients, or 23% of the total. Mortality during follow-up was 43% for patients with a history of hypertension vs. 37% for normotensive patients. Relative risk of death associated with trandolapril treatment was 0.59 in hypertensive patients vs. 0.85 in normotensive patients (Fig 1). The mortality benefit of trandolapril for hypertensive patients was still apparent after multivariate analysis for potential confounders. In addition, patients with higher blood pressures at the time of randomization received greater benefit from trandolapril treatment. The analysis revealed significant interactions between

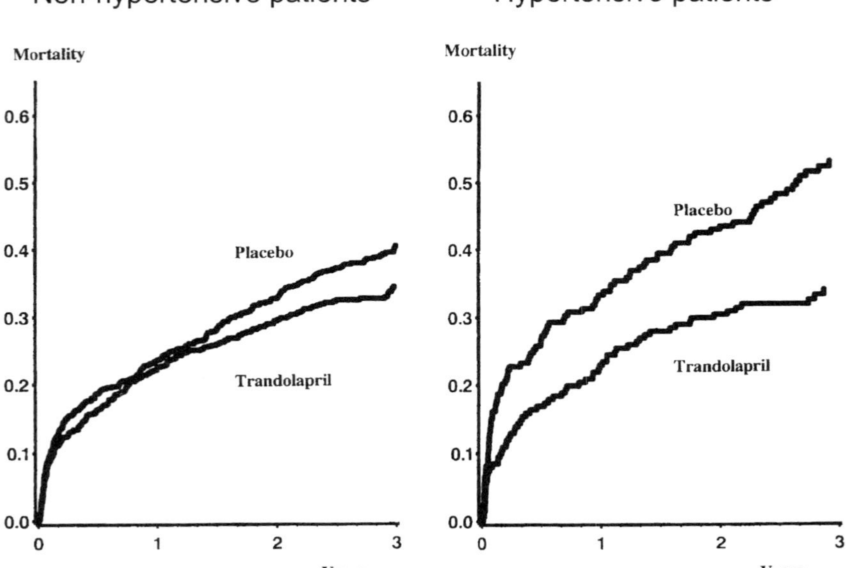

FIGURE 1.—Total mortality (time-to-event curves) for normotensive patients and for patients with a history of arterial hypertension. (Courtesy of Gustafsson F, for the Trandolapril Cardiac Evaluation Study: Influence of a history of arterial hypertension and pretreatment blood pressure on the effect of angiotensin converting enzyme inhibition after acute myocardial infarction. *J Hypertens* 16:65S-70S, 1998.)

benefit from ACE inhibitor treatment and history of hypertension, and systolic and diastolic blood pressure.

Conclusions.—Among patients with AMI and left ventricular dysfunction, the benefits of ACE inhibition may be more pronounced for those with arterial hypertension or high pretreatment blood pressure. The increased benefit is apparent not only in mortality but also in sudden and cardiovascular death rates. More research is needed to confirm the clinical importance of these findings.

▶ These data suggest that the protection provided by the use of ACE inhibitors in patients who have an AMI may be even greater in those who have preexisting hypertension. The implications are significant: at least one third of patients who have AMI have preexisting hypertension and without ACE inhibitor therapy, their prognosis is worse than that of normotensive patients. ACE inhibitors are clearly indicated for AMI patients, particularly if systolic dysfunction is present. If these preliminary data are substantiated in additional larger studies, their use will be recognized to be even more critical in hypertensives who have an AMI.

N.M. Kaplan, M.D.

Time Course of Complete Normalization of Left Ventricular Hypertrophy During Long-term Antihypertensive Therapy With Angiotensin Converting Enzyme Inhibitors

Franz I-W, Tönnesmann U, Müller JFM (Klinik Wehrawald de BfA, Todtmoos, Germany)
Am J Hypertens 11:631-639, 1998

1–39

Background.—Available data suggest that treatment with angiotensin-converting enzyme (ACE) inhibitors is more effective in reducing left ventricular hypertrophy (LVH) than other first-line antihypertensive therapies. The average duration of the studies performed to date has been approximately 6 months, whereas maximal regression of LVH is known to take several years. This study analyzed the time course and degree of reversal of LVH during ACE inhibitor therapy, including the likelihood of complete normalization.

Methods.—The prospective study included 23 patients (15 men), aged a mean of 46 years, with previously untreated hypertension and echocardiographically demonstrated LVH. The men, had a left ventricular mass index (LVMI) greater than 125 g/m^2, and the women had an LVMI greater than 100 g/m^2. All patients received 3 years of treatment with quinapril, at a dose of 10 mg/day in 9 patients and 20 mg/day in 12; in addition, 5 patients received hydrochlorothiazide, 25 mg/day. The patients were followed up using echocardiography for changes in LVMI, relative wall thickness, left atrial size, fractional shortening, and diastolic function. In addition, they underwent ambulatory blood pressure monitoring and exercise testing every 6 months.

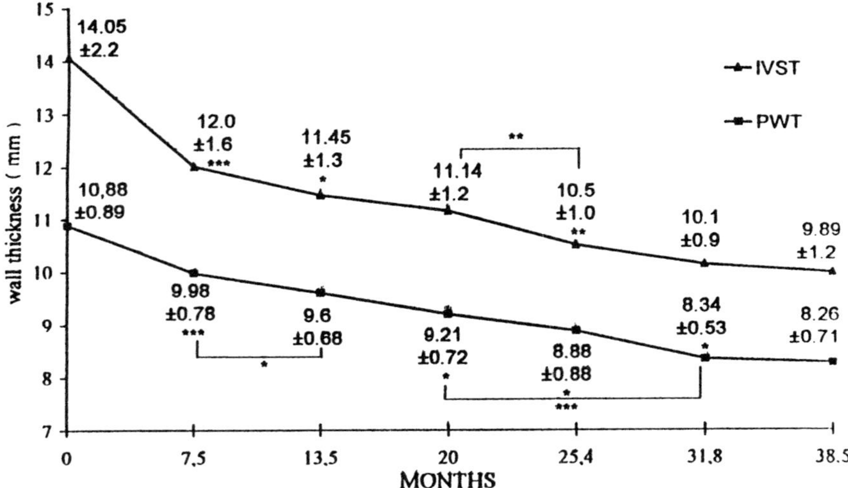

FIGURE 3.—Top, Regression of interventricular septal (*IVST*) and posterior wall (*PWT*) thickness during antihypertensive long-term treatment with quinapril in 21 previously untreated patients. Significances refer to preceding values for wall thickness and to baseline for relative wall thickness (*P <0.05; †P <0.01; ‡P <0.001). (Courtesy of Franz I-W, Tönnesmann U, Müller JFM: Time course of complete normalization of left ventricular hypertrophy during long-term antihypertensive therapy with angiotensin converting enzyme inhibitors. *Am J Hypertens* 11:631-639, 1998. Reprinted by permission of Elsevier Science Inc., copyright 1998 by American Journal of Hypertension, Inc.)

Results.—Mean reduction in LVMI was 17.5% at 7.5 months and 38.6% at 38 months. Complete normalization of LVH was achieved in 90.5% of patients. A peak increase of 14.6% in fractional shortening was achieved at 38 months. Peak early/atrial velocity increased to its maximum at 7.5 months, with no subsequent change. Similarly, most of the reduction in left atrial dimension occurred within 7.5 months. Significant reductions were also achieved in intraventricular septal and posterior wall thickness (Fig 3, top).

Conclusions.—In hypertensive patients receiving ACE inhibitor therapy, reversal of LVH is a prolonged process. Antihypertensive therapy should seek not only to reduce but also to normalize left ventricular mass, left atrial size, and diastolic dysfunction. The findings suggest that treatment periods of longer than 1 year are needed to assess the effects of antihypertensive drugs on LVH and other cardiac structural abnormalities.

▶ Previous abstracts described the immediate and long-term consequences of LVH in hypertensive patients (Grimelli, Abstract 5–31; Verdecchia, Abstract 5–2). As noted in Abstract 5–6 (Ofili), regression of LVH has been seen with virtually all antihypertensive agents, and such regression is increasingly being used as a surrogate endpoint for coronary protection by therapy.

The article by Franz et al. is another of this group of investigators' almost unique and important studies on the time course of regression and is the first to analyze the long-term effects of an ACE inhibitor. It is obvious that regression is not complete in the 6- to 12-month intervals used in most published studies. Normalization requires years of effective therapy.

Nonetheless, most regression of LVH and improvement in diastolic function occur within 1 year and in most series is related to the degree of blood pressure reduction.[1] The pressure of LVH may be predicted by the finding of higher levels of plasma renin activity,[2] but it is not associated with blood pressure variability[3] and a considerable proportion of differences of left ventricular mass cannot be explained by known variables.[4]

N.M. Kaplan, M.D.

References

1. Vyssoulis GP, Trikas AG, Paleologos AA, et al: Significance of blood pressure levels achieved with felodipine anti-hypertensive treatment on cardiovascular structure and function changes. *J Human Hypertens* 12:427-432, 1998.
2. Koga M, Sasaguri M, Miura S, et al: Plasma renin activity could be a useful predictor of left ventricular hypertrophy in essential hypertensives. *J Human Hypertens* 12:455-461, 1998.
3. Schillaci G, Verdecchia P, Borgioni C, et al: Lack of association between blood pressure variability and left ventricular mass in essential hypertension. *Am J Hypertens* 11:515-522, 1998.
4. de Simone G, Devereux RB, Kimball TR, et al: Interaction between body size and cardiac workload. *Hypertens* 31:1077-1082, 1998.

Antihypertensive Efficacy of Angiotensin Converting Enzyme Inhibition and Aspirin Counteraction
Guazzi MD, Campodonico J, Celeste F, et al (Istituto di Cardiologia dell'Università degli Studi, Milano, Italy)
Clin Pharmacol Ther 63:79-86, 1998

1–40

Objective.—Because prostaglandins may be involved with angiotensin II and the kinins in the antihypertensive activity of angiotensin-converting enzyme (ACE) inhibitors, the potential antagonistic effects of aspirin need to be considered in patients taking ACE inhibitors. The minimal dosage of aspirin that exerts antagonistic activity against the antihypertensive properties of ACE inhibitors, and the incidence of aspirin counteraction in relation to hypertension severity and the combination of ACE inhibitors with other antihypertensive drugs were investigated.

Methods.—Two days after admission, 52 previously untreated or poorly regulated patients were started on a constant isocaloric diet with 30 mEq sodium and 100 mEq potassium. Group 1 patients (n = 26), with mild to moderate hypertension, received 20 mg twice daily of enalapril, and group 2 patients (n = 26), with severe primary hypertension, received enalapril plus 30 mg/day of long-acting nifedipine and 50 mg/day of atenolol. Aspirin at either 100 or 300 mg/day was administered for 5 days either alone or with the antihypertensive agents. Those patients whose response to enalapril was attenuated by more than 20% were classified as responders.

Results.—Aspirin at 100 mg had no antagonistic effect, but aspirin at 300 mg produced an antagonistic effect in 57% of group 1 patients and 50% of group 2 patients. The average efficacy of enalapril upon reduction of mean blood pressure was diminished by 63% in group 1 and by 91% in group 2 by the concomitant administration of 300 mg of aspirin.

Conclusions.—Whereas 100 mg/day of aspirin had no antagonistic effect, 300 mg/day of aspirin significantly attenuated the antihypertensive effect of inhibition probably by inhibiting prostaglandins.

▶ Interference of the antihypertensive effects of various drugs by nonsteroidal anti-inflammatory drugs (NSAIDs) has long been recognized and is likely responsible for a significant portion of apparently resistant or refractory hypertension.

This study broadens the interaction to standard 300-mg daily doses of aspirin commonly taken for protection against vascular thrombosis and heart attack. The degree of interference—from 63% to 91% of the antihypertensive effect of a fairly large dose of an ACE inhibitor in more than 50% of patients—should be taken as a warning by all who prescribe and use these exceedingly popular drugs.

The anti-inflammatory properties for which NSAIDs are typically prescribed can be provided by acetaminophen without interfering with the efficacy of various antihypertensive drugs. However, larger doses of antihypertensives (or the substitution of calcium antagonists, which seem not to be blocked) may be needed if large doses of aspirin are to be used for cardioprotection. Fortunately, no significant interaction was seen with 100 mg of aspirin, which should be enough to provide most if not all its vascular protection.

N.M. Kaplan, M.D.

Comparative Efficacy of Two Angiotensin II Receptor Antagonists, Irbesartan and Losartan, in Mild-to-Moderate Hypertension
Kassler-Taub K, for the Irbesartan/Losartan Study Investigators (Bowman Gray School of Medicine, Winston-Salem, NC)
Am J Hypertens 11:445-453, 1998   1–41

Introduction.—Pharmacologic differences that could result in different efficacy and tolerability profiles exist among the angiotensin II type 1 (AT_1) blockers. Irbesartan is a competitive antagonist and is a long-acting AT_1 blocker that does not require biotransformation for its pharmacologic activity. Losartan is a competitive antagonist with a pharmacokinetic profile that is different from irbesartan, and is the first orally available AT_1 blocker that was developed for clinical use. Maximal reductions in blood pressure were estimated to occur at 50 to 100 mg using once-daily doses of losartan up to 150 mg, whereas in studies using once-daily doses of irbesartan ranging from 1 to 900 mg, doses above 300 mg provided little additional benefit. The antihypertensive efficacy and tolerability of 150-mg and 300-mg irbesartan once daily vs. 100-mg losartan daily was explored.

Methods.—The study included 567 patients with mild-to-moderate hypertension who were randomized to once-daily therapy with 300-mg irbesartan, 100-mg losartan, 150-mg irbesartan, or placebo for 8 weeks. The treatment groups had similar demographic and baseline characteristics.

Results.—There were greater reductions with 300-mg irbesartan from baseline in trough (24 ± 3 hours after medication)-seated diastolic blood pressure and trough-seated systolic blood pressure than with 100-mg losartan after 8 weeks of treatment. The reduction was 3.0 mm Hg for trough-seated diastolic blood pressure and 5.1 mm Hg for trough-seated systolic blood pressure. At weeks 1 and 4, larger reductions were demonstrated. At week 1, normalization rates were 48% with 300-mg irbesartan and 31% with 100-mg losartan, and at week 8, they were 52% with 300-mg irbesartan and 42% with 100-mg losartan (Fig 2). There was no significant difference in the antihypertensive effect between 150-mg irbesartan and 100-mg losartan. Patients tolerated all therapies well. The lowest incidence of adverse events and discontinuations because of adverse events were associated with the 300-mg dose of irbesartan.

Conclusion.—Clinically significant differences in blood pressure reductions may result with the maximally effective once-daily doses of 2 different AT$_1$ receptor antagonists. The potential importance of the pharmaco-

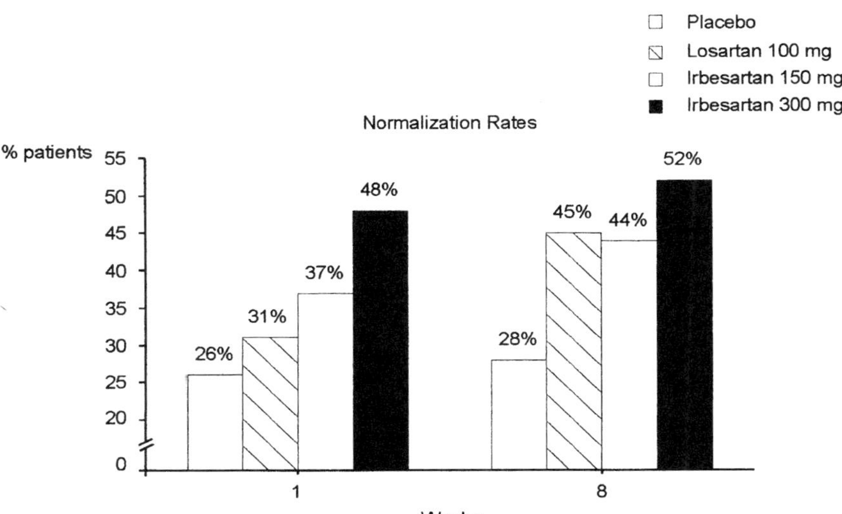

FIGURE 2.—Normalization rates (trough-seated diastolic blood pressure < 90 mm Hg) at weeks 1 and 8. (Courtesy of Kassler-Taub K, for the Irbesartan/Losartan Study Investigators: Comparative efficacy of two angiotensin II receptor antagonists, irbesartan and losartan, in mild-to-moderate hypertension. *Am J Hypertens* 11: 445-453, 1998. Reprinted by permission of Elsevier Science Inc., copyright 1998 by American Journal of Hypertension, Inc.)

kinetic and pharmacodynamic differences between these 2 members of this class is highlighted.

▶ Now that 4 or 5 different AT_1 receptor blockers are being marketed in the United States and more are likely on the way, pharmaceutical companies are trying to prove that theirs is better than others. These data do suggest that the largest recommended dose of irbesartan is more effective, particularly in the first week, than the largest recommended dose of losartan, but the 8-week response rates were little different.

Obviously, AT_1 receptor blockers largely avoid the most common side effect of ACE inhibitors, a dry hacking cough[1] and they really may be associated with fewer adverse effects than any other class of hypertensives[2]. However, until they are shown to be as effective as ACE inhibitors in preventing morbidity and mortality, they should be used mainly in those who develop a cough on an ACE inhibitor.

N.M. Kaplan, M.D.

References

1. Mimran A, Ruilope L, Kerwin L, et al: A randomised, double-blind comparison of the angiotensin II receptor antagonist, irbesartan, with the full dose range of enalapril for the treatment of mild-to-moderate hypertension. *J Human Hypertens* 12:203-208, 1998.
2. Pool JL, Guthrie RM, Littlejohn TW, et al: Dose-related antihypertensive effects of irbesartan in patients with mild-to-moderate hypertension. *Am J Hypertens* 11:462-470, 1998.

Evaluation of Changes in Sympathetic Nerve Activity and Heart Rate in Essential Hypertensive Patients Induced by Amlodipine and Nifedipine
Hamada T, Watanabe M, Kaneda T, et al (Tottori Univ, Japan)
J Hypertens 16:111-118, 1998
1–42

Background.—Evaluation of antihypertensive drug treatment must consider not only the effects on diurnal patterns of blood pressure but also of heart rate and sympathetic activity. Dihidropyridine-based calcium antagonists (CAs) such as nifedipine are widely used, although their effects on long-term cardiovascular mortality are debatable. The newer classes of dihydropyridines, such as amlodipine, permit once-daily dosing without fluctuating plasma levels and unwanted side effects. The effects of these 2 antihypertensive drugs on heart rate, sympathetic nerve activity, and cardiovascular outcomes were evaluated.

Methods.—The randomized, single-blind study included 45 patients with essential hypertension. Each underwent 24-hour ambulatory ECG and blood pressure monitoring. The patients were assigned to 4 weeks of treatment with amlodipine, 5 mg/day (after breakfast); slow-release nifedipine, 10 mg twice daily (after breakfast and dinner); or short-acting nifedipine, 10 mg after each meal. Plasma and urinary catecholamine levels

TABLE 3.—Plasma and Urinary Concentrations of Norepinephrine and Epinephrine Before and After the Start of Treatments With Amlodipine, Slow-release Nifedipine, and Short-acting Nifedipine

	Control	Acute	Chronic
Urinary norepinephrine (µg/day)			
Amiodipine	65.1 ± 10.3	69.2 ± 11.8	50.5 ± 4.3
Slow-release nifedipine	47.4 ± 7.1	78.1 ± 21.1	55.8 ± 7.7
Nifedipine	50.0 ± 12.7	92.5 ± 14.7	67.5 ± 12.5
Plasma norepinephrine (pg/mL)			
Amlodipine	271 ± 31	249 ± 43	213 ± 17*
Slow-release nifedipine	212 ± 30	245 ± 29	259 ± 40
Nifedipine	221 ± 40	398 ± 60*	309 ± 51
Urinary epinephrine (µg/day)			
Amiodipine	5.61 ± 0.66	6.04 ± 1.06	5.03 ± 1.12
Slow-release nifedipine	6.15 ± 1.52	8.56 ± 2.65	7.24 ± 1.86
Nifedipine	6.01 ± 1.86	7.82 ± 2.10	7.80 ± 2.48
Plasma epinephrine (pg/mL)			
Amlodipine	25 ± 5	19 ± 4	19 ± 2
Slow-release nifedipine	19 ± 4	25 ± 6	26 ± 6
Nifedipine	20 ± 6	26 ± 7	29 ± 8

Note: Values are expressed as means ± SD.
*$P < 0.05$, vs. control.
(Courtesy of Hamada T, Watanabe M, Kaneda T, et al: Evaluation of changes in sympathetic nerve activity and heart rate in essential hypertensive patients induced by amlodipine and nifedipine. *J Hypertens* 16:111-118, 1998.)

were measured before treatment and again after 1 day and 4 weeks of treatment. Heart rate power spectral analysis was performed to assess the low-frequency and high-frequency power spectral densities and low-frequency/high-frequency ratio.

Results.—During the chronic treatment period, the 3 groups showed similar and significant reductions in blood pressure. The total QRS count per 24 hours remained at a constant level during treatment with slow-release nifedipine, increased during treatment with short-acting nifedipine, and decreased by nearly 3% during treatment with amlodipine. Amlodipine treatment was also associated with reductions in plasma and urinary norepinephrine levels, which were increased in the short-acting nifedipine group and unchanged in the slow-release nifedipine group (Table 3). Nifedipine treatment was associated with increases in the low-frequency/high-frequency ratio, significant in the short-acting nifedipine group. This ratio was decreased by amlodipine treatment during both the acute and chronic periods.

Conclusions.—In patients with essential hypertension, chronic treatment with amlodipine does not lead to increased sympathetic nerve activity. Thus, continued benefits of amlodipine can be expected after long-term administration. Reflex sympathetic activation is milder with slow-release nifedipine than with the short-acting preparation.

▶ These data provide additional evidence to explain what has become increasingly obvious: the possible cardiovascular disturbances attributed to short-acting CAs do not occur with long-acting CAs. In the 4 years since Psaty et al.[1] reported an increase in myocardial infarctions among hypertensives treated with a short-acting CA compared with those treated with other classes of antihypertensive agents in a retrospective case-control study, a steadily expanding body of data from prospective, randomized, controlled trials have shown less, not more, coronary disease among hypertensives treated with long-acting dihydropyridine CAs.[2-4] Excellent protection against coronary mortality was shown in the Hypertension Optimal Therapy (HOT) trial based on another long-acting dihydropyridine CA (see Abstract 1–31).

Clearly, as shown by Hamada et al., long-acting CAs do not produce the marked activation of the sympathetic nervous system provoked by the abrupt lowering of the blood pressure induced by short-acting CAs. Short-acting CAs should be avoided if at all possible; long-acting CAs can be used when indicated without concern about coronary (or cancer) danger.

N.M. Kaplan, M.D.

References

1. Psaty BM, Heckbert SR, Koepsell TD, et al: The risk of myocardial infarction associated with anti-hypertensive drug therapies. *JAMA* 274:620-625, 1995.
2. Gong L, Zang W, Zhu Y, et al: Shanghai trial of nifedipine in the elderly (STONE). *J Hypertens* 14:1237-1246, 1996.
3. Staessen J, Fagard R, Thijs L, et al: Randomised double-blind comparison of placebo and active treatment for older patients with isolated systolic hypertension. *Lancet* 30:757-764, 1997.
4. Hansson L, Zanchetti A, Carruthers SG, et al: Effects of intensive blood-pressure lowering and low-dose aspirin in patients with hypertension: Prinicpal results of the Hypertension Optimal Treatment (HOT) randomised trial. *Lancet* 351:1755-1762, 1998.

Cancer Risk of Hypertensive Patients Taking Calcium Antagonists

Hole DJ, Gillis CR, McCallum IR, et al (Univ of Glasgow, Scotland; Ruchill Hosp, Glasgow, Scotland; CSC Computer Sciences Ltd, Paisley, Scotland)
J Hypertens 16:119-124, 1998   1–43

Objective.—The possible relationship between increased incidence of cancer among elderly patients taking calcium antagonists (CAs) is controversial. The rates of incident and fatal cancer in hypertensive patients taking CAs compared with 3 control groups was investigated retrospectively.

Methods.—The 134 incident cancers among 2,297 patients at the Glasgow Blood Pressure Clinic were compared with those in 2,910 clinic patients taking other antihypertensive drugs, a middle-aged population of Renfrew and Paisley towns, and the general population of the west of Scotland. Outcomes measured were relative risk of cancer—the ratio of observed to expected cancers in the CA group using expected values based on the 3 control groups.

Results.—Between 1980 and 1995, the relative risk was 1.02 for cancer among CA users (134 deaths) compared with controls using non-CA medications, 1.01 compared with populations in Renfrew and Paisley, and 1.02 compared with west of Scotland (Fig 1).

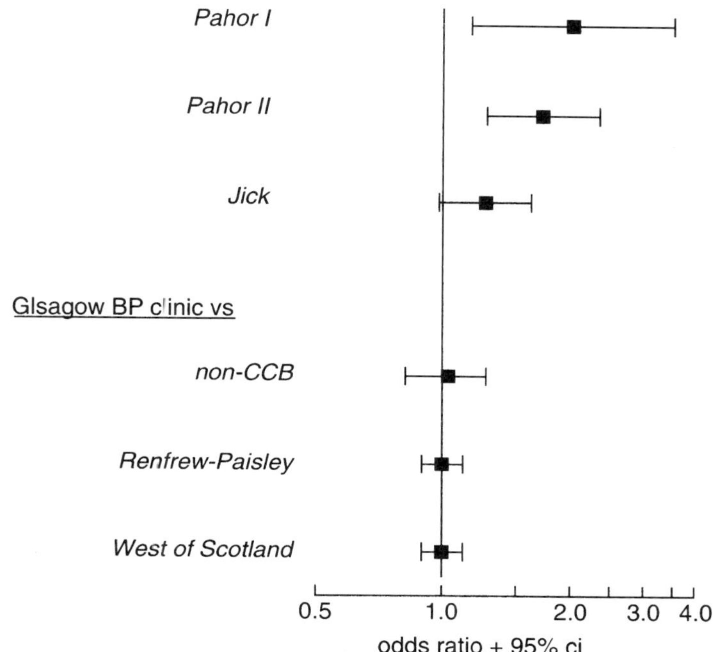

FIGURE 1.—Relative risk (odds ratio) with 95% confidence intervals for incident cancer in the calcium antagonist (*CCB*) group of 3 previous studies (Pahor et al. and Jick et al.) and in 3 analyses from the Glasgow Blood Pressure (*BP*) Clinic: with noncalcium antagonist group as controls and with Renfrew-Paisley and West of Scotland controls. (Courtesy of Hole DJ, Gillis CR, McCallum IR, et al: Cancer risk of hypertensive patients taking calcium antagonists. *J Hypertens* 16:119-124, 1998.)

Conclusions.—Cancer mortality among CA users was not increased compared with users of non-CA antihypertensive medications.

▶ One of the major claims made by Pahor and associates against CAs is that they cause an increased incidence of various cancers.[1,2] Since their claims (based on case-control data with literally no documentation of the actual intake of CAs by the victims), a number of larger, better controlled and documented studies have shown no such connection. The data from the 5,000 patients in this carefully observed population can be added to those of Rosenberg et al.[3] involving more than 1,500 individuals, which also found absolutely no increase in cancer in those using CAs.

The best data of all come from the largest prospective, randomized, controlled trial comparing a placebo to a long-acting dihydropyridine CA in more than 4,600 elderly hypertensives followed up for more than 4 years.[4] A 15% lesser incidence in cancer was observed in those on the CA. Once again, spurious claims turn out to be spurious, so hopefully the scare mongers will back off.

N.M. Kaplan, M.D.

References

1. Pahor M, Guralnik JM, Salive ME, et al: Do calcium channel blockers increase the risk of cancer? *Am J Hypertens* 9:695-699, 1996.
2. Pahor M, Guralnik JM, Ferrucci L, et al: Calcium-channel blockade and incidence of cancer in aged populations. *Lancet* 348:493-497, 1996.
3. Rosenberg L, Rao RS, Palmer JR, et al: Calcium channel blockers and the risk of cancer. *JAMA* 279:1000-1004, 1998.
4. Staessen JA, for the Systolic Hypertension–Europe (Syst-Eur) Trial Investigators: Morbidity and mortality in the placebo-controlled European Trial on Isolated Systolic Hypertension in the Elderly. *Lancet* 350:757-764, 1997.

Comparison of the Fixed Combination of Enalapril/Diltiazem ER and Their Monotherapies in Stage 1 to 3 Essential Hypertension

Cushman WC, for the Enalapril/Diltiazem ER Comparison to Monotherapies Group (Univ of Tennesee, Memphis; et al)
Am J Hypertens 11:23-30, 1998   1–44

Introduction.—There are many options for effective drug monotherapy in patients with hypertension. Two frequently used options, both individually and in combination, are the angiotensin-converting enzyme (ACE) inhibitors, such as enalapril, and the calcium channel blockers, such as diltiazem. A fixed combination product of enalapril and diltiazem extended release (ER) for once-daily dosing is now available. Two fixed-dose combinations were compared with their corresponding monotherapies and with placebo for the treatment of patients with stage 1 to 3 hypertension.

Methods.—The multicenter, randomized trial included 891 patients with sitting diastolic blood pressures of 95 to 115 mm Hg. They were assigned to 12 weeks of treatment with enalapril 5 mg, diltiazem ER 120 mg, diltiazem ER 180 mg, enalapril 5 mg plus diltiazem ER 120 mg, enalapril 5 mg plus diltiazem ER 180 mg, or placebo. This blinded phase was followed by a 36-week open-label phase, during which 562 patients received the fixed combination, titrated to maintain sitting diastolic pressure at less than 90 mm Hg. At the end of each phase, trough sitting blood pressure was measured to assess treatment efficacy. Patient symptoms, laboratory tests, and ECG results were used to assess patient safety.

Results.—Trough systolic blood pressure was significantly reduced by the 2 fixed combinations, compared with their monotherapies and compared with the 2 diltiazem ER monotherapies. Values were 7.6-9.0 mm Hg lower with the fixed combinations. However, all active treatments reduced blood pressure compared with placebo. During the open phase, the fixed combination effectively reduced sitting diastolic and systolic measurements. The various groups were similar in their incidence of adverse effects, including the combination groups vs. the monotherapy groups. The most common adverse events were headache, edema/swelling, dizziness, asthenia/fatigue, cough, rash, and impotence.

Conclusions.—For patients with stage 1 to 3 hypertension, fixed combinations of enalapril and diltiazem are generally well tolerated. These combinations appear more effective in reducing blood pressures than their individual components. The fixed combinations will help to increase drug compliance in patients requiring enalapril and diltiazem, thus leading to better long-term blood pressure control.

▶ There's nothing very exciting or unexpected in this multicenter parallel study of an ACE inhibitor, enalapril, and a calcium antagonist, diltiazem ER, separately and in 2 fixed combinations. The results were as expected: additive antihypertensive efficacy with the combination with no significant increase in side effects.

The rationale for its inclusion is to recognize the growing availability and likely increasing use of low-dose fixed combinations for treatment of hypertension. The major difference in the new combinations from those previously available is their low dosage, thereby providing additional efficacy while minimizing dose-dependent side effects. Truly low doses of hydrochlorothiazide, 6.25 mg/day, are available with a β-blocker (Ziac) or an ACE inhibitor (Lotensin-HCT). These are appropriate for initial therapy. Other low-dose combinations such as enalapril plus diltiazem are usually indicated as second steps in therapy but may be suitable for initial choice as well.

N.M. Kaplan, M.D.

The Effect of an Endothelin-Receptor Antagonist, Bosentan, on Blood Pressure in Patients With Essential Hypertension
Krum H, for the Bosentan Hypertension Investigators (Monash Univ, Prahran, Victoria, Australia; et al)
N Engl J Med 338:784-790, 1998   1–45

Background.—The endothelium-derived peptide endothelin-1 has potent vasoconstrictor effects, and may play a role in the pathogenesis of hypertension and chronic heart failure. It may also play a role in blood pressure elevation; however, the effects of treatment with endothelin-receptor antagonists on blood pressure control in hypertensive patients are unknown. The endothelin receptor antagonist bosentan was studied for its effects on blood pressure and heart rate in patients with essential hypertension.

Methods.—Participants were 293 adult patients with essential hypertension, defined by average diastolic pressure of 95 to 115 mm Hg after a 4-week placebo run-in period. The patients were randomly assigned to receive bosentan in a dosage of 100, 500, or 1,000 mg once daily or 1,000 mg twice daily; enalapril, 20 mg once daily; or placebo. The blood pressure response to treatment was analyzed, along with the effects on cardiovascular neurohormonal status. Sympathetic nervous system activation was assessed by measurement of plasma norepinephrine level, and renin-angiotensin system activation by measurement of plasma renin activity and angiotensin II.

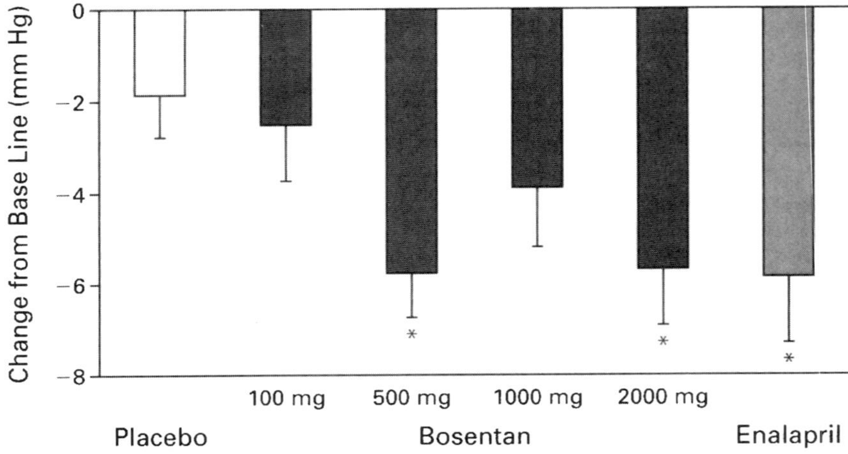

FIGURE 1.—Mean (±SE) change from baseline in diastolic pressure in patients with mild-to-moderate hypertension assigned to receive placebo, bosentan (100, 500, 1,000, or 2,000 mg daily), or enalapril (20 mg daily). Measurements were made while the patients were sitting upright. *Asterisks* denote $P < 0.05$ for the comparison with placebo. $P = 0.02$ by the trend test for the comparison of the 4 doses of bosentan. (Reprinted by permission of *The New England Journal of Medicine*, from Krum H, for the Bosentan Hypertension Investigators: The effect of an endothelin-receptor antagonist, bosentan, on blood pressure in patients with essential hypertension. *N Engl J Med* 338:784-790. Copyright 1998, Massachusetts Medical Society. All rights reserved.)

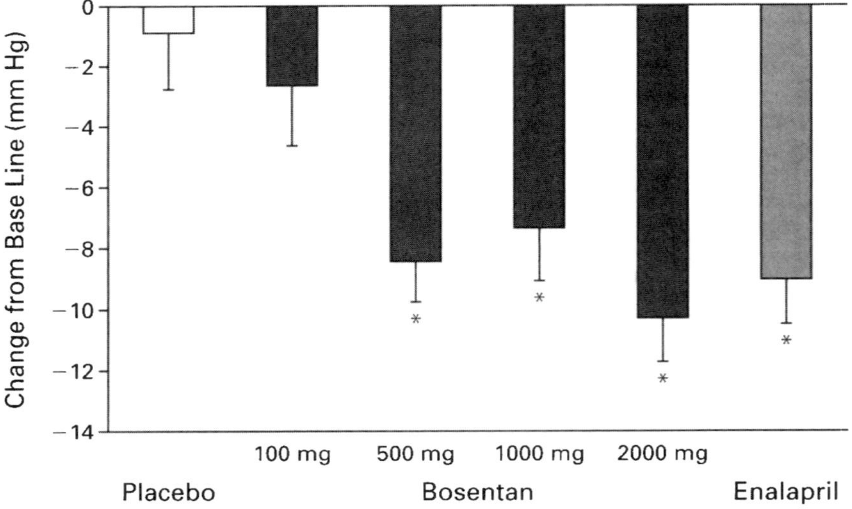

FIGURE 2.—Mean (±SE) change from baseline in systolic pressure in patients with mild-to-moderate hypertension assigned to receive placebo, bosentan (100, 500, 1,000, or 2,000 mg daily), or enalapril (20 mg daily). Measurements were made while the patients were sitting upright. *Asterisks* denote $P < 0.05$ for the comparison with placebo. $P = 0.001$ by the trend test for the comparison of the 4 doses of bosentan. (Reprinted by permission of *The New England Journal of Medicine*, from Krum H, for the Bosentan Hypertension Investigators: The effect of an endothelin-receptor antagonist, bosentan, on blood pressure in patients with essential hypertension. *N Engl J Med* 338:784-790. Copyright 1998, Massachusetts Medical Society. All rights reserved.)

Results.—Compared with placebo, diastolic blood pressure was reduced by approximately 6 mm Hg with bosentan 500 or 2,000 mg/day or with enalapril (Fig 1). Similar effects were noted on systolic blood pressure (Fig 2). Heart rate was unaffected by treatment. Treatment with bosentan did not produce activation of the sympathetic nervous system or renin-angiotensin system.

Conclusions.—Endothelin receptor antagonism with bosentan significantly lowers blood pressure in patients with essential hypertension. The findings support the role of endothelin-1 in blood pressure elevation. Bosentan's beneficial effect on hypertension occurs in the absence of reflexive neurohormonal activation.

▶ In a very short time since its discovery in 1988, the endothelium-derived vasoconstrictor has been found to be involved in normal growth and development and cardiovascular homeostasis, and to play a likely role in the pathophysiology of hypertension, heart failure, stroke, and renal parenchysmal disease.[1]

The availability of an orally active endothelin receptor antagonist, bosentan, provides a pharmacologic tool to learn more about the role of this peptide.[2] The results found in this well-conducted, large clinical trial suggest that such agents may become the next new class of antihypertensive drugs. An even more exciting role may be found for the treatment of heart failure.[3]

Keep tuned in.

N.M. Kaplan, M.D.

References

1. Webb DJ, Monge JC, Rabelink TJ, et al: Endothelin: New discoveries and rapid progress in the clinic. *Trends Pharmacol Sci* 19:5-8, 1998.
2. Webb DJ, Strachan FE: Clinical experience with endothelin antagonists. *Am J Hypertens* 11:71S-79S, 1998.
3. Brunner HR: Endothelin inhibition as a biologic target for treating hypertension. *Am J Hypertens* 11:103S-109S, 1998.

Secondary Hypertension

Risk of Morbidity From Renovascular Disease in Elderly Patients With Congestive Cardiac Failure

MacDowall P, Kalra PA, O'Donoghue DJ, et al (Hope Hosp, Salford, UK)
Lancet 352:13-16, 1998
1–46

Purpose.—Atheromatous renovascular disease is a frequent and important problem in the elderly and often goes unrecognized until serious complications occur. Patients with congestive heart failure probably have increased rates of renovascular disease. These patients often receive angiotensin-converting enzyme (ACE) inhibitors, which may be associated with renal impairment. The prevalence of renovascular disease in elderly patients with heart failure was studied.

Methods.—The study included 86 patients with heart failure from 1 English town. The patients were aged a mean of 77.5 years and were referred for intention-to-treat with ACE inhibitors. All patients were screened for renovascular disease using captopril renography. If this study was abnormal, renal artery magnetic resonance angiography was also performed. The same angiographic study was performed in 40% of patients with normal renograms, who served as negative control subjects. Patients with occlusion or greater than 50% stenosis of the renal artery were considered to have severe renovascular disease.

Results.—Thirty-four percent of patients proved to have severe renovascular disease. The sensitivity of captopril renography in detecting renovascular disease was estimated at 79%, with a specificity of 94%, positive predictive value of 90%, and negative predictive value of 88%. Mean creatinine was 201 µmol/L for patients with renovascular disease, compared with 135 µmol/L for normal subjects. Patients with disease were aged a mean of 81 years compared with normal subjects aged a mean of 77 years. Many patients with renovascular disease had peripheral arterial disease as well.

Conclusions.—This study identifies severe renovascular disease in nearly one third of patients with congestive heart failure being considered for ACE inhibitor therapy. Such patients should be evaluated for potential risk of renal impairment. Risk factors include widespread atheromatous disease, particularly peripheral vascular disease; impaired renal function; and advanced age.

▶ These data add to the considerable evidence that patients with any form of atherosclerotic-induced cardiovascular disease are more likely to have renovascular disease than would be found in nonafflicted patients. In this study, ischemic heart disease was the underlying cause of heart failure in three quarters of the patients with or without renovascular disease. Interestingly, only one third were hypertensive.

This last fact immediately brings up the question as to whether the renal artery disease, here defined as a greater than 50% stenosis on magnetic-resonance angiography, was hemodynamically important, that is, responsible for renovascular hypertension. In most patients, it likely was not.

Nonetheless, the authors correctly warn about potential problems when ACE inhibitors are routinely given to treat heart failure without recognition of underlying renovascular disease. Obviously, if the patient has a significant rise in serum creatinine or a marked fall in blood pressure, functionally significant renovascular disease must be looked for.

In addition, recurrent acute heart failure, that is flash pulmonary edema, has been recognized as a manifestation of renovascular disease[1]—more reason to consider the combination.

N.M. Kaplan, M.D.

Reference

1. Pickering TG, Herman L, Devereaux RB, et al: Recurrent pulmonary edema in hypertension due to bilateral renal artery stenosis: Treatment by angioplasty or surgical revascularization. *Lancet* 2:551-552, 1988.

Blood Pressure Outcome of Angioplasty in Atherosclerotic Renal Artery Stenosis: A Randomized Trial
Plouin P-F, for the Essai Multicentrique Medicaments vs Angioplastie (EMMA) Study Group (Hôpital Broussais, Paris)
Hypertension 31:823-829, 1998   1–47

Objective.—Renovascular hypertension results from renal artery stenosis (RAS), most often caused by atherosclerosis; renal insufficiency can occur as well. Renal artery stenosis can be treated by surgery or balloon angioplasty, in the hope of avoiding the need for antihypertensive therapy and progressive renal ischemia. However, few controlled studies have evaluated the effects of renal artery balloon angioplasty on blood pressure. The efficacy and safety of balloon angioplasty for blood pressure reduction in patients with RAS caused by atherosclerosis were assessed.

Methods.—Participants were 49 patients referred for management of hypertension and confirmed unilateral atherosclerotic RAS. After a 2- to 6-week run-in period to standardize the antihypertensive regimen, the patients were randomly assigned to undergo immediate angioplasty or to continue antihypertensive treatment, adapted as necessary. Measurements of 24-hour ambulatory blood pressure were done at baseline and at study termination—either 6 months after randomization or at the development of refractory hypertension. Patients assigned to angioplasty stopped taking antihypertensive drug treatment, which was restarted if hypertension persisted after the procedure. Treatment score and incidence of complications were used as secondary end points.

Results.—Procedural complications occurred in 6 patients in the angioplasty group vs. 2 in the control group. For 7 patients in the control group, study participation was terminated early because of refractory hypertension. Seventeen of 23 patients assigned to angioplasty had to restart antihypertensive therapy. At the time of study termination, mean ambulatory blood pressure was 140/81 mm Hg in the angioplasty group and 141/84 mm Hg in the control group. Patients in the angioplasty group were 60% less likely to have a treatment score of 2 or greater at the time of study termination. One patient in the angioplasty group had dissection with segmental renal infarction; 3 more had restenosis. There were no cases of renal artery thrombosis.

Conclusions.—For patients with hypertension and unilateral atherosclerotic RAS, renal artery balloon angioplasty reduces the need for antihypertensive drug treatment. However, the procedure carries significant morbidity. The ability of angioplasty to reduce blood pressure has been overestimated, based on uncontrolled and unblinded studies. Pending analyses of the long-term cardiovascular outcomes, the risks and benefits of angioplasty should be considered individually for each patient, taking patient preference into account.

▶ Despite the fact that many thousands of patients have been treated with 1 of 3 modalities (medical, surgical, or angioplasty) for renovascular hypertension during the past 30 years, this is the first properly performed comparison between medical therapy and angioplasty. One other small trial found that surgery was more successful than angioplasty in keeping the vessels open but provided little better effect on blood pressure at 2 years.[1]

The results of this study are surprising in the relative lack of success of angioplasty, which in itself connotes the need for such controlled studies early in the use of various procedures. On the other hand, stents are now being used to improve both the initial and long-term success rates of angioplasty,[2] so better results are likely possible than what Plouin et al. noted.

N.M. Kaplan, M.D.

References

1. Weibull H, Bergquist D, Bergentz SB: Percutaneous transluminal angioplasty versus reconstruction of atherosclerotic renal artery stenosis. *J Vasc Surg* 18:841-852, 1993.
2. Blum D, Krumme B, Flugel P: Treatment of ostial renal-artery stenoses with vascular endoprostheses after unsuccessful balloon angioplasty. *N Engl J Med* 336:459-465, 1997.

The Prevalence of Obstructive Sleep Apnea in Hypertensives

Worsnop CJ, Naughton MT, Barter CE, et al (Austin and Repatriation Med Centre, Heidelberg, Victoria, Austria)
Am J Respir Crit Care Med 157:111-115, 1998   1–48

Introduction.—Previous studies have demonstrated an association between systemic hypertension and obstructive sleep apnea (OSA). However, it remains unclear whether this relationship is causative or reflects confounding factors. The prevalence of OSA was compared in patients with treated and untreated hypertension and in normotensive individuals, with adjustment for possible confounders.

Methods.—Thirty-four patients with untreated hypertension, 34 with treated hypertension, and 25 without hypertension were studied. Mean ages were 58, 61, and 55 years, respectively. All patients were free of known disorders. Blood pressure was measured by 24-hour ambulatory monitoring; hypertension was defined as a mean 24-hour blood pressure of greater than 140/90. All patients underwent full polysomnography to determine the presence of OSA. The relationship between OSA and hypertension was assessed, with adjustment for body mass index, age, sex, and alcohol consumption.

Results.—An apnea-hypopnea index of greater than 5 was recorded for 38% of patients with untreated hypertension and 38% of those with treated hypertension, compared with 4% of normotensive individuals. Factors significantly associated with OSA on logistic regression analysis were body mass index, age, sex, and hypertension, whether treated or untreated. Alcohol consumption was not related to OSA. The relationship between OSA and hypertension was still apparent after adjustment for confounding variables.

Conclusions.—A relationship between OSA and hypertension exists. This association is partially explained by confounding variables—particularly body mass index but also age and sex. However, the relationship persists after controlling for these factors.

▶ The association between daytime hypertension and nighttime disturbed sleep from OSA has been repeatedly documented. The prevalence of the association seen in this small but carefully studied population—38% of both treated and untreated hypertensve patients had significantly high apnea-hypopnea indices—is in keeping with other reports. Moreover, the association between sleep apnea and hypertension persists when obesity and age are allowed for.

Of interest, the prevalence of hypertension was found to be even greater among nonobese sleep apneics than among obese sleep apneics in a large population study.[1] Because sleep apnea may be a major factor in the hypertension found in more than 1 million Americans, a careful history of sleep-disordered breathing (from both the patients and bed partner) should be obtained and if positive, appropriate sleep studies obtained.

N.M. Kaplan, M.D.

Reference

1. Young T, Peppard P, Palta M, et al: Population-based study of sleep-disordered breathing as a risk factor for hypertension. *Arch Intern Med* 157:1746-1752, 1997.

Preeclampsia Selectively Impairs Endothelium-dependent Relaxation and Leads to Oscillatory Activity in Small Omental Arteries
Pascoal IF, Lindheimer MD, Nalbantian-Brandt C, et al (Univ of Chicago)
J Clin Invest 101:464-470, 1998
1–49

Background.—In patients with preeclampsia, blood pressure is increased as the result of increases in systemic vascular resistance, in the presence of normal or reduced cardiac output. It has been suggested that the vascular pathophysiology of preeclampsia involves endothelial dysfunction, apparent mainly as deficient nitric oxide (NO) synthesis. Contraction and dilation were studied in small resistance-size omental arteries from women with preeclampsia.

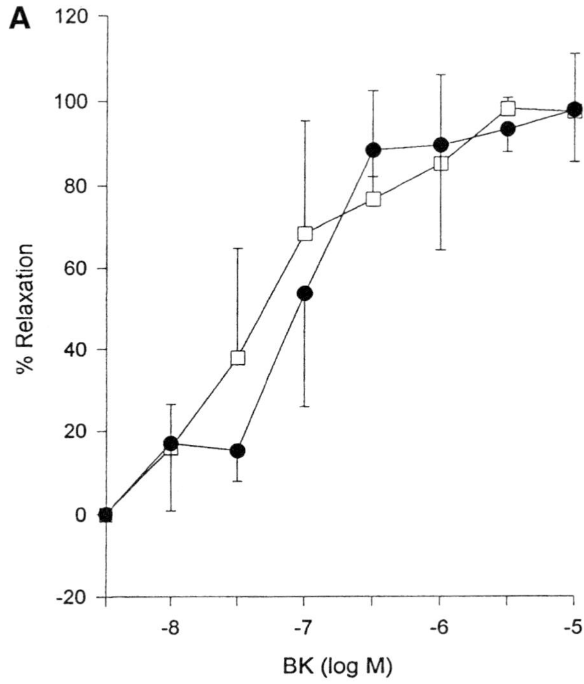

FIGURE 4.—Dose-response curves for percent relaxation vs. log concentration of bradykinin (*BK*) (**A**) or acetylcholine (*ACh*) (**B**). Data from normal gravidas (*open squares*) and preeclamptic women (*closed circles*) are shown (± SD). Dose-dependent BK-induced relaxation did not differ between groups. ACh-induced relaxation was selectively ablated in vessels from preeclamptic women. (Reproduced from *The Journal of Clinical Investigation* from Pascoal IF, Lindheimer MD, Nalbantian-Brandt C, et al: Preeclampsia selectively impairs endothelium-dependent relaxation and leads to oscillatory activity in small omental arteries. *J Clin Invest* 101:464-470. Copyright 1998, by copyright permission of Rockefeller University Press.)

(*Continued*)

Methods.—Small resistance-size omental arteries were obtained at surgery from women with preeclampsia. For comparison, vessels from normotensive gravidas, pregnant women with chronic hypertension, pregnant women with chronic hypertension and superimposed preeclampsia, and premenopausal, nonpregnant controls were studied. All vessels, with internal diameters of approximately 200 μm, were studied in vitro with a Mulvany-Halpern myograph. Contraction was studied in response to potassium chloride (KCl) and arginine vasopressin (AVP); dilation was studied in response to acetylcholine (ACh) and bradykinin. It was hypothesized that vessels from preeclamptic women would show increased contraction and decreased endothelium-dependent relaxation as an effect of decreased NO production.

Results.—The vessels from patients with preeclampsia did show significantly increased contraction in response to both KCl and AVP. Both endothelium- and cyclooxygenase-dependent phasic oscillations were apparent in vessels from the preeclamptic group, whereas all other groups

FIGURE 4 (cont.)

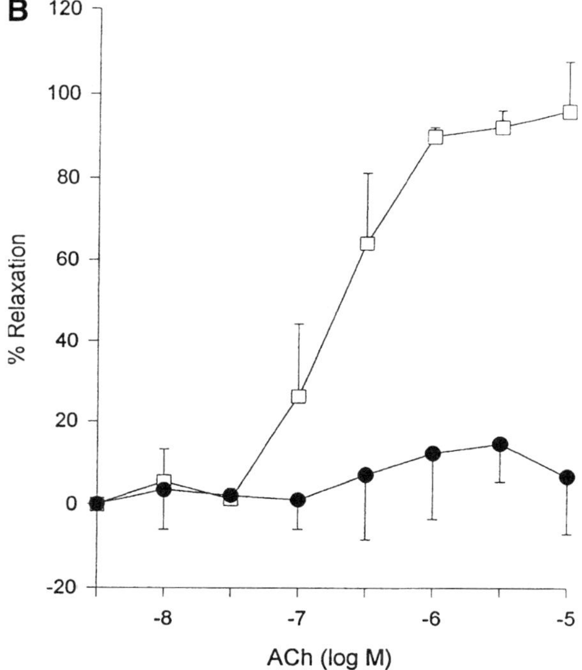

showed tonic contractions only. Relaxation in response to ACh and bradykinin was both dose and endothelium dependent, and was unaffected by inhibitors of NO synthesis. There was no difference in the bradykinin response of vessels from normal pregnant women vs. women with preeclampsia. In contrast, vessels from preeclamptic women showed no response to acetylcholine (Fig 4).

Conclusions.—Omental resistance arteries from women with preeclampsia show augmented contraction, exaggerated vasomotion, and selective loss of ACh-induced relaxation. These findings suggest that preeclampsia is related to a selective endothelial cell dysfunction. If this vascular abnormality is operative in vivo, it may provide an effector mechanism leading to the characteristic hypertension and pathologic vasospasm of preeclampsia.

▶ The basic cause of preeclampsia continues to be elusive, in part because it is not reproducible in animal models and it cannot be adequately studied in pregnant women. The studies reported here on omental vessels obtained during surgery on women near the end of either normotensive or preeclamptic pregnancies are about as close as investigators can get. The results support a number of defects in the responses of the endothelium of resistance arteries but not in the classic. NO system, which is thought to be the major endothelium-derived relaxation pathway.

Others have presented evidence of defective implantation of placental tissue as the basic defect, which in turn could lead to the elaboration of local or humoral factors that could affect overall endothelial function. Regardless, the promise that low-dose aspirin could serve as a preventative, likely by blocking synthesis of vasoconstricting prostaglandins, seems not to have been fulfilled.[1] Thus, the search for both cause and prevention of preeclampsia must go on.

N.M. Kaplan, M.D.

Reference

1. CLASP Collaborative Group: CLASP: A randomised trial of low-dose aspirin for the prevention and treatment of pre-eclampsia among 9364 pregnant women. *Lancet* 343:619-629, 1994.

Transdermal Oestrogen Reduces Daytime Blood Pressure in Hypertensive Women

Manhem K, Ahlm H, Milsom I, et al (Sahlgrens Univ, Göteborg, Sweden)
J Hum Hypertens 12:323-327, 1998   1–50

Purpose.—Menopause is believed to be associated with an increase in blood pressure, although the specific effect of menopause has been difficult to determine. It is unclear whether estrogen treatment reduces blood pressure in postmenopausal women. The effects of transdermal estrogen on blood pressure in postmenopausal women with hypertension were assessed.

Ambulatory Diastolic Blood Pressure, daytime

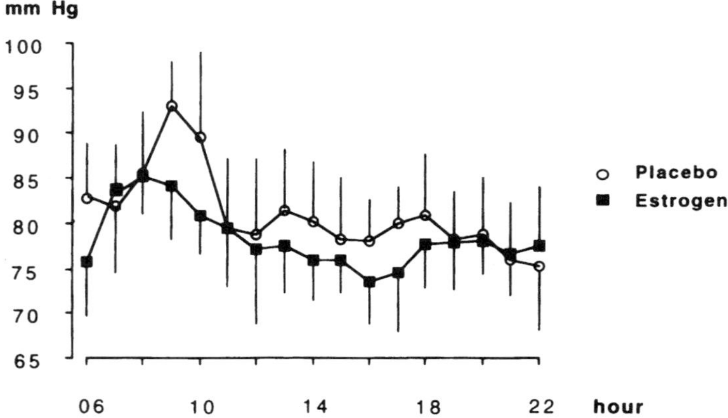

FIGURE 2.—**Bottom,** Daytime (6:00 AM-11:00 PM) ambulatory recordings of diastolic BP (mean and SEM) during placebo (*circles*) conditions and estrogen (*squares*) treatment in 13 hypertensive women. (Courtesy of Manhem K, Ahlm H, Milson I, et al: Transdermal oestrogen reduces daytime blood pressure in hypertensive women. *J Hum Hypertens* 12:323-327, 1998.)

Methods.—The placebo-controlled, crossover trial included 13 postmenopausal women, mean age 62 years, who were receiving antihypertensive therapy. None had ever received any type of hormone replacement therapy. The patients underwent two 24-hour blood pressure and heart-rate recordings, performed at least 1 week apart. One study was performed during treatment with a 17-β-estradiol patch, delivering 100 μg every 24 hours, and 1 with treatment with a placebo patch. The acute effects of the 2 treatments were compared.

Results.—Serum estradiol level was 139 pg/mL during active treatment compared with 40.5 pg/mL during placebo treatment. Office and ambulatory blood pressure measurements found no significant increase in blood pressure. However, a 3-mm Hg reduction in daytime blood pressure was noted while the women were wearing the estradiol patch; the difference was significant for diastolic blood pressure. No accompanying change in heart rate was seen. Placebo treatment was associated with nighttime dipping in systolic and diastolic blood pressure; these dips were not more pronounced during active treatment (Fig 2, bottom).

Conclusions.—Transdermal estrogen does not cause any acute elevation in blood pressure among postmenopausal women with hypertension. Instead, it may produce a mild reduction in daytime blood pressure, with no change in heart rate. Estrogen therapy does not appear to blunt or increase nocturnal dipping of blood pressure in this group of patients. Randomized trials are needed to assess the long-term effects of estrogen therapy on blood pressure.

▶ This is only the latest of a number of articles that show either no change or a slight fall in blood pressure with estrogen replacement therapy (ERT). It is included because of its careful documentation of the blood pressure by ambulatory monitoring, its inclusion of hypertensive women, and its clean design of using either a placebo or an estrogen patch for only 1 week. Most of the previous papers have looked at routinely measured blood pressure after variable periods of oral estrogen.

The importance of these data is that they give additional assurances of the safety of postmenopausal ERT relative to its effect on blood pressure, particularly because estrogen in larger amounts in oral contraceptives almost always raises pressure. Long observed in animals[1] and more recently in people,[2] estrogen given to the estrogen-deprived causes vasodilatation likely by activating synthesis of nitric oxide by the vascular endothelium. This vasodilatory effect and slight fall in blood pressure could contribute to the well-recognized cardioprotective effect of ERT.

N.M. Kaplan, M.D.

References

1. Magness RR, Rosenfeld CR: Local and systemic estradiol-17 beta: Effects on uterine and systemic vasodilation. *Am J Physiol* 256:536-542, 1989.
2. Gilligan DM, Badar DM, Panza JA, et al: Acute vascular effects of estrogen in postmenopausal women. *Circulation* 90:786-791, 1994.

2 Pediatric Cardiovascular Disease

Introduction

The emphasis again is on surgical therapy and follow-up or outcome studies in the 1999 YEAR BOOK. In our specialty, we continue to deal with more and more complex patients for whom palliative or reparative surgical therapy is possible and outcomes are improving. However, there are less-than-optimal outcomes in many conditions; thus, follow-up and outcome studies become extremely important for advancements in this field. In addition to these reports, there continue to be outstanding results in interventional catheterization techniques, particularly in the areas of stenting. Arrhythmia treatment with radio-frequency ablation is also extremely successful in children, with very low morbidity and rates of recurrence.

Among the improved outcomes in surgery are results for the infant with hypoplastic left heart syndrome and for the patient awaiting aortic valve surgery who is a candidate for a Ross procedure. We have moved from a condition with a 93% mortality to one with a 50% to 60% survival in a relatively short time for the infant with hypoplastic left heart syndrome. Another change is the increasing popularity of the Ross procedure, which postoperatively has an improved hemodynamic profile from prosthetic valves and the lack of need for long-term anticoagulation. Hopefully, the long-term outcomes will be as good as the midterm outcomes in both of these conditions.

Thomas P. Graham, M.D.

Acquired Heart Disease

Fatal Kawasaki Disease With Coronary Arteritis and No Coronary Aneurysms

Burke AP, Virmani R, Perry LW, et al (Armed Forces Inst of Pathology, Washington, DC; Georgetown Univ, Washington, DC; Univ of Maryland, Baltimore)
Pediatrics 101:108-111, 1998   2–1

Introduction.—Among Japanese patients, coronary artery aneurysms have been reported in all but the early stages of Kawasaki disease. The 2 patients described here show that localized aneurysmal dilatation is not, however, a constant feature of fatal forms of the disease.

Case Reports.—Two boys, ages 4 years and 20 months, experienced episodes of fever, conjunctivitis, and pharyngitis. The 4-year-old (case 1) also had a rash and mild lymphadenopathy; the younger child (case 2) was found to have palpable submandibular, axillary, inguinal, and occipital adenopathy. In case 1, development of abdominal pain led to a tentative diagnosis of ulcerative colitis; Kawasaki disease was not suspected and no cardiac evaluation was undertaken. A sedimentation rate of 94 mm/hr and a platelet count of 946,000 were present in case 2, and Kawasaki disease was diagnosed. The 4-year-old boy was admitted for abdominal pain and apnea, then evaluated for porphyria and heavy metal poisoning. Both toxicologic screening and neurologic evaluations were normal. He died suddenly before a scheduled upper gastrointestinal series. Autopsy revealed a heart weight of 155 g (vs. 53-115 g for body weight of 17 kg). His left ventricular lateral wall showed gross evidence of fibrosis or necrosis. In the second case, the patient was treated for Kawasaki disease but continued to have symptoms of an inflammatory process. Approximately 1 year after the initial illness, the boy died of cardiac arrest during an examination by a neurologist. The boy had never shown ECG evidence for a myocardial infarction. At autopsy, the heart weighed 69 g (at the upper range of normal for body size). Coronary arteries showed diffuse intimal thickening and ongoing arteritis.

Conclusion.—In both of these cases, death was the result of diffuse fibrointimal proliferation involving all epicardial arteries. Both differed clinically and pathologically from cases of typical Kawasaki disease. Patients with possible mucocutaneous lymph node syndrome should undergo tests other than echocardiography in order to determine coronary artery involvement.

▶ This brief article reporting 2 cases of presumed Kawasaki disease, arteritis, and severe fibrointimal proliferation with coronary involvement raises the specter of diffuse coronary disease without echo evidence of aneurysm as another manifestation, albeit rare, of this childhood disease. Although these patients did not have classic features of Kawasaki disease, there were enough signs and symptoms to make this a possible cause and to alert pediatric cardiologists to the possibility of such a problem in patients with "atypical Kawasaki disease."

T.P. Graham, M.D.

Prognostic Value of Dipyridamole-Thallium Myocardial Scintigraphy in Patients With Kawasaki Disease

Miyagawa M, Mochizuki T, Murase K, et al (Ehime Natl Hosp, Japan; Ehime Univ, Japan; City of Yawatahama, Ehime, Japan)
Circulation 98:990-996, 1998   2–2

Introduction.—Coronary arterial aneurysms can develop during the acute stage of Kawasaki disease. Most of these lesions regress spontaneously, but others progress to obstructive coronary lesions. The progress of the lesions can be difficult to monitor, as coronary angiography (CAG) is not a frequently repeatable procedure, particularly in infants. Dipyridamole-thallium single-photon emission CT (SPECT) was evaluated for use in the long-term follow-up of children with Kawasaki disease.

Methods.—Four hundred fifty-nine patients with Kawasaki disease were admitted over a 5-year period. Of these, 90 were found to have coronary aneurysms by cross-sectional echocardiography during the acute stage, a rate of 20%. Sixty-one patients were boys and 29 were girls. They underwent paired studies of selective CAG and dipyridamole-thallium SPECT, performed within 1 month of each other. The patients were then examined for 8 years or longer for the occurrence of cardiac events. The prognostic value of dipyridamole-thallium SPECT was analyzed.

Results.—Fifteen cardiac events occurred during follow-up, including 7 cases of unstable angina, 5 myocardial infarctions, 2 coronary artery bypass graft operations, and 1 death. All but 1 of these 15 patients had thallium redistribution on the SPECT scan. The sensitivity of this finding was 93%, with a specificity of 83%, a positive predictive value of 52%, and a negative predictive value of 98%. Thallium redistribution was the best independent predictor of late cardiac events on multivariate analysis. The ability to predict late cardiac events was little improved by addition of the number of aneurysms detected on CAG.

Conclusion.—In children with Kawasaki disease, dipyridamole-thallium SPECT scanning is a safe procedure that is useful for risk stratification and long-term follow-up of coronary aneurysms. The finding of thallium redistribution is the best independent predictor of late cardiac events. Dipyridamole-thallium SPECT is a noninvasive procedure that can be successfully carried out, even in patients less than 3 years of age.

▶ These authors show an incredibly high relative risk for future cardiac events in patients with Kawasaki disease and aneurysms when dipyridamole-thallium myocardial scintigraphy shows thallium redistribution. Thallium redistribution was much more predictive of future cardiac events than was the number of aneurysms, presence of coronary stenosis, or maximal size of aneurysms. There are many different ways to study patients with Kawasaki disease and aneurysms to try to detect occult myocardial ischemia. These include CAG, treadmill testing, dobutamine stress testing with echocardiographic monitoring for wall motion abnormalities, and radionuclide studies. This particular scintigraphic technique appears highly predictive and certainly deserves further study in patients with significant aneuryms.

T.P. Graham, M.D.

Idiopathic Dilated Cardiomyopathy in Children: Prognostic Indicators and Outcome

Arola A, Tuominen J, Ruuskanen O, et al (Univ of Turku, Finland)
Pediatrics 101:369-376, 1998
2–3

Introduction.—Prognosis is generally poor for patients with idiopathic dilated cardiomyopathy (IDCM), but the clinical course can vary considerably. To determine factors that might be useful as prognostic indicators in children with IDCM, a group of Finnish children and adolescents was retrospectively analyzed.

Methods.—The 62 children and adolescents ranged in age from 1 day to 20 years (median 13 months at diagnosis). All were seen between 1980 and 1991 and met strict inclusion criteria for DCM. Their medical histories were reviewed, together with laboratory studies, treatment, and findings at follow-up examinations.

Results.—During the study period, approximately 5 new cases per year were diagnosed in an age-specific population of 1.4 million. Ten patients (16%) had familial cardiomyopathy and 29 (47%) were reported to have a recent upper respiratory or gastrointestinal illness at initial examination. Forty-five patients (73%) were admitted with clinical features of fulminant congestive heart failure. Ten other patients were seen with symptoms such as arrhythmias, chest pain, and feeding problems. During a mean follow-up of 3.9 years, 31 patients (50%) had died, 17 had residual disease, 10 recovered, and 4 underwent heart transplantation. Infants younger than 1 year and boys aged 15 years and older with progressing symptoms of left ventricular failure after starting medical therapy tended to have the poorest outcomes. Multivariate analysis, however, identified 3 significant predictors of long-term outcome: histologic evidence of endocardial fibroelastosis (EFE), an initial finding of right ventricular failure, and the need for anticoagulation therapy during follow-up. All patients with EFE were younger than 2 years and died soon after diagnosis. Five-year survival rates tended to be better for patients who had IDCM diagnosed in the second half of the study period.

Conclusions.—The underlying cause of DCM is unknown in most cases, and outcome can vary from full recovery to death. Overall outcome was poor; half of the patients died. Yet some, mainly infants, recovered completely. Patients determined to be at high risk for poor outcome should be assessed for cardiac transplantation, which has offered 1- and 3-year survival rates as high as 95% and 87%, respectively.

▶ It has been difficult to find precise indicators of 1- and 2-year survival in children with cardiomyopathy, so that transplantation can be offered at the appropriate time—that is, not too early and not too late. In this study of 62 Finnish patients, those patients who had histologic evidence of endocardial fibroelastosis, clinical signs of right ventricular failure at presentation, those who were adolescent males, or who failed to show improvement of fractional shortening over the first 6 to 12 months were more likely to die or require heart transplantation during 12 to 24 months of follow-up. These risk factors for poor outcome should be weighed heavily when managing these patients.

T.P. Graham, M.D.

Left Ventricular Geometry and Severe Left Ventricular Hypertrophy in Children and Adolescents With Essential Hypertension

Daniels SR, Loggie JMH, Khoury P, et al (Univ of Cincinnati, Ohio)
Circulation 97:1907-1911, 1997
2–4

Objective.—Although the relationship of obesity and elevated blood pressure to increased left ventricular (LV) mass index is well established in adults, the importance of these factors for determining LV mass in children is uncertain. The cut-off point establishing excessive LV mass for body size and associated with increasing morbidity is an LV mass index of 51 $g/m^{2.7}$. Severe LV hypertrophy and LV geometry were evaluated in children and adolescents with essential hypertension.

Methods.—LV mass was determined using echocardiography in 130 patients (25% female), aged 6 to 23, who had essential hypertension, defined as systolic or diastolic pressure greater than the 90th percentile for a minimum of 3 months. Body mass index, dietary sodium intake, lipids, and lipoproteins were determined. In a graded bicycle ergometer test, patients performed at 50%, 75%, and 100% of predicted maximum workload.

Results.—Approximately half the patients were white and half were black. LV mass index exceeded 51 $g/m^{2.7}$ in 11 patients (2 female, 5 white). A total of 19 patients had an LV mass index higher than the 99th percentile. Of 61 patients with an LV mass index greater than the 95th percentile, 22 (17%) had concentric hypertrophy and 32 had eccentric hypertrophy. In adults, concentric hypertrophy is associated with increased risk of cardiovascular disease. No other differences between groups were noted. Stepwise multiple regression analysis revealed that male sex, increased heart rate at maximum exercise, and increased body mass index were significant and independent predictors of severe LV hypertrophy.

Conclusion.—Young people with essential hypertension and a high body mass index are more likely to have severe LV hypertrophy. However, there were no significant and consistent determinants of LV geometry that could be identified in children with essential hypertension.

▶ Pediatric cardiologists frequently are asked to assess hypertensive patients, either as part of general management or to determine how the hypertension has affected the heart. This article indicates that a significant number of patients with essential hypertension and very few, if any, symptoms have LV hypertrophy, which appears to be related to, among other variables, gender and body mass index. Weight loss is an important component of therapy, but obviously very difficult to achieve in this group. Early pharmacological treatment and serial cardiac assessment are important parts of lifelong management of this common condition.

T.P. Graham, M.D.

Diagnosis and Management of Stenotic Aorto-Arteriopathy in Childhood
D'Souza SJA, Tsai W-S, Silver MM, et al (Univ of Toronto)
J Pediatr 132:1016-1022, 1998   2–5

Background.—Patients with stenotic aorto-arteriopathy (SAA), an uncommon group of vascular diseases, have segmental stenoses of the aorta and its branches. The most common type is middle aortic syndrome, characterized by severe stenosis of the thoracic and abdominal descending aorta. The differential diagnosis includes mainly Takayasu arteritis (TA) and fibromuscular dystrophy or other noninflammatory aortic-arterial diseases. An experience with the management of SAA in childhood is reviewed, including the results of several different management approaches.

Patients.—The 16-year experience included 14 children and adolescents with acquired SAA. There were 7 boys and 7 girls, aged 4 to 18 years. Most patients were asymptomatic, with hypertension noted at routine examination. Clinical findings included abdominal bruits in 8 patients, mixed absent/diminished and normal pulses in 8, and leg claudication in 4. On angiography, 13 of 13 patients showed involvement of the abdominal or descending thoracic aorta. A midthoracoabdominal coarctation was detected in most patients. Eleven patients received a diagnosis of TA. It was difficult to distinguish TA and fibromuscular dysplasia on clinical or angiographic grounds.

Treatment and Outcomes.—Treatment started with antihypertensive therapy, usually with an arteriolar vasodilator followed by β-adrenergic blockade. In patients with TA, prednisone did not reverse the aortic disease, but it did worsen hypertension. Six patients underwent percutaneous transluminal balloon angioplasty of renal artery stenosis, but the renal arteries usually restenosed. Renal autotransplantation—excision of the stenotic area of the affected artery, with reimplantation of the kidney onto a disease-free vessel—was performed in 5 patients. This provided temporary improvement in blood pressure in most patients; 1 patient had renal artery thrombosis with deteriorating renal function. Three patients underwent abdominal aorta enlargement with percutaneously implanted balloon expandable stents. In 1 case, this was successfully followed by renal autotransplantation. There were 3 deaths.

Conclusions.—This experience illustrates the difficulties in diagnosis and management of SAA in children. Pathologic information is important, but it is difficult to obtain a representative specimen. Most patients are first seen in the chronic vaso-occlusive phase, when TA is usually not progressive. The distinction from fibromuscular dysplasia may be irrelevant to treatment. The goal of treatment is to minimize end-organ damage, and to manage sequelae.

▶ SAA rarely occurs in pediatric patients, but early recognition of the extent of obstruction is necessary to minimize end-organ damage. It is interesting that 7 of these patients had no symptoms and were identified only because of moderate or severe hypertension. Presence of an abnormal bruit or abnormal pulses can bring attention to this condition and lead to diagnostic angiography and treatment.

T.P. Graham, M.D.

Medical Therapy

Guidelines for Antithrombotic Therapy in Pediatric Patients
Andrew M, Michelson AD, Bovill E, et al (Hamilton Civic Hosps Research Centre, Hamilton, Ont; Hosp for Sick Children, Toronto; Univ of Massachusetts, Worcester; et al)
J Pediatr 132:575-588, 1998   2–6

Purpose.—Recent years have seen a sharp increase in the use of antithrombotic agents in pediatric patients. Although guidelines for use of these agents in adults are well established, they cannot simply be extended to infants and children. These authors reviewed the literature on antithrombotic therapy in pediatric patients and sought to provide general guidelines for such therapy.

Antithrombotic Therapy in Children.—The most frequent congenital prethrombotic disorders are activated protein C resistance and deficiency of protein C, protein S, or antithrombin. The most common of these is activated protein C resistance. It is caused by a point mutation in factor V, called factor V Leiden. Homozygous deficiencies of protein C or S may be manifest within hours after birth. By far, most acquired venous thromboembolic events in pediatric patients are related to serious primary disorders. The main cause is the presence of a central venous line, most often in the upper venous system. Other conditions include right atrial thrombus, renal vein thrombosis, and portal vein thrombosis. Venous thromboembolic events in children can have a number of different complications, including pulmonary embolism, recurrent thrombosis, postphlebitic syndrome, and death. Acquired arterial thrombotic events may be related to cardiac catheterization, prosthetic heart valves, Blalock-Taussig shunts, or the Fontan procedure. Antithrombotic therapy in children may consist of heparin, including low–molecular-weight heparin; oral anticoagulants, such as warfarin; antiplatelet agents, such as aspirin; and various thrombolytic agents. Variables affecting the activity of each of these agents were presented.

Recommendations.—Based on a review of the literature and a consensus conference of the American College of Chest Physicians, guidelines for the use of antithrombotic therapy in children were presented. Conditions addressed were venous thromboembolism in children; venous/arterial thromboembolism in newborns; heparin prophylaxis for patients undergoing cardiac catheterization; mechanical and biological prosthetic heart valves in children; Kawasaki disease; Fontan operation; Blalock-Taussig shunts; and homozygous protein C and S deficiency. The recommendations were classified according to the strength of the evidence on which they are based.

Discussion.—Despite the differences in thromboembolic disorders between children and adults, most previous guidelines on the use of antithrombotic therapy in pediatric patients have been extrapolated from guidelines for adults. The new recommendations are based on the best available data, although the authors underscore the lack of data on the risk-benefit ratio of the interventions and on the long-term outcomes. They call for clinical trials to clarify the management of thromboembolic disorders in infants and children. They also discuss the need for development of the new field of childhood thrombophilia.

▶ With increasing surgical success in the treatment of very complex congenital cardiac defects, more and more patients, with their associated central venous lines, are spending significant time in the ICU before and after operations. The incidence of thrombosis in these patients is extremely high and, unfortunately, US can be misleading for determining the presence or extent of thrombosis, because of the development of large collateral vessels that can be mistaken for normal central venous structures. The early use of angiography is needed in these patients. The prevention of thrombosis should be the mainstay for this group, with most patients needing more heparin than is frequently used. The guidelines for the use of heparin, warfarin, and antiplatelet and thrombolytic therapy in this review are excellent and hopefully, can be used to decrease the incidence of patient morbidity and mortality from severe thromboembolic complications.

T.P. Graham, M.D.

Beta-Blocker Therapy of Severe Congestive Heart Failure in Infants With Left to Right Shunts
Buchhorn R, Bartmus D, Siekmeyer W, et al (Georg-August-Univ, Göttingen, Germany)
Am J Cardiol 98:1366-1368, 1998   2–7

Objective.—Congestive heart failure (CHF) often develops in infants with left and right shunts as a result of congenital heart disease. Most surgical and medical therapeutic approaches have led to less than satisfactory results. Because of the success of various selective and nonselective β-blockers on the neurohumoral state and clinical outcome in adults, infants with CHF were treated with propranolol.

Methods.—Between July 1996 and June 1997, 6 consecutive infants with CHF as a result of left to right shunt, who had failed conventional therapy, were treated with a 1 mg oral dose of propranolol increasing, if tolerated, to 1 mg/kg per day and then by 1 mg every 3 days to a maximum of 2 mg/kg per day. Plasma renin activity, aldosterone, and catecholamine levels were measured at baseline and at the end of the propranolol titration period.

Results.—Respiratory and heart rates decreased significantly from 75 to 61 beats per minute and 139 to 117 beats per minute, respectively. Mean arterial pressure decreased significantly in 3 infants. Oxygen saturation was unchanged. At the end of the titration period, only 1 infant required furosemide. Infants gained an average of 130 g per week and the gastric tube could be removed from all infants. Heart failure scores decreased significantly from 9.8 to 2.7. Average plasma renin and aldosterone levels decreased significantly from 124 to 20 ng/mL/hr and 3,170 to 1,159 pg/L, respectively. Average norepinephrine levels declined from 1,270 to 709 ng/L. Average propranolol dose at discharge was 1.8 mg/kg per day.

Conclusion.—Propranolol appeared to have a beneficial effect on these 6 infants with CHF as a result of congenital left to right shunts.

▶ This study of a very small number of patients with severe CHF appears to show a beneficial effect of β-blockade similar to what has been shown in adults with heart failure from idiopathic or ischemic cardiomyopathy. Apparently angiotensin-converting enzyme inhibitors were not used before resorting to β-blocker therapy. These studies suggest that chronic low dose propranolol therapy can achieve deactivation of the renin-angiotensin system, and this therapy may be useful in pediatric patients with CHF not controlled by standard therapy.

T.P. Graham, M.D.

β-Blocker Therapy in Young Children With Congestive Heart Failure Under Consideration for Heart Transplantation

Shaddy RE (Univ of Utah, Salt Lake City)
Am Heart J 136:19-21, 1998   2–8

Introduction.—In adult patients with cardiomyopathy, β-blocker therapy can increase left ventricular ejection fraction while reducing symptoms and increasing survival. The authors have shown good results with β-blockers in adolescents with chemotherapy-induced cardiomyopathy. They reported on the use of β-blocker therapy in children with severe congestive heart failure being considered for heart transplantation.

Patients.—The 4 children, with a mean age of 8 years, all had New York Heart Association class IV symptoms related to borderline myocarditis, postoperative cardiomyopathy, Duchenne's muscular dystrophy, or idiopathic dilated cardiomyopathy. After receiving conventional therapy with digoxin, diuretics, and angiotensin-converting enzyme inhibitors without improvement, the children were considered for β-blocker therapy. All were given metoprolol starting at 0.1 mg/kg/dose twice daily and increased to a maximal dosage of 0.9 mg/kg/day. The mean follow-up was 13 months.

Results.—With β-blocker therapy, mean left ventricular fractional shortening increased from 14% to 26% and ejection fraction from 20% to 11%. In the 2 youngest patients, aged 4 and 5 years, dramatic echocardiographic and symptom improvement was noted within 7 weeks of starting therapy. The other 2 patients had a less dramatic response which began 3 months after starting metoprolol. One underwent heart transplantation at 18 months after starting metoprolol; the patient with Duchenne muscular dystrophy died after 17 months.

Conclusion.—For some young children with cardiomyopathy and congestive heart failure, β-blocker therapy may improve ejection fraction and symptom status. More study is needed to determine which children can benefit the most from β-blocker therapy and which medications are the most effective.

▶ The use of β-blocker therapy for heart failure is not a strategy that most cardiologists would have intuitively arrived at. Fortunately, some bright people treating adults have realized that the intensive sympathomimetic and renin-angiotensin–mediated stimulation of the heart which occurs with congestive failure can be detrimental in the long run and that both angiotensin-converting enzyme inhibition therapy and β-blockade may prove useful in adult patients with severe congestive heart failure from both dilated and ischemic cardiomyopathy. There are only a few small reports of children with β-blocker therapy in this setting, but there appears to be a beneficial effect in the small number of patients studied, including a small number of infants with large left-to-right shunts and severe congestive heart failure. More studies are needed. Hopefully, we can add this therapy to the growing list of effective treatments for heart failure in children.

T.P. Graham, M.D.

Surgical Therapy

Geometric Mismatch of Pulmonary and Aortic Anuli in Children Undergoing the Ross Procedure: Implications for Surgical Management and Autograft Valve Function

Reddy VM, McElhinney DB, Phoon CK, et al (Univ of California, San Francisco)

J Thorac Cardiovasc Surg 115:1255-1263, 1998

2–9

Introduction.—Many children treated with the Ross procedure for congenital heart lesions have a significant discrepancy between the pulmonary and aortic anuli. No systematic study has examined whether such a mismatch presents a contraindication to the procedure. A review of 41 children who underwent the Ross procedure focuses on the surgical management of geometric mismatch and the effects of mismatch on autograft valve function.

Methods.—Patients had a mean age of 7.8 years. The diameter of the pulmonary valve was greater by ≥3 mm than that of the aortic valve in 20 cases, equal (within 2 mm) in 12 cases, and less by ≥3 mm in 9 cases: differences ranged from +10 to −12 mm. Aortoventriculoplasty was used to correct the mismatch in the 12 children with a larger pulmonary anulus. In those with a larger aortic anulus, the correction was made by a gradual adjustment along the circumference of the autograft. Patients were followed (median, 31 months) for autograft valvular regurgitation.

Results.—Two patients required reoperation on the neoaortic valve for moderate regurgitation. In the remaining 38 survivors, autograft regurgitation was absent or trivial in 30, mild in 7, and moderate in 1. Regurgitation showed no correlation with age of the child, geometric mismatch, or previous or concurrent procedures. No patient had evidence of significant autograft root dilatation.

Conclusion.—Geometric mismatch is not a contraindication to the Ross procedure in children. Autograft regurgitation is likely to result from subtle technical factors that may distort the valve complex.

▶ In most cases, the techniques illustrated here and a successful Ross procedure can overcome a prominent geometric mismatch between the aortic root and the pulmonary artery root. In the hands of an experienced surgeon, this technique looks good from the start and, hopefully, will stand the test of time.

T.P. Graham, M.D.

The Ross Operation in Children: 10-Year Experience

Elkins RC, Knott-Craig CJ, Ward KE, et al (Univ of Oklahoma, Oklahoma City)
Ann Thorac Surg 65:496-502, 1998   2–10

Introduction.—The Ross operation for aortic valve replacement in children has been performed for 30 years, but its widespread acceptance was delayed because of the procedure's technical demands and the need to place 2 valves at risk. With modification of operative techniques, the Ross operation is now the operation of choice for children and young adults who require aortic valve replacement.

Methods.—Researchers reviewed the records of 150 consecutive patients to provide additional long-term follow-up of the Ross operation. There were 112 boys and 38 girls in the study group; their median age was 12 years. Primary diagnoses were aortic stenosis in 40, aortic insufficiency in 29, and a combination of these lesions in 80. Most had undergone other procedures before the Ross operation. Echocardiographic assessment was available on 91% of patients within 2 years of study closure.

Results.—Eight-year survival was 97.3%. Six patients required reoperation with restitution of autograft function and 2 with late autograft valve dysfunction required a replacement procedure. At 8 years, freedom from reoperation for autograft dysfunction was 90%, freedom from reoperation for homograft obstruction was 94%, and freedom from reoperation on the homograft or a gradient of 40 mm Hg was 89%. All patients enjoy a normal, active life, unencumbered by the need for anticoagulants.

Conclusion.—The Ross operation in children has an excellent rate of success and a low operative risk. Valve-related complications are not life-threatening, and long-term satisfactory autograft valve function can be achieved.

▶ Dr. Elkins has pioneered the use of the Ross operation in children and has very good medium-term results. Most patients achieve a very good early result. Significant aortic regurgitation is rare early after repair, although it can be more prevalent with increasing time. Hopefully, results will continue to improve since freedom from residual obstruction is usually much improved with this therapy over any alternative therapy.

T.P. Graham, M.D.

The Double Switch Procedure for Anatomical Repair of Congenitally Corrected Transposition of the Great Arteries in Infants and Children

Reddy VM, McElhinney DB, Silverman NH, et al (Univ of California, San Francisco)
Eur Heart J 18:1470-1477, 1997   2–11

Introduction.—There is no evidence that anatomical repair for congenitally corrected transposition of the great arteries (CCTGA) will enhance long-term ventricular function in patients without a compromised right ventricle. Recent data suggest that midterm systemic ventricular performance in patients with a double switch might be somewhat better than in patients who have undergone conventional repair. A double switch procedure may be effective in the presence of tricuspid regurgitation and in preventing regurgitation in patients with tricuspid valvar abnormalities likely to lead to dysfunction. The outcome of the double switch procedure was examined in infants and children with CCGTA.

Methods.—Seventeen patients underwent surgery for CCGTA between September 1993 and August 1996. Of these, 11 patients with a median age of 3.2 years (range, 4.8-7.8 years) underwent double switch procedure. Six patients did not undergo the double switch procedure because of unfavorable anatomy (2 patients), earlier conduit repair (2 patients), biventricular dysfunction (1 patient), and an isolated complete atrioventricular blockage (1 patient). All 11 patients who underwent the double switch procedure had a type of defect that involved malalignment of the ventricular septum. Nine patients had pulmonary outflow tract obstruction, and 5 had significant tricuspid valve pathologic conditions or dysfunction.

Results.—Patients underwent anatomical repair with either a Senning or Mustard procedure combined with an arterial switch operation plus a ventricular septal defect procedure or a Rastelli procedure with left ventricle to aortic baffle and right ventricle to pulmonary artery conduit. There was 1 early death in a patient who had undergone Senning repair and an arterial switch, with Aubert's procedure instead of simple coronary transfer. The cause of death was multi-organ failure and brain death secondary to mediastinal hemorrhaging and cardiac tamponade. There were no episodes of surgical complete atrioventricular blockage. There were no late deaths in this cohort at a median follow-up of 22 months. Two patients needed 3 late reoperations. All patients had normal biventricular function, were asymptomatic, and were taking no medications at a final follow-up.

Conclusion.—The double switch procedure may be performed to achieve anatomical repair of corrected transposition and has low rates of early mortality and surgical heart blockage and favorable midterm outcome. Long-term follow-up is now needed to determine whether this approach improves outcome compared with less aggressive surgical approaches that leave the right ventricle in the systemic circulation.

▶ There is increasing interest in the double switch procedure for patients with CCTGA and large ventricular septal defects. There are 2 different double switch procedures that probably should be reported and followed separately in terms of their midterm and long-term results. The first is the atrial (Mustard or Senning repair) plus arterial switch and ventricular septal defect closure, which is performed in patients without pulmonary stenosis either at a relatively early age (as it was performed in 3 patients in this report) or in the occasional older patient with a pulmonary artery band whose proximal pulmonary artery is still suitable for becoming the neoaorta. The second operation has been called the "Mustarelli" and involves an atrial switch (Mustard or Senning), ventricular septal defect closure, and conduit connection of the anatomical right ventricle to the pulmonary artery. Both of these operations are long and arduous. In this series of 17 patients, 11 had the double switch procedure, and there was only 1 early death and no late deaths. This is a reasonable choice for patients who have no left ventricular dysfunction and in whom the anatomy seems favorable.

T.P. Graham, M.D.

Primary Arterial Switch Operation for Transposition of the Great Arteries With Intact Ventricular Septum in Infants Older Than 21 Days
Foran JP, Sullivan ID, Elliott MJ, et al (Great Ormond Street Hosp for Children, London)
J Am Coll Cardiol 31:883-889, 1998   2–12

Introduction.—Infants with transposition of the great arteries with intact ventricular septum (TGA/IVS) usually undergo an arterial switch operation (ASO) within 2-3 weeks after birth. Beyond this period, some surgeons advocate an atrial switch operation or a 2-stage procedure using a pulmonary artery band to prepare the left ventricle for a later ASO. An experience with performing a primary ASO in older (3 weeks to 2 months) infants with TGA/IVS was reported.

Methods.—During a 7-year period (1990 through 1996), 37 infants underwent ASO for TGA/IVS between 21 and 61 days of age (late ASO group). From the group of 156 infants who underwent ASO in the first 21 days of life (early ASO group), 37 were randomly selected for comparison of surgical outcome. The procedure was performed on cardiopulmonary bypass under profound hypothermia. Postoperative data recorded included duration of ventilatory support and of inotropic support, and time spent in the cardiac ICU.

Results.—One infant (2.7%) died in-hospital in the late ASO group, whereas 13 infants (8.3%) died in-hospital in the early ASO group. Each group also had 1 late death. Comparisons of the late ASO group and the early ASO subgroup of 37 patients showed no significant differences in ventilation requirements, duration of IV inotropic or vasodilator support, or time spent in the cardiac ICU. These outcomes and mortality rates could not be predicted by patient age, left ventricular (LV) mass index, LV posterior wall thickness index, LV volume index, LV mass/volume ratio, pattern of LV geometry, the presence of a patent arterial duct, or pattern of coronary artery anatomy.

Discussion.—The upper age limit for a primary ASO in TGA/IVS remains controversial. There is concern that after 3 weeks of age, regression of the LV myocardial mass will leave the left ventricle incapable of coping with the acutely increased work of systemic perfusion. Although the upper age limit is not yet defined, infants older than 3 weeks can benefit from primary ASO.

▶ Shortly after the ASO for TGA was proven feasible in young infants, the conventional wisdom was that these patients should have the ASO performed in the first 2 to 3 weeks of life. The concern was that regression of LV mass would render the left ventricle incapable of performing systemic work after the ASO if the infants were older and had been subjected to a relatively low LV pressure. Despite abnormal echocardiograms indicating low LV pressure and low LV volumes and mass in a number of patients, there was no significant difference in mortality or morbidity in patients who underwent early vs. late ASOs. These authors have definitely extended the age range in which primary ASO can be offered to infants with transposition. The upper limit of age remains an individual clinical decision, with factors such as individual surgical results and echocardiographic findings playing a role in making the final management decision.

T.P. Graham, M.D.

One-Lung Fontan Operation: Hemodynamics and Surgical Outcome
Zachary CH, Jacobs ML, Apostolopoulou S, et al (Children's Hosp of Philadelphia)
Ann Thorac Surg 65:171-175, 1998   2–13

Introduction.—The outcomes of 7 patients with acquired atresia of 1 main branch pulmonary artery who underwent the Fontan operation were reviewed. No previous study has addressed the morbidity, the mortality, and the physiology of Fontan completion in this patient subgroup.

Methods.—The 7 patients (1-lung group) underwent a completion Fontan operation between 1991 and 1995. Before completion, all had a left pulmonary artery that was hypoplastic and discontinuous from the right pulmonary artery. The preoperative and postoperative data of these patients were compared with those of 65 patients with continuous pulmonary arteries (2-lung group) who underwent a completion Fontan procedure at the study institution after 1991.

Results.—The 2 groups did not differ significantly in preoperative right atrial pressure, aortic saturation, ventricular end-diastolic pressure, pulmonary artery pressure, pulmonary blood flow, or pulmonary vascular resistance. Analysis of postoperative data yielded no significant differences between groups in mean values for heart rate, urine output, and pulmonary venous pressure in the first 24 hours. Mean hospital stay was longer in the 2-lung group (40.7 vs. 27.4 days), but the difference was not significant. The difference in overall mortality did not reach a level of significance (28.6% in the 1-lung and 13.8% in the 2-lung group). Postoperative systemic arterial saturation was lower in the 1-lung group. Five of the 7 patients in the 1-lung group are long-term survivors.

Conclusions.—Patients with a hypoplastic and discontinuous left pulmonary artery can successfully undergo a completion Fontan procedure. The patients described had preoperative hemodynamics comparable to those of patients with continuous pulmonary arteries. Except for a lower systemic arterial saturation, postoperative hemodynamics were also similar in the 2 groups.

▶ The successful completion of a Fontan in 7 patients with a single pulmonary artery with 5 long-term survivors is both surprising and encouraging. It had been my bias that this operation would not work effectively with 1 lung unless the pulmonary artery was quite large and pulmonary resistance quite low. No data are given regarding pulmonary artery size, but obviously it was adequate in this group of patients. It will be of interest to note whether these patients have more problems with morbidity in the next 10 years vs. their cohorts with flow to both lungs.

T.P. Graham, M.D.

Primum Atrial Septal Defect in Children: Early Results, Risk Factors, and Freedom From Reoperation
Najm HK, Williams WG, Chuaratanaphong S, et al (Univ of Toronto)
Ann Thorac Surg 66:829-835, 1998   2–14

Objective.—Children with congestive heart failure who are undergoing repair of primum atrial septal defect (ASD-I) are at increased risk of early death. Early mortality and incidence of reoperation in children undergoing ASD-I repair were retrospectively analyzed.

Methods.—Between July 1982 and December 1996, 180 consecutive children (83 boys), aged 1 month to 16.4 years, underwent repair of ASD-I. Of the 177 survivors, follow-up information was available on 171. The average age at surgery was 4.6 years, although 23 children were aged less than 1 year. ASD-I was diagnosed using echocardiography. Symptoms were mild or absent in 80% of children, whereas 20% had congestive heart failure, and 57% had associated anomalies. Outcomes were analyzed for children aged 1 year or less and for those who were older.

Results.—There were 3 in-hospital deaths, 2 with congestive heart failure in the 1 year or less age group. Ten-year survival was 98% with all children in the New York Heart Association functional class I or II. The only significant predictor of death, according to univariate and multivariate analyses, was age 1 year or less. Children aged 1 year or less had a significantly higher risk of mortality and reoperation than did older children. Of the 17 children requiring reoperation, including 5 who were aged 1 year or less, 5 had subaortic obstruction and 12 had left atrioventricular valve (LAVV) regurgitation. The average interval to reoperation was 3.2 years. Age 1 year or less and moderate-to-severe preoperative LAVV regurgitation predicted reoperation (Fig 2). Postoperative LAVV regurgitation was absent or mild in 124 children, moderate in 20, and severe in 2. Patients with incomplete closure of the cleft were significantly more likely to have moderate-to-severe LAVV regurgitation postoperatively.

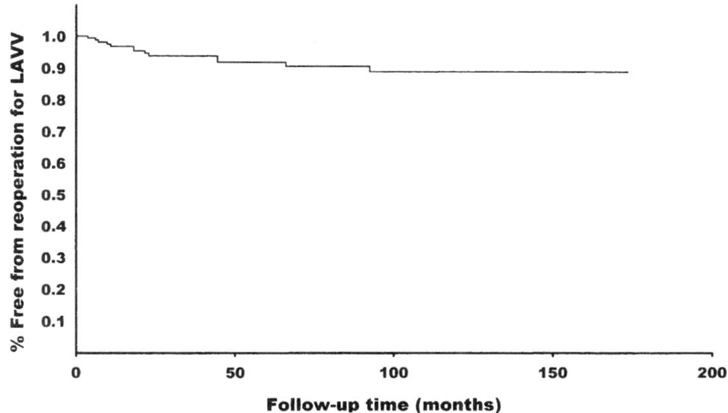

FIGURE 2.—Freedom from reoperation for left atrioventricular valve (*LAVV*) regurgitation. (Reprinted with permission from the Society of Thoracic Surgeons from Najm HK, Williams WG, Chuaratanaphong S, et al: Primum atrial septal defect in children: Early results, risk factors, and freedom from reoperation. *Ann Thorac Surg* 66:829-835, 1998.)

Conclusion.—Mortality is low for children undergoing ASD-I repair. Age 1 year or less is a risk factor for mortality. Reoperation does not pose a significant risk for mortality.

▶ These data highlight how well this condition can usually be treated, with excellent results during long-term follow-up, with freedom from reoperation for the LAVV regurgitation in the majority of patients. Subaortic stenosis requiring reoperation occurred in only 5 patients. This complication occurs more commonly with partial atrioventricular septal defect than with a complete defect. The 3 causes for subaortic stenosis include a discrete fibromuscular ring, tunnel-like constriction, and left valvular and subvalvular tissue attached to the outflow tract. Management of this complication requires careful tailoring of treatment to the cause; transesophageal echocardiography before and after surgery is useful to assess the results and to be sure that obstruction is corrected as completely as possible and that the mitral valve is not injured. Unfortunately, recurrent subaortic stenosis still occurs in these patients, as it does in those without a primum atrial septal defect, despite the use of multiple methods to resect obstruction completely at the time of surgery.

T.P. Graham, M.D.

Reconstructive Surgery in Congenital Mitral Valve Insufficiency (Carpentier's Techniques): Long-term Results

Chauvaud S, Fuzellier JF, Houel R, et al (Hôpital Broussais, Paris)
J Thorac Cardiovasc Surg 115:84-93, 1998   2–15

Introduction.—Reports of outcome after surgical correction of congenital mitral valve insufficiency (MVI) have concluded that results are good initially, but reoperation rates are high. The authors describe their own 10-year experience with Carpentier's techniques in a group of 145 children with congenital MVI.

Methods.—Patients were 74 boys and 71 girls, ranging in age from 2 months to 12 years. According to Carpentier's classification, 31 children were type I (mitral valve incompetence with normal leaflet motion), 79 were type II (leaflet prolapse), and 35 were type III (restricted leaflet motion). Among those with type III, papillary muscles were abnormal in 20 and normal in 15. Fifty-one children (35%) had associated lesions; 43 children had these lesions corrected in the primary procedure. In all but 7 cases (95%), a conservative approach was possible. Seventy patients required a prosthetic annuloplasty, and 21 underwent valve extension with a pericardial patch. Valve replacement was performed in the remaining 7 patients.

Results.—Seven patients with a mean age of 3.7 years died during repair of MVI. Mortality was highest (13%) in patients with type III, but functional type and hospital mortality had no statistically significant correlation. With an average follow-up of 9.3 years, 6 patients in the repair group (4%) and 3 (43%) in the replacement group died. Ten-year survival for the entire cohort was 86%. Most patients (85%) were in New York Heart Association class I after repair. Reoperation was required in 21 (15%) patients, at a mean of 5.8 years after the initial repair, and in 2 (28%) after valve replacement. The most common cause of reoperation was recurrent MVI. No thromboembolic event occurred in any group.

Conclusion.—Carpentier's techniques can be used successfully in most patients with congenital MVI, and long-term results of the procedure are excellent. Favorable outcome is attributed, in most cases, to use of a prosthetic ring to remodel the anulus.

▶ This article presents 145 children younger than 12 years who underwent mitral valve repair for congenital MVI. Specifically excluded were patients with atrioventricular septal defect, atrioventricular discordance, straddling mitral valve, acquired valvular disease, or Marfan syndrome. A number of different techniques were used. The actual freedom from reoperation was 68% at 15 years, which represents an excellent long-term result in this complex group. I hope these techniques can be used for most children needing mitral valve surgery.

T.P. Graham, M.D.

Techniques and Results in the Management of Multiple Ventricular Septal Defects
Kitagawa T, Durham LA III, Mosca RS, et al (Univ of Michigan, Ann Arbor)
J Thorac Cardiovasc Surg 115:848-856, 1998   2–16

Introduction.—Specific management guidelines for patients with multiple ventricular septal defects (VSDs) have yet to be defined, and morbidity and mortality in such cases remain high. A review of patients with multiple VSDs describes the surgical techniques used and examines patient and procedural risk factors.

Methods.—Twenty-one of the 33 patients who underwent repair between January 1988 and October 1996 had pulmonary artery hypertension (group 1) and 12 had pulmonary stenosis (group 2). In most cases, closure was achieved by a right atriotomy alone. Group 1 patients had a mean age of 5.9 months at repair; 6 had coarctation; Group 2 had a mean age of 6.6 years at repair; major associated anomalies included tetralogy of Fallot in 2 cases. Reoperation for residual VSD was required in 2 group 1 and 3 group 2 patients.

Results.—No early or late deaths occurred in group 1 patients, and there were no cases of heart block or of significant residual VSDs. At a mean follow-up of 23.4 months, all were free of significant residual cardiovascular conditions and 14 were free of symptoms and of medication. There was 1 early death in group 2, a child with double outlet right ventricle and left ventricle hypoplasia. Two patients had complete heart block, 1 required late mitral valve replacement, and 2 had transplantation for left ventricular failure.

Conclusion.—Primary repair for infants with multiple VSDs can yield good long-term results. The right atrial approach is usually satisfactory, with the exception of defects in the apical muscular portion of the septum.

▶ The authors show reasonably good results for repair of multiple VSDs using several different techniques. Apical defects continue to be problematic with the data unclear as to whether left ventricular incisions will lead to late ventricular dysfunction.

T.P. Graham, M.D.

A Modified Repair Technique for Tricuspid Incompetence in Ebstein's Anomaly

Hetzer R, Nagdyman N, Ewert P, et al (Deutsches Herzzentrum Berlin)
J Thorac Cardiovasc Surg 115:857-868, 1998   2–17

Background.—In Ebstein's anomaly, the septal or posterior leaflets of the tricuspid valve are deformed and fail to attach normally to the tricuspid valve anulus. The leaflets are displaced into the right ventricle, and typically the valve is incompetent. Some authors support valve replacement, whereas others perform valve repair. The results of tricuspid valve repair in Ebstein's anomaly are reported.

Methods.—The research subjects were 19 patients (7 males and 12 females; mean age, 21 years; age range, 2-54 years) with Ebstein's anomaly and incompetent tricuspid valves (grade II in 2 patients, grade III in 14, and grade IV in 3). All patients had some degree of congestive heart failure that prompted the surgical repair. The surgical approach used the most mobile tricuspid valve leaflet for valve closure, without plication of the atrialized chamber. This approach basically restructured the valve mechanism at the level of the true tricuspid anulus. All but 1 of the patients also had associated congenital malformations (mainly interatrial communication), which were also repaired. Follow-up continued for a median of 28 months (range, 10-103 months).

Findings.—None of the patients died during surgery, and none of the patients experienced late death; however, 1 patient died 2 months after surgery as a result of recurrent sepsis. Two patients required pacemakers because of permanent third-degree atrioventricular blockage. Preoperatively, all patients with intracardiac communication had cyanosis at rest or during exercise (mean oxygen saturation, 86%); after surgery, oxygen saturation values were normal. Functional capacity (as determined by New York Heart Association classes) improved after surgery, from a mean of 2.8 preoperatively to 1.9 postoperatively. Furthermore, tricuspid incompetence (as determined by grades 0-4) decreased after surgery, from a mean of 3.1 preoperatively to 0.9 postoperatively. Echocardiography revealed that the tricuspid valve function remained patent (inflow velocities from 0.5 to 1.3 m/sec), and the unplicated atrialized ventricular chamber did not enlarge.

Conclusions.—This surgical approach provided excellent repair of the incompetent tricuspid valve. Functional capacity improved, cyanosis resolved, and the repaired valve remained patent. There has been no valve deterioration in up to 103 months of follow-up. Also, there have been no negative sequelae from the unplicated atrialized chamber.

▶ These techniques use the most mobile tricuspid leaflets for valve closure without plication of the atrialized chamber. The early results are favorable, and it is hoped that this type of repair may be useful for more patients so that valve replacement can be minimized in patients whose atrialized ventricular portion had been so large that valvuloplasty previously was not believed to be feasible and tricuspid valve replacement was then used. As mentioned in the discussion section of this article, some patients can have the combination of a Glenn shunt performed with this operation to achieve adequate pulmonary blood flow without overloading the right ventricular chamber.

T.P. Graham, M.D.

Trends in the Management of Truncal Valve Insufficiency
McElhinney DB, Reddy VM, Rajasinghe HA, et al (Univ of California, San Francisco)
Ann Thorac Surg 65:517-524, 1998   2–18

Introduction.—Patients with truncus arteriosus often have a dysplastic or dysfunctional single semilunar valve. Truncal valve insufficiency in children with truncus arteriosus is a difficult surgical problem, associated with increased rates of early and late mortality. The records of patients who underwent treatment for truncal valve insufficiency were reviewed to determine whether outcome has improved in recent years.

Patients and Methods.—Patients included in the review were seen at the study institution between 1975 and 1995 with a diagnosis of truncus arteriosus and truncal valve insufficiency. Repair was performed in 77 of 89 patients. Eight patients died before repair was possible and 4 underwent pulmonary artery banding. The median age at repair was 3.2 months, decreasing from 4 months between 1975 and 1985 to 1 month between 1986 and 1995. Truncal valve insufficiency was characterized as mild or moderate in most cases. Ten infants had truncal valve replacement and 5 underwent valve repair.

Results.—The infants treated with pulmonary artery banding all died. Hospital mortality in the repair group was 34%. Eleven of 51 hospital survivors died during follow-up (median, 10 years). Overall 1- and 10-year actuarial survival rates were 56% and 48%, respectively. Patients with severe truncal valve insufficiency had lower survival rates. Twenty-one patients required late truncal valve replacement; the incidence of replacement was significantly higher in patients with moderate or severe truncal insufficiency than in those with mild truncal insufficiency preoperatively. Four late deaths were related directly to reoperation for truncal valve replacement or to prosthetic valve dysfunction. Among infants who received allograft root replacement, 3 died within 7 months of repair and 1 required replacement when severe allograft valve insufficiency developed.

Conclusion.—One-year mortality remains high for infants with truncus arteriosus and truncal valve insufficiency, but most late deaths are related to reoperation, especially during the first 6 months after repair. Although outcome has improved over time, results remain disappointing for patients with severe insufficiency and those with allograft truncal valve root replacement.

▶ Repair of truncus arteriosus in the infant remains a difficult task, particularly for patients with moderate or severe truncal insufficiency. Because the volume load is much decreased after operation, it is not necessary to attain perfect or near perfect repair of the truncal valve. However, if moderate or severe insufficiency is present postoperatively, a favorable outcome is unlikely. Prebypass and postbypass transesophageal echo has become an important part of trying to minimize valvular insufficiency before the patient leaves the operating room.

T.P. Graham, M.D.

Effects of Modified and Classic Blalock-Taussig Shunts on the Pulmonary Arterial Tree
Godart F, Qureshi SA, Simha A, et al (Guy's Hosp, London)
Ann Thorac Surg 66:512-518, 1998   2–19

Introduction.—Systemic-pulmonary arterial shunting may be performed for surgical palliation of newborns and children with reduced pulmonary artery blood flow. There is debate regarding the effects of shunting on the pulmonary arteries, with concern over the possibility of distortion, stenosis, and asymmetric growth. The long-term effects of the classic and modified Blalock-Taussig shunts on the growth and development of the pulmonary arterial tree were evaluated.

Methods.—The retrospective study included 78 children who underwent Blalock-Taussig shunting between 1980 and 1992 and for whom postoperative angiograms were available. A classic Blalock-Taussig shunt was performed in 25 patients and a modified shunt in 71. The mean postoperative interval was 51 months. The late effects of the shunts on the pulmonary arterial tree were analyzed, with particular attention to growth and development of stenosis and distortion.

Results.—Pulmonary artery diameter at the level of the anastomosis was reduced in 49% of shunts. Fourteen percent of shunts showed major stenosis, i.e., greater than 50% luminal narrowing, whereas 19% showed distortion of the pulmonary artery. These late effects were similar for modified and classic shunts. Patients who were younger at the time of surgery were significantly more likely to have pulmonary artery distortion.

Conclusion.—In patients undergoing Blalock-Taussig shunting, growth of the pulmonary artery after shunting does not exceed the normal growth of the pulmonary arterial tree. Some shunt procedures are associated with long-term distortion and stenosis of the pulmonary artery. These late effects could significantly affect the options for future corrective surgery. The findings of this retrospective study support the use of early surgical repair for correctable congenital cardiac defects. Because growth is poor after implantation of smaller shunts, 4-mm shunts should be used only in patients for whom complete repair is expected within 1 to 2 years after shunt implantation.

▶ The classic or modified Blalock-Taussig shunt continues to provide effective early palliation of patients with complex congenital heart disease. Fortunately, it is now seldom needed for patients with classic tetralogy of Fallot or even for pulmonary atresia with ventricular septal defect when the main pulmonary artery and branches are present and reasonably sized. Nevertheless, a large number of patients still require this operation and problems of stenosis and distortion of pulmonary arteries continue as shown in this report. These problems are not infrequent in patients with hypoplastic left heart syndrome in which it is frequently difficult to get equal flow to both lungs, and left pulmonary artery stenosis, distortion, and/or hypoplasia post first-stage palliation are common.

Early postoperative catheterization is needed in most patients to try to avoid progressive, detrimental changes in pulmonary artery size and configuration. Often the first shunt can set the stage for either a smooth or a rocky long-term outcome for patients with complex anatomy. The case is strong for these first operations to be done by surgeons with considerable experience in congenital heart disease.

T.P. Graham, M.D.

Hematologic and Economic Impact of Aprotinin in Reoperative Pediatric Cardiac Operations
Miller BE, Tosone SR, Tam VKH, et al (Emory Univ, Atlanta, Ga)
Ann Thorac Surg 66:535-541, 1998   2–20

Purpose.—Studies have shown that aprotinin reduces blood loss and transfusion requirements in adult patients after cardiopulmonary bypass. However, studies of aprotinin in children have yielded inconsistent results. This prospective study evaluated the effects of aprotinin in children undergoing cardiopulmonary bypass for repeat cardiac surgical procedures.

Methods.—The study included 45 children, aged 5.5 months to 14.5 years, undergoing reoperative cardiac surgical procedures. They were randomized into 3 groups: 1 group received low-dose aprotinin (loading dose of 20,000 kallikrein inhibiting units (KIU)/kg before skin incision, 20,000 KIU/kg in the pump prime, and an infusion of 10,000 KIU/kg/hr during surgery); 1 group received high-dose aprotinin (loading dose of 40,000 KIU/kg, 40,000 KIU/kg in the pump prime, and an infusion of 20,000 KIU/kg/hr during surgery); and a control group received no aprotinin. The effects on postbypass coagulopathies were assessed by comparing platelet counts, fibrinogen levels, and thromboelastographic values at baseline and after protamine sulfate administration. The 3 groups were also compared for transfusion requirements and chest tube drainage at 6 and 24 hours. The cost effects of aprotinin were assessed by evaluating the time to skin closure after protamine administration and the length of ICU and hospital stays.

Results.—Fibrinolysis was rarely detected on coagulation testing performed after protamine administration. However, significantly reduced platelet and fibrinogen levels and function were apparent. Platelet function was preserved in the aprotinin-treated groups, as evidenced by thromboelastographic testing. Aprotinin treatment was also associated with reduced transfusion requirements, reduced skin closure times, and reduced ICU and hospital stays. High-dose aprotinin reduced patient charges by an average of nearly $3,000.

Conclusion.—Aprotinin treatment can reduce postbypass coagulopathies in children undergoing repeat cardiac surgical procedures. Aprotinin reduces transfusion requirements while improving patient outcomes and reducing patient charges. High-dose aprotinin appears to offer greater clinical and cost benefits. More study is needed to establish the ideal aprotinin dose.

▶ Aprotinin has been shown to reduce blood loss and transfusion requirements after cardiopulmonary bypass in adults by multiple mechanisms, including inhibition of fibrinolysis and preservation of platelet function through its antagonism of the actions of plasmin and kallikrein. Studies in children have previously shown conflicting results, but this study showed a beneficial effect in terms of decreased blood product transfusions, shortened skin closure times, shorter durations of intensive care, shorter hospital stays, and a marked reduction in hospital charges. If this drug can be proven safe, and to definitely attenuate the hemocellular components of an inflammatory response to cardiopulmonary bypass, it could well prove useful for pediatric cardiac operations. Further studies are needed to determine optimal dose and whether there are significant risks or side effects of this therapy.

T.P. Graham, M.D.

Pediatric Cardiac Surgery: The Effect of Hospital and Surgeon Volume on In-Hospital Mortality

Hannan EL, Racz M, Kavey R-E, et al (State Univ of New York, Albany; SUNY, Syracuse; Columbia-Presbyterian Hosp, New York; et al)
Pediatrics 101:963-969, 1998
2–21

Background.—An inverse relationship between adverse outcomes for certain types of patients and the amount of experience of health care providers in treating such patients has been documented. The relationship between in-hospital mortality and provider (surgeon and hospital) volume for pediatric cardiac surgery in New York State between 1992 and 1995 was retrospectively analyzed.

Study Design.—Information was obtained from the part of New York's Cardiac Surgery Reporting System (CSRS) database dedicated to pediatric cardiac surgery, which comprises all 7,169 pediatric cardiac surgeries performed from 1992 to 1995 in New York State in the 16 hospitals with certificate of need approval. The risk-adjusted mortality rates for hospital and surgeon volume ranges were calculated with adjustments made for severity of illness.

Findings.—After controlling for severity of illness, hospitals with annual pediatric cardiac surgery volumes of fewer than 100 cases had significantly higher mortality rates than hospitals with volumes of 100 or more. Surgeons with annual volumes of fewer than 75 cases had significantly higher mortality rates than surgeons with annual volumes of 75 or more.

Conclusions.—Both the annual hospital and surgeon volume were found to be significantly related to in-hospital mortality of pediatric cardiac surgery patients, even after controlling for patient age, procedure complexity, and other clinical risk factors. These differences persisted even when only low-complexity pediatric cardiac procedures were considered.

▶ This study from New York where access to clinical data is readily available shows significantly higher mortality for pediatric cardiac surgery in hospitals with relatively low surgery volumes vs. those with higher volumes. Similar data were obtained for surgeons with relatively low volumes vs. those with higher volumes. The differences were more significant in the group of infants younger than 90 days and also in the group aged 90 days to 1 year. These differences persist both for high-complexity and low complexity disease, and further support the need for regionalization of pediatric cardiac surgery.

T.P. Graham, M.D.

Follow-up & Outcome Studies

Intermediate Survival in Neonates With Aortic Atresia: A Multi-institutional Study

Jacobs ML, Blackstone EH, Bailey LL, et al (Deborah Heart and Lung Ctr, Browns Mills, NJ; Univ of Alabama, Birmingham; Loma Linda Univ)
J Thorac Cardiovasc Surg 116:417-431, 1998   2–22

Objective.—Aortic valve atresia is the most frequent cause of hypoplastic left heart syndrome in neonates. Because there is no general agreement on therapeutic intervention, a 21-institution, nonrandomized, prospective study was undertaken to examine the various treatment strategies and outcomes and to identify the factors responsible for the success or failure of each.

Methods.—Between January 1994 and January 1997, 323 neonates, aged less than 30 days, with aortic valve atresia were treated with either staged reconstructive surgery (n = 253), heart transplantation (n = 49), or nonsurgical management (n = 21). Patients were studied through March 1997. There were 158 survivors, and 149 of those could be located. Survivors were studied for an average of 21 months. Left ventricular size and structure and patency of the mitral valve were estimated from echocardiographic reports. Outcomes by procedure were evaluated statistically, and a Competing Risks of Events Analysis was performed.

Results.—Survival for all patients was calculated (Fig 1). Risk factors for death were lower birth weight, nonwhite race, and presence of another cardiac abnormality. When protocols were compared, patients receiving no treatment or those receiving staged reconstructive surgery had a significantly higher risk of death than those undergoing heart transplantation. Of the 4 institutions with higher and similar survival rates, 2 used the staged reconstructive protocol and 2 used the heart transplantation protocol. Survival rates for 113 patients at these institutions were 77%, 70%, 64%, 62%, and 61% at 1, 3, 12, 24, and 36 months, respectively.

Conclusion.—Neonates with aortic valve atresia had higher survival rates if treated surgically with heart transplantation or staged reconstruction. Risk factors for death included lower birth weight, associated cardiac abnormality, entry into a nonsurgical protocol, and staged reconstruction.

▶ The treatment of neonates with hypoplastic left heart occupies a large part of the personnel and resources at centers that treat many infants with complex congenital heart disease. This collaborative article shows the 1, 2, and 3 year survival is about 50% for all patients entered in this series. For 2 institutions with heart transplant protocols and 2 with staged reconstructive protocols that have achieved superior results, the 1, 2, and 3 year mortalities are 64%, 62%, and 61%, respectively. At least 4 of 21 institutions that have

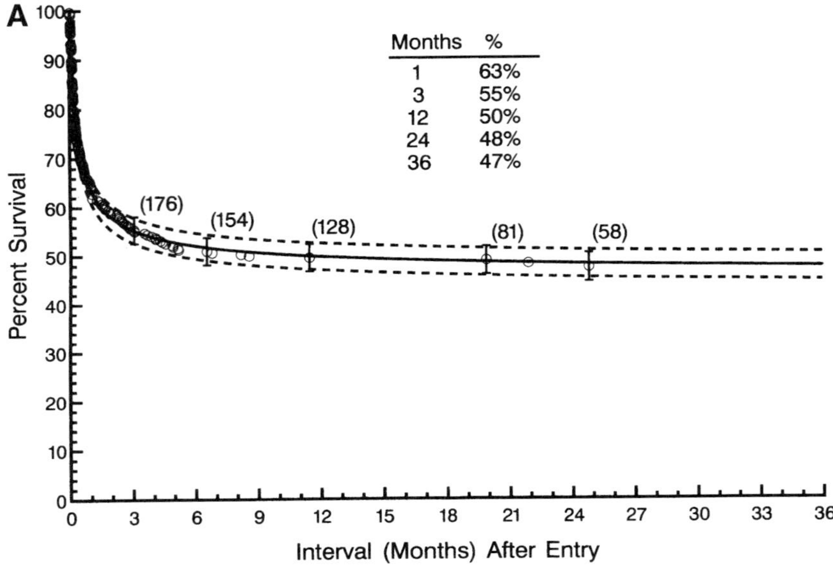

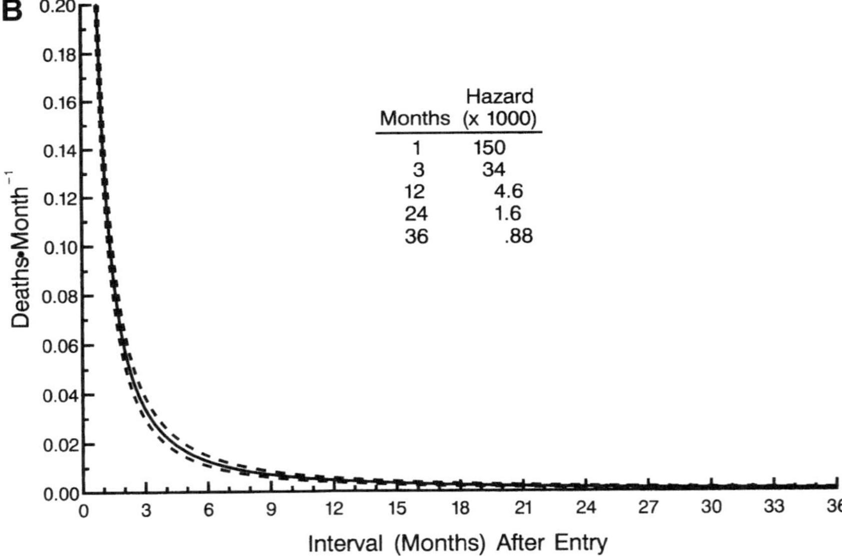

FIGURE 1.—Non–risk-adjusted survival and hazard function for death for all 323 patients in the study. A, survival after entry (at time zero). Each *circle* represents an actual death, positioned at the time of death along the *horizontal axis* and actuarially along the *vertical axis*. The *vertical bars* depict ± 1 standard error. The *numbers* indicate the number of patients remaining at risk at the time of the estimate. The *solid line* is the parametric estimate of survival, and the *dashed lines* enclose the 70% confidence intervals. B, hazard function for death. (Courtesy of Jacobs ML, Blackstone EH, Bailey LL, et al: Intermediate survival in neonates with aortic atresia: A multi-institutional study. *J Thorac Cardiovasc Surg* 116:417-431, 1998.)

confined their approach to 1 strategy (that is, to transplant or staged reconstruction) appear to have achieved the best outcomes. The current overall survival, almost 50% at 3 years, for these 21 institutions represents a major achievement over the last 10 to 15 years for treatment of this complex anomaly that 20 years ago had very few survivors. Improving on the current 40% to 50% mortality will continue to be a real challenge, because many of these patients represent the smallest, most critically ill infants.

T.P. Graham, M.D.

Protein-losing Enteropathy After the Fontan Operation: An International Multicenter Study

Mertens L, Hagler DJ, Sauer U, et al (UZ Leuven, Belgium; Mayo Clinic, Rochester, Minn; Deutsches Herzzentrum, München, Germany; et al)
J Thorac Cardiovasc Surg 115:1063-1073, 1998   2–23

Introduction.—Protein-losing enteropathy (PLE) occurs as a rare but life-threatening complication in patients who have undergone the Fontan operation. Reports on successful management of PLE are limited. A retrospective study analyzed data on 114 patients drawn from 35 participating centers.

Methods.—During the study, 3,029 Fontan operations were performed. The incidence of PLE among survivors was 3.7%. The median time interval between surgery and diagnosis of PLE was 2.7 years. Common findings were edema (79%) and effusions (75%). Patients were studied for the effects of treatment on PLE.

Results.—The mean right atrial pressure in the group with PLE was 17 mm Hg; mean cardiac index was 2.4 L/min/m². After medical treatment only, 46% of patients died, 29% had no improvement, and 25% achieved complete resolution of symptoms. Surgical treatment brought relief of PLE in 19% of cases and no improvement in 19%; 62% of patients died. Sixteen percutaneous interventions in 13 patients yielded symptomatic improvement after 12 interventions and no improvement after 4.

Discussion.—The prognosis of patients with PLE after Fontan operation remains poor, whatever treatment method is used. The mortality rate was particularly high after surgery. As soon as the diagnosis is suspected, an immediate, careful, complete hemodynamic evaluation with catheterization is required. Heart transplantation should be considered before chronic PLE develops when other options have failed.

▶ Although the incidence of PLE after Fontan operation is low, current management can be difficult. Appropriate treatment for any obstruction to pulmonary flow with balloon dilatation or stenting to lower right atrial pressure is the first step in treatment. Some patients also may benefit from creation or enlargement of an atrial fenestration to lower right atrial pressure. Finally, corticosteroid therapy has been useful in a few patients, as has intravenous heparin. Heart transplantation is the fallback strategy when all of these interventions fail.

T.P. Graham, M.D.

Biventricular Systolic Function and Mass Studied with MR Imaging in Children With Pulmonary Regurgitation After Repair for Tetralogy of Fallot
Niezen RA, Helbing WA, van der Wall EE, et al (Leiden Univ, The Netherlands)
Radiology 201:135-140, 1996   2–24

Introduction.—Pulmonary regurgitation may occur after surgical correction of tetralogy of Fallot. With the trend toward earlier correction of this congenital condition, there is a longer follow-up period for measurement of pulmonary regurgitation (PR) and biventricular function to evaluate the results of surgery. This study examined the effects of PR on biventricular function and mass in patients undergoing early surgical correction of tetralogy of Fallot.

Methods.—The study included 19 children who had undergone surgical correction of tetralogy of Fallot at a mean age of 1.5 years. Doppler echocardiography revealed residual PR in each patient. A group of healthy controls was studied for comparison. The mean age was 12 years in both groups. The subjects underwent transverse gradient-echo MRI of both ventricles, including creation of MR velocity maps of the pulmonary artery. Measurements of biventricular volumes, ejection fraction and myocardial mass, and pulmonary flow volumes were made. In addition, 17 patients underwent exercise testing.

Results.—The patients with corrected tetralogy of Fallot had lower right ventricular ejection fraction (54% vs. 66%) and higher right ventricular mass than controls. Left ventricular ejection fraction was also significantly lower in the patients, 52% vs. 68% and was significantly correlated with PR. An inverse correlation between exercise performance and PR was noted as well.

Conclusion.—In patients with residual PR after surgical correction of tetralogy of Fallot, MRI can provide a complete evaluation of cardiac biventricular volumes and mass, as well as pulmonary artery flow. Residual PR has adverse effects on right ventricular and left ventricular function and exercise performance in these patients. The presence of right ventricular hypertrophy demonstrates the possibility of persistently increased right ventricular mass after this surgery.

▶ Many years ago, it was shown that right ventricular volume was markedly increased and ejection fraction decreased in patients with tetralogy of Fallot who had required a transannular patch for repair of that condition. Most of those patients had undergone repair in midchildhood to late childhood. This study reports on patients operated on at a mean age of 18 months and shows quite similar findings, with markedly increased volume and decreased ejection fractions of right and left ventricles in patients undergoing tetralogy of Fallot repair. As might be expected, these findings are particularly marked in those patients who required a transannular patch. To achieve an adequate repair in many patients with tetralogy of Fallot, a transannular patch is needed. The art of surgery involves minimizing the right ventricular incision, the size of the outflow patch, and the degree of PR while achieving minimal or no outflow gradient. Frequently, the best congenital heart disease surgeons can be judged by the almost normal physical examination results in their postoperative tetralogy of Fallot patients.

T.P. Graham, M.D.

Right Ventricular Function and Exercise Performance Late After Primary Repair of Tetralogy of Fallot With the Transannular Patch in Infancy
Singh GK, Greenberg SB, Yap YS, et al (St Louis Univ; St Christopher Hosp for Children, Philadelphia; Southampton Gen Hosp, England)
Am J Cardiol 81:1378-1382, 1998   2–25

Objective.—Current surgical repair of tetralogy of Fallot (TOF) involving reconstruction of the right ventricle (RV) usually results in chronic pulmonary insufficiency. Exercise performance and RV systolic and diastolic functions in a group of patients with chronic pulmonary regurgitation late after early primary repair of TOF in infancy was assessed with cine magnetic resonance imaging and compared with results in normal individuals.

Methods.—Ten New York Heart Association (NYHA) class I (n = 7) or II (n = 3) patients with chronic pulmonary regurgitation for an average of 13.6 years after surgery for primary repair of TOF at an average age of 6.9 months had reconstruction of the RV outflow tract with a transannular patch. Cine magnetic resonance imaging was performed using a spoiled, gradient-recalled acquisition in the steady-state technique and flip angle of 30 degrees, acquiring 6 to 10 contiguous 8-mm slices with an interslice gap of 1 mm. Ventricular volume and function indices were calculated and compared with those of 7 age- and sex-matched healthy controls.

Results.—Patients had RV enlargement despite normal cardiac output at rest. RV enlargement and left ventricular ejection fraction during exercise were correlated with the extent of pulmonary regurgitation. Patients also had abnormal ventricular function, abnormal filling characteristics, a reduced early diastolic filling fraction, a reduced RV peak filling rate, increased RV end-diastolic and end-systolic volumes, and a significantly decreased ejection fraction. Peak filling rate was negatively correlated with the extent of pulmonary regurgitation. Exercise capacity was decreased in patients.

Conclusion.—Early primary repair of TOF and RV outflow tract reconstruction in infancy does not necessarily prevent late RV diastolic dysfunction and decreased exercise capacity where chronic regurgitation occurs.

▶ It had been hoped that early repair of TOF would improve long-term outcome of RV function. The authors, however, show that when transannular patches are required for repair (as they are in most infants), the degree of RV dilatation and depressed ejection fraction are quite similar to data reported many years ago for older patients at the time of their initial repair. These patients were repaired in infancy and did not have clinical signs of right heart failure. Many probably will require pulmonary valve replacement at a later age because of the significant volume overload and the low RV ejection fractions shown here.

T.P. Graham, M.D.

A 26-Year Experience With Surgical Management of Tetralogy of Fallot: Risk Analysis for Mortality or Late Reintervention

Knott-Craig CJ, Elkins RC, Lane MM, et al (Univ of Oklahoma, Oklahoma City)
Ann Thorac Surg 66:506-511, 1998   2–26

Objective.—Since the early 1990s, the trend in correction of tetralogy of Fallot (TOF) has been toward primary repair and away from 2-stage repair. The results suggest that primary repair offers improved outcomes, although the long-term effects on survival and recurrent right ventricular outflow tract disease remain unclear. A 26-year experience with TOF repair was reviewed to analyze the effects of the trend toward earlier repair on early outcomes and recurrent right heart obstruction.

Patients.—From 1971 to 1997, the authors' institution performed TOF repair on 291 patients. Sixty-eight percent of patients underwent primary complete repair and 21% had a staged repair; the remainder had palliative surgery only. The pathology was complex in 23% of patients, most often including pulmonary atresia. Follow-up information was available on 90% of patients, with a median duration of follow-up of nearly 11 years.

Outcomes.—The overall in-hospital mortality rates were 11% for patients undergoing primary repair, 18% for those undergoing staged repair, and 16% for those undergoing palliative surgery only. During the 1990s, these mortality figures decreased to 2%, 12%, and 0%, respectively. Patient age at surgery was 0.6 year after 1990, compared with 2 years in the earlier part of the experience. Significant risk factors for in-hospital death on multivariate analysis were hypothermic circulatory arrest, pulmonary artery patch angioplasty, earlier year of surgery, and closure of the foramen ovale.

Among patients who survived to hospital discharge, the 20-year survival rate was 98% for those with TOF and pulmonary stenosis vs. 88% for those with TOF and pulmonary atresia. Fourteen percent of patients required reoperation on the right ventricular outflow tract. The 20-year rate of freedom from such intervention was 86% for patients with TOF and pulmonary stenosis compared with 43% for those with TOF and pulmonary atresia. Among the latter group, the rate of freedom from reintervention was 85% after primary repair vs. 91% after staged repair. Patients aged 1 year or less at the time of surgery were somewhat less likely to remain free from intervention, although the difference was not significant.

Conclusion.—This long-term retrospective study suggests that survival after primary repair of TOF has improved significantly over the years. Patients undergoing primary repair have an excellent chance of long-term survival. Performing primary repair during infancy is not associated with an increased risk of reintervention on the right ventricular outflow tract. The authors, therefore, favor early primary repair, with staged repair being performed only in patients with complex pathology or serious noncardiac co-morbidity.

▶ This report gives 20-year survival rates after repair for patients with both classical TOF and TOF with pulmonary atresia after the initial operative mortality. Reintervention for the classic tetralogy group was relatively rare. There are no data on how many patients required pulmonary valve replacement, but apparently this intervention, as well as reoperation or catheter intervention for pulmonary artery stenosis, was rare in this cohort. I seem to be seeing more adult postoperative TOF patients who have unsuspected left pulmonary artery stenosis requiring stenting or operative arterioplasty and then pulmonary valve replacement.

T.P. Graham, M.D.

Progressive Tricuspid Valve Disease in Patients With Congenitally Corrected Transposition of the Great Arteries
Prieto LR, Hordof AJ, Secic M, et al (Columbia Univ, New York; Cleveland Clinic Found, Ohio)
Circulation 98:997-1005, 1998   2–27

Introduction.—Patients with corrected congenital transposition of the great arteries (CTGA) are commonly found to have morphologic abnormalities of the tricuspid valve, with 20% to 50% having clinically significant tricuspid insufficiency (TI). The progression of tricuspid valve disease in patients with CTGA is unclear. A long-term follow-up study of patients with CTGA, with and without open heart surgery, was reported, with special attention to the significance of TI or intrinsic right ventricular dysfunction.

Methods.—The study included 40 patients with CTGA seen at 1 medical center since 1958. Twenty-seven patients were male and 13 were female. The mean follow-up was 20 years. Potential risk factors for poor outcome were evaluated, including age, open heart surgery, TI, cardiac rhythm, pulmonary overcirculation, and right venticular dysfunction.

Results.—Twenty-one patients underwent intracardiac repair, whereas 19 had no surgery or had closed-heart procedures only. The only independent prognostic factor for death was moderately severe or worse TI (TI$_s$), as demonstrated by echocardiography and/or angiography. Furthermore, the only factor that independently predicted the presence of TI$_s$ was morphologic abnormalities of the tricuspid valve. The 20-year survival rate decreased from 93% for patients without TI$_s$ to 49% for those with TI$_s$. All but 1 poor long-term postoperative outcome were ascribed to TI$_s$. For patients undergoing surgery, the 20-year survival rate was 34% for patients with TI$_s$ and 90% for those without. Among patients who did not have surgery, the 20-year survival rate was 60% with TI$_s$ and 100% without, regardless of whether an attempt was made to repair the TI.

Conclusion.—In patients with CTGA, the main risk factor for poor outcomes is TI$_s$. When right ventricular dysfunction occurs, it is nearly always related to long-standing TI. When deciding as to whether surgery should be performed in a patient with CTGA, whether or not associated lesions are present, the status of the tricuspid valve must always be considered.

▶ The question continues to plague cardiologists as to whether progressive tricuspid regurgitation develops in patients with CTGA because of right ventricular dysfunction or whether moderate-to-severe tricuspid regurgitation is a major risk factor for the development of progressive right ventricular dysfunction. These authors show data supporting the latter hypothesis. Although, the numbers are small, those patients who do not have moderate or severe tricuspid regurgitation, as defined by the authors from echocardiograms or angiograms, have a much better prognosis than those who have moderate or severe tricuspid valve abnormalities. In addition, patients with tricuspid valve abnormalities tolerate open heart surgery poorly, with most having a deterioration of right ventricular function and the onset or worsening of clinical heart failure after operation.

T.P. Graham, M.D.

Recurrent Aortic Coarctation: Is Surgical Repair Still the Gold Standard?
Sakopoulos AG, Hahn TL, Turrentine M, et al (Indiana Univ, Indianapolis)
J Thorac Cardiovasc Surg 116:560-565, 1998   2–28

Objective.—Coarctation of the aorta is a congenital condition that leads to premature death through progressive hypertension. Although balloon angioplasty is a popular alternative to surgery for managing aortic coarctation, angioplasty can result in complications and has a high recurrence rate. The complication rates, mortality, and morbidity of balloon angioplasty and surgery were compared, through a retrospective chart review, in the management of coarctation of the aorta.

Methods.—Between January 1970 and 1996, 56 children (25 girls, aged 2 months to 18 years) of 645 children treated at Riley Children's Hospital in Indianapolis had recurrent coarctation. For most patients, a collagen-impregnated, knitted, diamond-shaped Dacron graft was used for repair.

Results.—Only 10 patients had repair after 6 months of age. Cardiac defects were seen in 33 children, (59%) defects including patent ductus arteriosus in 19 children (34%), ventricular septal defect in 15 children (27%), and atrial septal defect and patent foramen ovale in 7 children (13%). There were recurrences in 18 children (33%) within 2 years and in 28 children (50%) in 7 to 15 years. The mean age in the early recurrence group was 15 days, whereas the mean age in the late recurrence group was 67 days. Subclavian flap repair was performed in 55% of the early repair group compared with 16% of the entire study group. Resection and end-to-end anastomosis were performed in 30 (53%) patients and prosthetic patch angioplasty in 13 (23%) of the primary group, whereas 4% and 80% of patients with recurrence received resection and end-to-end anastomosis and prosthetic patch angioplasty.

Conclusion.—Surgical repair of recurrent aortic coarctation is safe and effective.

▶ These authors demonstrate excellent results in 56 patients undergoing surgical repair for recurrent coarctation; prosthetic patch angioplasty was used in the majority. Complications with the second or third operations were extremely rare. The technique of prosthetic patch angioplasty has been associated with a relatively high incidence of aneurysm formation, but no aneurysm formation is reported in this group. Controversy still exists about the best method for treatment of recurrent coarctation: repeat surgery, percutaneous balloon dilatation, and balloon dilatation with stent placement all have their advocates. Unfortunately, most series do not have the same criteria for determining residual obstruction, aneurysm formation, persistent hypertension, or complications of the procedure. There is a real need for a careful perspective comparison of different techniques for management of this problem, a comparison clearly defining criteria for early and late success.

T.P. Graham, M.D.

Management and Outcomes of Right Atrial Isomerism: A 26-Year Experience

Hashmi A, Abu-Sulaiman R, McCrindle BW, et al (Hosp for Sick Children, Toronto)
J Am Coll Cardiol 31:1120-1126, 1998   2–29

Background.—Infants with right atrial isomerism usually have other cardiac malformations, and the associated mortality is high. In years past, surgery was not considered an option; however, more recent studies have reported successes with a 1-ventricular (Fontan) or biventricular repair. A 26 year's experience with managing right atrial isomerism was reviewed to identify factors associated with mortality.

Methods.—Between January 1970 and March 1996, 91 patients (54 males and 37 females) received diagnoses of right atrial isomerism. When records included the information, their age at presentation was noted, as were associated congenital cardiac abnormalities.

Findings.—In 56 of 90 cases (62%), right atrial isomerism was noted at birth; by 1 month of age, most cases (80 of 90, or 89%) had been established. The longest delay between birth and presentation was 7.7 months. About two thirds of patients (58 of 87, or 67%) had cyanosis, and 40 of 79 (51%) required prostaglandin infusion to maintain oxygen saturation. Levocardia was present in 56 of 89 patients (63%), and dextrocardia was found in 33 of 89 (37%). A common atrium (76 of 91, or 84%) and a common atrioventricular (AV) valve (74 of 91, or 81%) were conditions seen in most patients. Other pervasive cardiac anomalies were abnormal ventriculoarterial connections (87 of 91, or 96%), anomalous pulmonary venous drainage (77 of 89, or 87%), obstruction of the pulmonary outflow tract (76 of 91, or 84%), ventricular hypoplasia or a single ventricle (66 of 90, or 73%), and obstruction of the pulmonary vein (25 of 84, or 30%). All but 5 patients had asplenia, and one third had gastrointestinal anomalies. Overall, 63 of 91 patients (69%) died; patients whose surgery was performed at more than 4 weeks of age had significantly better survival rates than those who were operated on during the neonatal period (mortality rates 51% vs. 75%). Of the 22 patients in whom no cardiovascular surgical interventions were planned or performed, 21 died (95%) at a median age of 4 days. Of the 69 patients who underwent cardiovascular surgical interventions, 20 patients underwent pulmonary vein repair, and 19 (95%) died. Of the remaining 49 patients undergoing various shunt procedures and ventricular repair, 23 died (47%). Survival estimates at 1 month were 71%; at 1 year, they were 49%; and at 5 years, they were 35%. Cox proportional hazards modeling revealed that independent risk factors for a shorter time to death were pulmonary vein obstruction (relative risk, 5.43), a major AV valve anomaly (relative risk, 5.23), and the absence of pulmonary outflow obstruction (relative risk, 2.23).

Conclusions.—Patients with right atrial isomerism continue to be a management challenge, and despite surgical intervention, only 1 of 3 neonates will likely live to 5 years of age. Their course is complicated by significant associated cardiac abnormalities and asplenia. Unfortunately, a comparison of early vs. more recent experience indicates that mortality rates are actually becoming worse. Select patients might benefit more from heart transplantation than from the current management strategies.

▶ This review of a large cohort of patients with asplenia and congenital heart disease includes the typical finding that the majority of patients have large ventricular septal defects *or* a single ventricle, a common AV valve, transposition of the great arteries, pulmonary outflow obstruction, and anomalous pulmonary venous connection. The outlook is poor when taken in the aggregate and, unfortunately, does not seem to have improved in the last several years. My bias is that outcome in this condition has improved recently, and many more of these patients are proceeding from palliative shunts to successful Fontan procedures. I hope that new treatment strategies for early intervention will prove my bias to be correct.

T.P. Graham, M.D.

Outcome in Cyanotic Neonates With Ebstein's Anomaly

Yetman AT, Freedom RM, McCrindle BW (Univ of Toronto)
Am J Cardiol 81:749-754, 1998   2–30

Background.—In Ebstein's anomaly, different patients have different degrees of inferior displacement of the proximal attachments of the tricuspid valve leaflets from the atrioventricular ring. Such differences, plus other associated cardiac lesions and the presence of cyanosis, help account for the large range of reported mortality rates for these infants (27% to 48%). Patient characteristics of neonates with Ebstein's anomaly and cyanosis were reviewed to determine possible risk factors for mortality.

Methods.—Between 1954 and 1996, 46 neonates with Ebstein's anomaly and cyanosis (mean systemic oxygen saturation, 62%) were identified. Clinical records and echocardiograms were analyzed, and the ratio of the combined area of the right atrium and atrialized right ventricle to the combined area of the functional right ventricle and left heart in a 4-chamber view at end-diastole was calculated. This ratio was used to define 4 grades of severity: grade 1, a ratio of less than 0.5; grade 2, a ratio of 0.5-0.99; grade 3, a ratio of 1-1.49, and grade 4, a ratio of 1.5 or greater. A 4-chamber view was used to assess the degree of tricuspid valve displacement and tricuspid regurgitation (assessed as mild, moderate, or severe).

Findings.—For two thirds of the patients, Ebstein's anomaly was diagnosed at birth (in utero in 3 cases). Twenty patients (40%) had an atrial septal defect 4 mm or larger. Ten patients (22%) had a patent connection between the right ventricle and the pulmonary artery, and 35 (88%) had atresia (functional in 25, anatomical in 11). Fifteen patients (35%) underwent surgery (including tricuspid valve repair, Blalock-Taussig shunt, and pulmonary valvotomy), and 7 survived. Overall, 32 (70%) of these patients died (compared with only 14% of neonates with Ebstein's anomaly but without cyanosis). Deaths were a result of low cardiac output (20 patients), postoperative complications (8 patients), or sudden death (4 patients). Survival estimates at age 1 week were 61%; at age 1 month, they were 48%; at age 1 year, they were 36%; and at age 5 years, they were 36%. However, mortality rates in the past 10 years (47%) improved significantly from rates during the period 1954-1985 (81%). Multivariate regression indicated that anatomical pulmonary atresia (relative risk, 5.97), reduced left ventricular function (relative risk, 4.10), functional atresia (relative risk, 2.44), and an atrial septal defect 4 mm or larger (relative risk, 2.39) were independent predictors of mortality. Also, all patients with a severity ratio greater than 1 died.

Conclusions.—The prognosis for patients with Ebstein's anomaly and cyanosis remains poor, but it has improved in recent years. Most patients die within the first week, even with surgery, and late deaths are not uncommon. Independent risk factors exist, but the most telling sign is a severity ratio greater than 1: all patients whose ratio of the combined area of the right atrium and atrialized right ventricle to the combined area of the functional right ventricle and the left heart was greater than 1 died.

▶ Mortality remains high for infants with severe Ebstein's anomaly, in particular those infants whose cyanosis does not improve in the first week of life and whose echocardiographic ratio of the area of the combined right atrium and atrialized right ventricle to the area of the functional right ventricle and left heart is greater than 1. Options for these patients include potential cardiac transplantation or radical surgery that involves creating anatomical pulmonary atresia, resecting excessive right atrial tissue, performing a palliative systemic-to-pulmonary shunt, and setting them on the path for an eventual Fontan repair as suggested by Starnes et al.[1] More data are needed regarding outcome for either transplantation or this new radical surgical approach.

T.P. Graham, M.D.

Reference

1. Starnes VA, Pitlick PT, Bernstein D, et al: Ebstein's anomaly appearing in the neonate: A new surgical approach. *J Thorac Cardiovasc Surg* 101:1082-1087, 1991.

Fate of the Neopulmonary Valve After the Arterial Switch Operation in Neonates
Nogi S, McCrindle BW, Boutin C, et al (Univ of Toronto)
J Thorac Cardiovasc Surg 115:557-562, 1998   2–31

Introduction.—Neopulmonary valve (neo-PV) stenosis is unusual in patients who have undergone a 1-stage or 2-stage arterial switch operation (ASO) for transposition of the great arteries. The incidence, risk factors, and early outcome of acquired stenosis of the neo-PV after a neonatal arterial switch operation were assessed retrospectively.

Methods.—The preoperative and follow-up echocardiograms of 136 of 288 patients undergoing ASO were reviewed. Of 188 patients, 91 had intact ventricular septa, 39 had ventricular septal defects, 5 had aortic coarctation, and 1 had a double-outlet right ventricle. There were no patients with preoperative valvular abnormalities.

Results.—At a median follow-up of 18 months (range, 1-90 months), 32 patients (24%) had supravalvular pulmonary stenosis and 15 (11%) had associated pulmonary valve stenosis (group 1). Estimates for freedom from any intervention were 94% and 79% at 1 and 5 years, respectively. The valve anulus was significantly larger before ASO in patients for whom neo-PV stenosis did not develop (group 2) compared with group 1 patients for whom neo-PV stenosis did develop. The pulmonary valve anulus diminished significantly in diameter in group 1 patients and remained larger in group 2 patients compared with a normal diameter. Significant pulmonary valve hypoplasia developed in group 1 patients; group 2 patients had significantly larger valves compared with normal size.

Conclusion.—Neopulmonary valve stenosis may occur after ASO and is related to growth failure of the valve anulus often associated with supravalvular pulmonary stenosis.

▶ Neo-PV stenosis usually develops in the first year after repair if it is going to be a problem. This apparent growth failure of the valve anulus frequently is associated with supravalvular stenosis at the suture line or with the patch reconstruction of the sites where the coronary arteries have been removed.

T.P. Graham, M.D.

Influence of the Postoperative Period and Surgical Procedure on Ambulatory Blood Pressure–Determination of Hypertension Load After Successful Surgical Repair of Coarctation of the Aorta

Johnson D, Perrault H, Vobecky SJ, et al (Ste-Justine Hosp, Montreal; McGill Univ, Montreal)
Eur Heart J 19:638-646, 1998

2–32

Introduction.—The monitoring of arterial blood pressure after surgical correction of coarctation of the aorta is usually performed using sphygmomanometry. Ten to 40% of patients who undergo an apparently successful repair of coarctation of the aorta have hypertension 10 to 20 years later, according to office blood pressure measurements. The hypertension load was quantified using 24-hour ambulatory blood pressure monitoring both less than and more than 10 years after successful surgical repair of coarctation of the aorta. The type of surgical repair was also assessed.

Methods.—Ambulatory blood pressure recordings were taken using an Accutracker II monitor every 30 minutes in the daytime and every hour in the nighttime. Patients were grouped according to whether their coarctation period was less than 10 years (group 1) or 10 years or greater (group 2). A group of healthy adolescents acted as controls. Data from all patients were assessed according to the type of surgery: left subclavian flap angioplasty (9 patients) or end-to-end anastomosis (12 patients).

Results.—Compared with controls, all day and night systolic and diastolic values were higher in patients with successful repair of coarctation of the aorta. Blood pressure measurements were higher in group 1 than in group 2. Daytime systolic hypertension occurred in 20% of recordings from group 1 and in 49% of those from group 2. There was no diastolic hypertension. Systolic and diastolic blood pressure responses to daily activities were significantly greater in patients who had undergone repair of coarctation of the aorta than in controls and higher in group 2 than in group 1. Hypertension prevalence and blood pressure reactivity were not influenced by the type of surgery.

Conclusion.—Successful repair of coarctation of the aorta is associated with significantly higher systolic and diastolic blood pressure compared with healthy controls. The prevalence of hypertension rises markedly with time. These increases in ambulatory blood pressure readings may be predictive of a chronic hypertensive state. Patients undergoing successful surgery for repair of coarctation of the aorta should be closely monitored.

▶ Hypertension continues to be a problem in patients who have had surgical repair of coarctation even when the repair appears successful. Many times it is difficult to decide whether a small residual gradient is contributing significantly to the problem and whether balloon dilatation or stenting or surgical reoperation is in the patient's best interest. Exercise testing can help in this assessment, as can a trial of medical therapy. This study reemphasizes the need for these patients to have long-term follow-up and adequate management of their hypertension when it is diagnosed.

T.P. Graham, M.D.

Neurodevelopmental Outcomes in Children With Fontan Repair of Functional Single Ventricle

Uzark K, Lincoln A, Lamberti JJ, et al (Children's Heart Inst, San Diego, Calif)
Pediatrics 101:630-633, 1998   2–33

Introduction.—Therapeutic advances have led to improved survival and surgical outcomes in children with congenital heart disease. Earlier reports showed that developmental delays and lower intelligence quotients (IQs) were common in the first 3 years of life, particularly in children who had cyanosis. The neurodevelopmental status of children after Fontan repair of a functional single ventricle was evaluated. The relationship between cognitive function and selected patient characteristics was assessed.

Methods.—Thirty-two children with complex single ventricles who underwent Fontan repair were assessed using the Stanford-Binet Intelligence (IQ) test and the Developmental Test of Visual Motor Integration (VMI). The age range was 26 months to 16 years. Patients were younger than 16 years at the time of surgery and were more than 6 months after Fontan repair. Mean scores and the distribution of IQ and VMI scores were compared with population norms. The association between test scores and patient characteristics was evaluated.

Results.—Most children had normal IQ scores. The VMI scores were below average in 21.4% of children. No significant relationship was found between intellectual function or visual motor integration ability and preoperative oxygen saturation or age at the time of the Fontan procedure. There was a tendency for children who had deep hypothermic circulatory arrest during an earlier Norwood procedure to have lower IQ scores.

Conclusion.—Children who undergo Fontan repair of complex heart defects usually have normal IQ scores. Visual motor integration deficits seem to occur more frequently in this population. The duration and degree of preoperative hypoxemia appeared to have no effect on cognitive function.

▶ The early outcomes at a mean age of 6 years in this small group of patients who had Fontan procedures is encouraging. The intellectional function was in the normal range, and the only below average scores were found in visual motor integration in 21% of children. In a small subgroup of 5 who had prior Norwood procedures, lower IQ scores were found. A problem with studies such as this 1 is the lack of a good chronic disease control group for comparison. In addition, a control cardiology group with a similar degree of severity of defects who did not have operative procedures requiring prolonged cardiopulmonary bypass and circulatory arrest would be of great interest.

T.P. Graham, M.D.

Doppler Echocardiography Studies

Echocardiographic Hemodynamic and Morphometric Predictors of Survival After Two-Ventricle Repair in Infants With Critical Aortic Stenosis
Kovalchin JP, Brook MM, Rosenthal GL, et al (Baylor College of Medicine, Houston; Univ of California, San Francisco)
J Am Coll Cardiol 32:237-244, 1998   2–34

Purpose.—The decision as to whether to perform 2-ventricle or 1-ventricle repair in an infant with critical aortic stenosis is an important one. Previously identified echocardiographic predictors of survival after 2-ventricle repair have been mainly morphometric in nature; there is little information on possible echocardiographic hemodynamic predictors. This study sought to identify useful echocardiographic variables, both hemodynamic and morphometric, for predicting the results of 2-ventricle repair in infants with critical aortic stenosis.

Methods.—The study included 28 infants with critical aortic stenosis; the infants had a mean age of 1 day. All underwent Doppler color flow mapping and pulsed Doppler scanning to measure hemodynamic flow in the ascending, transverse, and descending aorta; the ductus arteriosus; and across the aortic and mitral valves. Morphometric measurements were performed in the left heart as well. For both sets of variables, comparisons were made between infants who did and did not survive after surgery.

Results.—The initial attempt at surgery was a 2-ventricle repair in 19 patients; 9 underwent a Norwood (1-ventricle) procedure. Hemodynamic factors associated with survival in patients undergoing 2-ventricle repair included predominant or total antegrade flow in the ascending and transverse aorta. No significant predictive value was noted for aortic valve gradient, mitral valve inflow, or direction of flow in the ductus arteriosus and descending aorta. Significant morphometric variables in this group included the indexed aortic annulus, aortic root, ascending aorta, and left ventricular long-axis length. Outcome was unaffected by left ventricular volume, mass, ejection fraction, or mitral valve area.

Conclusion.—For patients with critical aortic stenosis undergoing 2-ventricle repair, survival is not significantly related to the presence of predominant or total antegrade flow in the ascending and transverse aorta. It can be very difficult to decide on a 1-ventricle or 2-ventricle repair for these infants. Hemodynamic data on the direction of aortic flow may be added to the known morphometric predictors in deciding which patients are candidates for the Norwood procedure.

▶ Most patients with critical aortic stenosis sort themselves out easily into those with clearly adequate left ventricular and aortic annulus size for biventricular repair and those with very small, obviously inadequate, left ventricles for this option. There remain, however, a significant number of patients who are in the borderline category, leaving open the question as to whether these ventricles with their associated "borderline" small mitral valve and subaortic, aortic and ascending aortic size will support the systemic circulation. Because 2-ventricle repair is usually a considerable improvement over a 3-stage Norwood-type series of operations, cardiologists tend to look for every possible positive sign indicating a feasible 2-ventricle repair. This study adds hemodynamic and Doppler data to the various morphometric factors that one must consider in making decisions regarding 2-ventricle repair. Predominant or total antegrade flow in the ascending aorta and transverse aorta correlated quite highly with survival. These data can help in making this difficult distinction between patients who are reasonable candidates for biventricular vs. single-ventricle repair.

T.P. Graham, M.D.

Development and Validation of an Echocardiographic Model for Predicting Progression of Discrete Subaortic Stenosis in Children
Bezold LI, Smith EO, Kelly K, et al (Harvard Med School, Boston; Baylor College of Medicine, Houston)
Am J Cardiol 81:314-320, 1998
2–35

Objective.—Discrete subaortic stenosis (DSS) is a progressive type of left ventricular outflow obstruction. It is difficult to predict the clinical course of the disease. A prediction model based on anatomic and Doppler echocardiographic features identifiable at diagnosis was developed and validated in 2 phases.

Methods.—In phase I, a multiple logistic regression model was developed to predict the clinical course of DSS, based on clinical and echocardiographic variables, in 52 children at Texas Children's Hospital. In phase

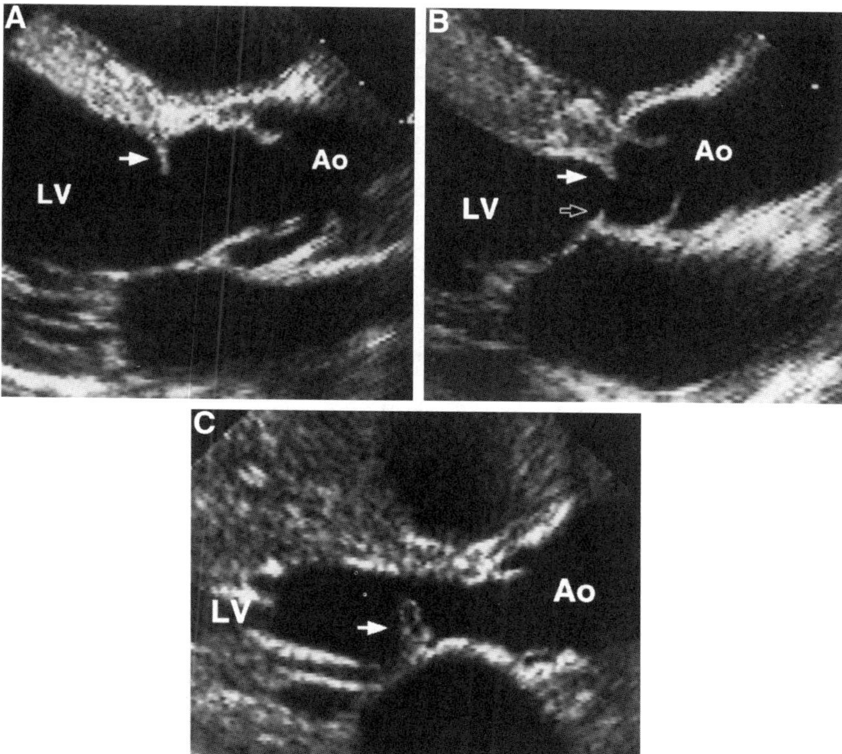

FIGURE 1.—Representative examples of subaortic membrane and left ventricular outflow tract morphology in the 3 study groups as seen from the parasternal long-axis view. **A**, nonprogressive group; low profile membrane at the crest of the ventricular septum (*arrow*) in a patient with a small membranous ventricular septal defect (not seen in this plane). Notice that the membrane is thin and is located 8 mm below the aortic valve. **B**, progressive group; thick protrusive membrane located 2 mm below the aortic valve (*solid arrow*) with involvement of the anterior mitral leaflet (*open arrow*). **C**, intermediate group; mild subaortic stenosis produced by accessory mitral valve tissue (*arrow*) attaching to the subaortic septum. *Abbreviations: Ao*, aorta; *LV*, left ventricle. (Reprinted by permission of the publisher from Bezold LI, Smith EO, Kelly K, et al: Development and validation of an echocardiographic model for predicting progression of discrete subaortic stenosis in children. *Am J Cardiol* 81:314-320. Copyright 1998 by Excerpta Medica, Inc.)

II, the model was tested in 48 children with DSS from Children's Hospital. Based on echocardiographic data, children were divided into 3 outcome groups: nonprogressive (Doppler gradient 20 mm Hg or less at last follow-up), progressive (Doppler gradient greater than 40 mm Hg at last follow-up), or intermediately progressive (Doppler gradient 20 to 40 mm Hg at last follow-up).

Results.—There were 33 patients in the nonprogressive group, 50 in the progressive group, and 17 in the intermediately progressive group. These groups were respectively characterized by significantly different initial gradients of 7, 16, and 26 mm Hg; significantly different final gradients of 11, 28, and 65 mm Hg; and by surgical resection % of 0, 0, and 74.

Multivariate analysis identified initial Doppler gradient, distance of subaortic obstruction from aortic valve, and involvement of the anterior mitral leaflet by the subaortic membrane as the 3 independent predictors of progressive disease (Fig 1). The probability of a patient having progressive or nonprogressive disease is $P = [1 + e^{-(-3.22 + 0.334X_1 + 4.06X_2 - 0.708X_3)}]^{-1}$, where X is the initial gradient in mm Hg, X_2 is the presence or absence of mitral leaflet involvement, and X_3 is the indexed distance between the aortic valve and the subaortic membrane in mm/body surface area$^{1/2}$. Phase II patients who progressed had at least a 58% probability of progression, whereas all patients with nonprogressive disease had a probability of progression of 0.29 or less. An estimated probability of progression of 0.55 or greater had a sensitivity, positive predictive value, specificity, negative predictive value, and accuracy of 100%.

Conclusion.—Progressive DSS can be distinguished from nonprogressive DSS by anatomic and echocardiographic features present at diagnosis.

▶ The progression or nonprogression of subaortic stenosis in young patients represents a fascinating pathophysiological phenomenon. These authors show that nonprogression of this lesion is associated with a thin, mobile membrane located at a greater distance from the aortic valve and usually lacking mitral valve involvement. Progressive subaortic stenosis is characterized by frequent involvement of the anterior mitral leaflet, close proximity to the aortic valve, and increased membrane thickness with decreased mobility. Accessory mitral tissue and chordal attachments to the ventricular septum were common in the intermediate group. Accessory mitral tissue can cause subaortic obstruction more frequently than we have appreciated.

T.P. Graham, M.D.

Interventional Catheterization

Early and Late Results and the Effects on Pulmonary Arteries of Balloon Dilatation of the Right Ventricular Outflow Tract in Tetralogy of Fallot
Godart F, Rey C, Prat A, et al (CHRU de Lille, France)
Eur Heart J 19:595-600, 1998
2–36

Objective.—Opinions differ about the safety and efficacy of balloon dilatation as palliative treatment of tetralogy of Fallot. Immediate and midterm results of balloon dilatation of the pulmonary valve in symptomatic infants with tetralogy of Fallot were evaluated retrospectively.

Methods.—Balloon dilatation of the pulmonary valve was performed in 33 infants (15 girls), aged 3 days to 11 months, between June 1990 and January 1997. Associated cardiac abnormalities were present in 21 infants.

Results.—Immediately, systemic oxygen saturation increased significantly, from 76% to 88%, and right ventricle to pulmonary artery pressure gradient decreased significantly, from 73 to 52 mm Hg. The procedure failed in 4 patients with predilatation spells, who required early surgical intervention. Two other patients required a modified Blalock-Taussig procedure 2 and 5 months after dilatation. Pulmonary annulus diameter increased significantly in 16 control patients, from 5.5 mm at baseline to 9.0 mm; right pulmonary artery diameter increased significantly, from 4.1 to 6.4 mm (mean z value from -3.0 to -1.9 standard deviation); and left pulmonary artery increased significantly, from 4.1 to 6.5 mm (mean z value from -2.7 to -1.6 standard deviation). At an average of 9 months after balloon dilatation, 28 patients underwent complete surgical repair. Twelve patients (43%) required pulmonary transannular patching. Four patients died of causes unrelated to dilatation.

Conclusion.—Balloon dilatation is an effective procedure for palliative treatment of tetralogy of Fallot, particularly in very young patients with numerous associated cardiac abnormalities, in whom complete repair carries a high risk of early death.

▶ A number of institutions are using balloon dilatation of the pulmonary valve as a palliative procedure in infants with severe cyanosis and tetralogy of Fallot. Many centers, however, reject this approach and proceed with surgery for cyanotic infants who need early intervention. Transannular patching was required in only 43% of these infants who underwent balloon dilatation treatment, and effective growth of the annulus and the right pulmonary artery was seen. The need for transannular patching in any patient with tetralogy is assessed at the time of surgery and obviously is individualized by the surgical team. Thus, whether more of these patients would have required transannular patching if they had gone straight to repair or had a palliative shunt before repair is not shown by this study. If balloon dilatation is used in this setting, it needs to be performed by teams with considerable expertise, so that the incidence of hypercyanotic spells during or after catheterization is minimized, and so that emergency surgery can be carried out promptly if necessary.

T.P. Graham, M.D.

Comparison of Cost and Clinical Outcome Between Transcatheter Coil Occlusion and Surgical Closure of Isolated Patent Ductus Arteriosus
Prieto LR, DeCamillo DM, Konrad DJ, et al (Cleveland Clinic Found, Ohio)
Pediatrics 101:1020-1024, 1998   2–37

Objective.—Transcatheter closure of the patent ductus arteriosus (PDA) using Gianturco coils was retrospectively compared to surgical repair at the Cleveland Clinic Foundation.

Methods.—Procedural and recovery costs for 36 patients, aged 13 months to 28 years, who underwent coil or surgical uncomplicated closure of PDA between August 1993 and June 1996 were determined. Patients were excluded if they had serious coexisting medical conditions.

Results.—The average cost of coil occlusion was a significant 38% lower than the cost of surgery ($5,273 vs. $8,509). Respective costs for inpatient hospital stays were $398 vs. $2,566 and for professional services were $1,506 vs. $2,782. Technical costs were similar even though hourly costs for the catheterization laboratory averaged twice those of the operating room. Median duration of the transcatheter coil occlusion was 150 minutes, and median duration of surgery was 165 minutes. Patient outcomes were similar in both groups, although 4 (17%) patients in the coil group vs. no patients in the surgery group had residual leaks, at an average of 6 months, as detected by echocardiography performed on all coil group patients and 5 (42%) surgery patients. There were no other short- or long-term complications in either group and no deaths.

Conclusion.—Transcatheter coil occlusion for PDA is as safe and effective as surgery and is much less expensive.

▶ Transcatheter coil occlusion of PDA has become the preferred treatment in many institutions. With improvements in technique, residual shunting and complications are uncommon and most patients can be sent home the day of the procedure or the following day. Early data indicate that obstruction to the left pulmonary artery and thromboembolic problems are exceedingly rare. In this comparison, the total cost was $3,236 less for coil closure than for surgical closure. Both surgical closure and coil occlusion provide excellent results for treatment of most patients with PDA. The limited thoracotomy approach to this lesion will undoubtedly lower the cost for a surgical approach in selected patients.

T.P. Graham, M.D.

Reopening After Successful Coil Occlusion for Patent Ductus Arteriosus
Daniels CJ, Cassidy SC, Teske DW, et al (Columbus Children's Hosp and Ohio State Univ, Columbus)
J Am Coll Cardiol 31:444-450, 1998   2–38

Introduction.—A study of children who had undergone successful coil occlusion for patent ductus arteriosus (PDA) was conducted to determine the frequency of PDA reopening and the factors that may predict reopening. Although the PDA minimal diameter has been associated with overall success of coil occlusion, researchers hypothesized that other factors are involved.

Methods.—The patients underwent percutaneous transarterial PDA coil occlusion between May 1995 and June 1996. Excluded from coil occlusion were children with additional cardiovascular abnormalities requiring surgery. A cineangiogram of the descending aorta determined PDA minimal diameter and PDA length. Doppler-echocardiography, performed within 24 hours of PDA coil occlusion, was used to document success, defined as the absence of a shunt into the main pulmonary artery. Patients were evaluated at 12 months.

Results.—Coil occlusion for PDA was attempted in 22 children with a median age of 4.9 years. Clinical success, with loss of a continuous murmur, was achieved in 20 patients (91%), and in 19 patients (90%) Doppler-echocardiography was negative for PDA shunting. Five patients were found to have reopening at follow-up. Compared with patients without reopening after successful coil occlusion, those with reopening had a larger PDA minimal diameter (1.4 vs. 1.2 mm) and a shorter PDA length (2.9 vs. 7.1 mm). The angiographic classification of the ductus arteriosus included 3 patients with type B PDA (conical with a short ductal ampulla); all of these patients were in the reopened group. A comparison of independent variables found only PDA length and type B PDA to predict reopening.

Conclusion.—Despite successful coil occlusion for PDA, reopening is not an uncommon occurrence. Previous reports have indicated that success is associated with the minimal diameter of the PDA. However, in this study only short PDA length and angiographic type B PDA were associated with reopening.

▶ This study suggests we should be a bit cautious before proclaiming transcatheter coil occlusion of the PDA as a virtually 100% successful long-term solution. In particular, the wide-diameter, short-length ductus may be difficult to achieve complete closure. Follow-up of these patients with Doppler studies will be needed, after presumed successful coil occlusion, to assess long-term results. I predict that the interventionalists will find a way to get complete closure in almost everyone.

T.P. Graham, M.D.

Intravascular Stents in Congential Heart Disease: Short- and Long-term Results From a Large Single-Center Experience
Shaffer KM, Mullins CE, Grifka RG, et al (Baylor College of Medicine, Houston; Texas Children's Hosp, Houston)
J Am Coll Cardiol 31:661-667, 1998   2–39

Introduction.—Intravascular stents for the treatment of patients with congenital heart disease and vascular stenoses were evaluated in Food and Drug Administration (FDA) phase 1 and 2 clinical trials at Texas Children's Hospital. Results of the only FDA-approved investigational device exemption study of balloon-expandable stents in patients with congenital heart disease and vascular stenoses were reported.

Methods.—All patients enrolled in the study had stenoses requiring treatment. Stents were placed in 3 groups of patients: those with postoperative pulmonary artery (PA) stenoses, congenital PA stenoses, or stenoses of systemic veins/venous anastomoses. A total of 347 stents was placed in 200 patients between September 1989 and June 1995. The Palmaz stent was used in all cases. Median patient age at implantation was 10.5 years. Data were collected before intervention, after stent implantation, and at follow-up catheterization.

Results.—All 3 groups of patients had a significant decrease in mean pressure gradients at stent implantation: from 46 to 10 mm Hg in postoperative PA stenoses; from 71 to 15 mm Hg in congenital PA stenoses; and from 7 to 1 mm Hg in stenoses of systemic veins/venous anastomoses. All 3 groups demonstrated a marked increase in mean vessel diameters: from 6 to 12 mm in postoperative PA stenoses; from 3 to 9 mm in congenital PA stenoses; and from 3 to 12 mm in stenoses of systemic veins/venous anastomoses. Right ventricular pressure decreased (right ventricular pressure indexed to femoral artery pressure ratio) in the postoperative (from 0.63 to 0.41) and congenital PA (from 0.71 to 0.55) stenoses groups. Perfusion to a single affected lung increased significantly from 31% to 46%. Little change was noted at recatheterization, performed at a mean of 14 months after stent implantation. There were 4 cases of stent migration early in the series but no late complications, and only 3 patients had significant restenosis. Two deaths were directly attributed to the stent procedure.

Conclusions.—Intravascular stents proved to be a safe and effective treatment for patients with congenital heart disease and vascular stenoses. Neither the device nor the procedure appeared to be associated with long-term morbidity, and the favorable results were seen immediately after implantation and at follow-up catheterization.

▶ Intravascular stents now play an increasingly important role in the therapy of patients with complex heart disease, particularly those with PA stenosis, narrowed systemic venous anastomoses, and older patients with coarctation. In the hands of experienced interventionalists, the implantation of stents is associated with very low morbidity and mortality. Data on whether intimal proliferation will result in stent failure long-term is still not available. It is encouraging that most stents can be redilated with low risk. This type of interventional care is mandatory for centers who deal with significant numbers of patients with congenital heart disease.

T.P. Graham, M.D.

Arrhythmia

Prolongation of the QT Interval and the Sudden Infant Death Syndrome
Schwartz PJ, Stramba-Badiale M, Segantini A, et al (Univ of Pavia, Italy; Univ of Milan, Italy; Ospedale Niguarda Ca' Granda, Milan, Italy; et al)
N Engl J Med 338:1709-1714, 1998   2–40

Background.—The cause of sudden infant death syndrome (SIDS) remains unknown. It is likely that a defect in neural control of either respiratory or cardiac function sets off a chain of events that may prove fatal. Previous research has suggested that a developmental abnormality in sympathetic innervation of the heart may prolong the QT interval and thus increase the risk of ventricular arrhythmias, which may lead to SIDS. This hypothesis was examined by reviewing ECGs of infants who died of SIDS and those of normal infants.

Methods.—Follow-up data at 1 year of age were available for 33,034 infants (16,538 boys and 16,496 girls) born during an 18-year period. Each neonate was assessed by ECG on day 3 or 4. The QT interval was assessed twice, once with and once without correction for heart rate (QTc).

Findings.—Mean heart rate, PR interval, duration of the QRS complex, and the QT interval were normal in this sample. A QTc value above the 97.5th percentile (440 msec), representing 2 SD above the mean, was considered prolonged. During 1 year of follow-up, 34 deaths occurred; 24 were caused by SIDS (incidence, 0.7/1,000 live births). Three fourths of these SIDS deaths occurred in infants 2 or 3 months old. The QTc interval was significantly longer in infants who died of SIDS (435 ± 45 msec) than in infants who died of other causes (393 ± 24 msec) and in those who survived (400 ± 20 msec). Half of the infants who died of SIDS had a prolonged QTc interval, whereas none of the children who died of other causes had a QTc greater than 440 msec. Even when absolute QT values were used in analysis, again half the infants who died of SIDS had a QT value above the 97.5th percentile. Infants with a normal QTc had a 0.037 absolute risk of SIDS; infants with a prolonged QTc had a 1.53 absolute risk of SIDS (odds ratio. 41.3).

Conclusions.—Sudden infant death syndrome was significantly more likely in infants with a prolonged QTc interval in the first week of life. In fact, the odds ratio for SIDS death associated with a prolonged QTc interval was higher than those of other risk factors, such as sleeping prone, maternal smoking, and bed sharing. Two mechanisms are proposed for prolongation of the QT interval: changes in cardiac sympathetic innervation that occur with development, and perhaps a genetic abnormality causing congenital long-QT syndrome. Although ECG screening could help identify infants at risk of SIDS caused by prolonged QT intervals, more data are needed to determine the cost-effectiveness of this approach. However, if infants at greater risk of SIDS could be identified, then perhaps administration of β-blockers during the first year of life could protect against sudden ventricular arrhythmias and, thus, SIDS.

▶ This association of prolongation of the QTc interval with SIDS is intriguing. The authors note that arrhythmias which are associated with a prolonged QTc interval frequently are triggered by increases in sympathetic activity. They postulate that in the first year of life, such an increase in sympathetic activity might be elicited by sudden noise, exposure to cold, rapid eye movements, sleep, or apnea leading to a chemoreceptor reflex and arousal. They also speculate that patients with prolonged QTc interval might be protected by the careful administration of β-blockers during the first year of life. This hypothesis would be extremely hard to prove because of the rarity of both SIDS and prolongation of the QTc interval. Hopefully, further population-based studies such as this one from Italy will be available to help in sorting out this problem.

T.P. Graham, M.D.

Five-Year Experience With Radiofrequency Catheter Ablation: Implications for Management of Arrhythmias in Pediatric and Young Adult Patients

Tanel RE, Walsh EP, Triedman JK, et al (Children's Hosp, Boston; Harvard Med School, Boston)
J Pediatr 131:878-887, 1997   2–41

Introduction.—The transcatheter delivery of radiofrequency energy has revolutionized the care of patients with most mechanisms of supraventricular or ventricular tachycardia. The first 5 years of experience with radiofrequency catheter ablation at a large pediatric referral center for patients with congenital heart disease and arrhythmias was retrospectively reviewed.

Methods.—A total of 410 radiofrequency catheter ablation procedures performed in 346 children for treatment of recurrent supraventricular or ventricular tachycardia were reviewed. The procedures were peformed during a 5-year period from March 1990 to February 1995.

Results.—The overall final success rate was 90% for all diagnoses. The success rate was higher in children with an accessory pathway (96%). With time the success rate improved, and rates of failure and late recurrence diminished. There was a 1.2% incidence of serious complications (1 late death, 1 ventricular dysfunction, 1 complete heart block, 1 cardiac perforation, and 1 cerebrovascular accident).

Conclusions.—The data from this large series of children who underwent radiofrequency catheter ablation confirm the safety and efficacy of this procedure. Specific technical, anatomical, and electrophysiologic variations in children that are crucial to the success of this procedure must be considered when it is used.

▶ This review of a large number of patients who had radiofrequency ablation indicates that in the majority of patients, there is a high success rate and a lack of serious complications, regardless of whether their rhythm disturbance is caused relatively by a simple or complex abnormal pathway. The incidence of serious complications is not zero, and these procedures should be undertaken only by physicians with training, experience, and proven competence in treating pediatric arrhythmias. As with most procedures in children, it appears that complications are more common in younger patients. Therefore, only after medical therapeutic options have been exhausted will these authors consider performing catheter ablation in infants younger than 1 year.

T.P. Graham, M.D.

Fetal Tachycardias: Management and Outcome of 127 Consecutive Cases

Simpson JM, Sharland GK (Guy's Hosp, London)
Heart 79:576-581, 1998   2–42

Background.—Fetal tachycardia is a significant cause of mortality. It can be diagnosed prenatally, but its treatment before birth is controversial. The treatment protocols for fetuses with tachycardia and their associated success rates and problems are described.

Methods.—Over 16 years, 127 fetuses (median gestational age, 32 weeks; range, 18-42 weeks) with fetal tachycardia were evaluated. The nature of the tachycardia (persistent vs. intermittent, supraventricular tachycardia vs. atrial flutter) was determined by echocardiography, and any hydropic infants were noted.

Findings.—Most of the fetuses (105, or 83%) had supraventricular tachycardia, and 22 (17%) had atrial flutter. Most of the fetuses (83, or 65%) had persistent tachycardia, and 44 (35%) had intermittent episodes. There were 75 fetuses without hydrops and 52 with hydrops; the median ventricular rates at baseline did not differ between the 2 groups (range, 210-300 beats per minute). Similarly, the response to drug therapy did not differ between fetuses with supraventricular tachycardia and atrial flutter in either the hydropic or nonhydropic groups. Sixty-three of the 75 fetuses without hydrops were treated prenatally; 39 of 63 (62%) treated with oral digoxin responded, 3 of 3 treated with oral flecainide responded, and 10 of 14 (71%) treated with maternal verapamil responded, which yielded a total of 52 responders (83%). Most of the fetuses without hydrops (73 of 75, or 97%) survived through the neonatal period, and 38 (52%) received neonatal antiarrhythmic agents.

Forty-seven of the 52 fetuses with hydrops were treated prenatally; only 1 of 5 (20%) treated with digoxin alone responded, 8 of 14 (57%) treated with digoxin and verapamil responded, 16 of 27 (59%) treated with flecainide acetate alone responded, and 6 of 9 (67%) treated with combinations of antiarrhythmics responded, which yielded a total of 31 responders (66%). Compared with the fetuses without hydrops, significantly fewer fetuses with hydrops survived through the neonatal period (39 of 52, or 75%), and significantly more received neonatal antiarrhythmic agents (31 of 39, or 79%). Also, after birth, pre-excitation was significantly more prevalent in the fetuses with hydrops than in the fetuses without hydrops (16% vs. 4%).

Conclusions.—Digoxin monotherapy successfully restored sinus rhythm in many of the treated fetuses without hydrops. Their prognosis after transplacental treatment is excellent. However, for the fetuses with hydrops, digoxin monotherapy was not very successful, and often a succession of antiarrhythmic agents was needed. Furthermore, despite prenatal control of the tachycardia, 25% of fetuses with hydrops died. Thus, the optimum approach to managing tachycardia in the fetus with hydrops remains to be established.

▶ One of the interesting aspects of this article is that maternal digoxin monotherapy seldom works for the fetus with severe tachycardia, and multiple drug therapy or flecainide acetate or both was needed in most of these patients. There has been a reluctance to use flecainide because of its proarrhythmic history. It is clear that fetuses with tachycardia and hydrops can benefit from referral to a high-risk perinatal unit, in which there is close collaboration between the obstetrician and a cardiologist with experience in fetal echocardiography and arrhythmia management.

T.P. Graham, M.D.

Permanent Junctional Re-entry Tachycardia: A Multicentre Long-term Follow-up Study in Infants, Children and Young Adults

Lindinger A, Heisel A, von Bernuth G, et al (Univ Children's Hosp, Homburg/ Saar, Germany; Univ Children's Hosp, Aachen, Germany; Univ Children's Hosp, Hannover, Germany; et al)
Eur Heart J 19:936-942, 1998   2–43

Background.—Permanent junctional reentry tachycardia (PJRT) is characterized by antegrade conduction through the atrioventricular node and retrograde conduction through an accessory pathway. The effects of drug therapy and ablation procedures on heart rates and left ventricular function were evaluated in patients with PJRT.

Methods.—The research subjects were 32 patients (12 males and 20 females) with PJRT (median age, 2 years; range, 27 weeks' gestation to 27 years). Patients were split into 3 groups based on New York Heart Association classifications of heart failure: group 1, no symptoms (20 patients); group 2, mild symptoms (8 patients); and group 3, severe symptoms (4 patients). Patients were treated either by conventional treatments (with or without antiarrhythmic drugs) or by ablation. Follow-up ranged from 1 to 31 years (mean, 10 years).

Findings.—At baseline, heart rates during PJRT were related to age; the highest rates (mean, 190-250 beats per minute) were in patients up to 1 year old and the lowest rates (mean, 110-160 beats per minute) were in patients older than 14 years. More than two thirds of the patients (69%) had PJRT for at least 50% of the day, but the daily frequency of PJRT episodes ranged from less than 10% to 100%. Nine patients (28%) had a tachycardia-related myopathy that reduced left ventricular function. Compared with group 1 patients, groups 2 and 3 patients had significantly more frequent PJRT episodes and significantly worse left ventricular function. Four patients had infrequent PJRT, and they required no treatment. During follow-up, 25 patients (78%) received antiarrhythmic drugs and 14 (56%) responded to this therapy. The most effective drugs were propafenone and flecainide. Eight of these 14 patients are continuing antiarrhythmic therapy and have no impairment of left ventricular function, have PJRT frequencies between 1% and 30% of the day, and have tachycardia rates from 170 to 250 beats per minute. Five of these 14 patients were able to discontinue therapy because of symptom improvement or resolution. One of these patients died at age 15 months as a result of a cause not related to the arrhythmia itself or to its therapy. The remaining 14 of 32 patients underwent ablation of the bypass tract, at a mean age of 17.8 (range, 4-31). Re-ablation was needed for 3 recurrences, which were successfully treated. Left ventricular function normalized a mean of 1.2 years (range, 6-24 months) after ablation.

Conclusions.—The clinical picture of PJRT is varied. Patients who have infrequent PJRT episodes may never have symptoms; thus, they may not need therapy. Younger patients who have frequent PJRT episodes, fast tachycardia rates, and left ventricular impairment should begin antiarrhythmic therapy as a first-line approach. The classic antiarrhythmic agents were most useful in treating PJRT, and no patient had major side effects from drug therapy. For younger patients whose conditions are refractory to drug therapy, and for older symptomatic patients, catheter ablation can be successfully used.

▶ This collaborative study clearly shows the relationship between time in PJRT and left ventricular shortening fraction. There can be devastating effects on ventricular function with this arrhythmia, which, fortunately, usually can be cured permanently with relief of the tachycardia. Ablation therapy appears to have promise as the treatment of choice for those who have symptoms despite medical treatment and who are outside the infant age range.

T.P. Graham, M.D.

Predictors of Early- and Late-Onset Supraventricular Tachyarrhythmias After Fontan Operation

Durongpisitkul K, Porter CJ, Cetta F, et al (Mayo Clinic and Found, Rochester, Minn)

Circulation 98:1099-1107, 1998

2–44

Objective.—Development of late-onset supraventricular tachyarrhythmias (SVTAs) after the Fontan operation continues to be a problem in patients with tricuspid atresia. The frequency of early and late clinically significant SVTA after the Fontan operation, the frequency of SVTA among various modifications of the operation, and the risk factors for SVTA after the Fontan operation were determined.

Methods.—Between January 1985 and January 1994, 499 patients (61.7% male), aged 8 months to 39 years, had a Fontan operation, including total cavopulmonary connection, atriopulmonary connection with or without lateral tunnel, heterotaxy surgery, intra-atrial conduit procedure, and others. Patients were studied for a minimum of 2 years.

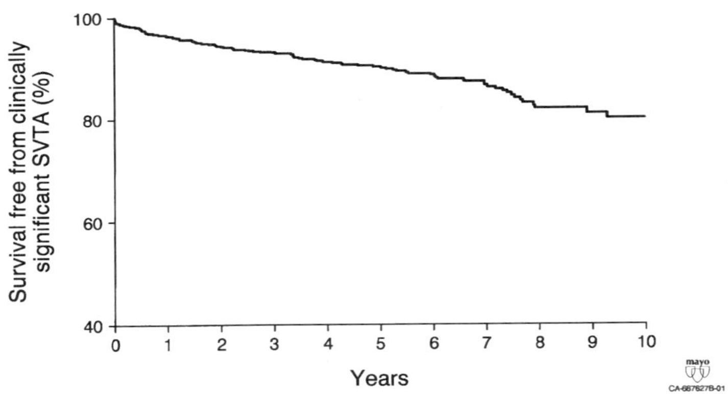

FIGURE 3.—Survival free of clinically significant supraventricular tachyarrhythmia (*SVTA*) (late onset) for 443 Fontan patients alive 30 days after operation. Time 0 indicates 30 days after operation. (Courtesy of Durongpisitkul K, Porter CJ, Cetta F: Predictors of early- and late-onset supraventricular tachyarrhythmias after Fontan operation. *Circulation* 98:1099-1107, 1998.)

Clinically significant SVTAs were those requiring antiarrhythmic drug treatment, synchronized direct current cardioversion, or atrial overdrive pacing and were recorded and divided into early (less than 30 days after surgery) and late onset (more than 30 days after surgery). Clinical histories were reviewed, patients and physicians were contacted, and a detailed health questionnaire was sent to survivors.

Results.—At last contact, there were 399 survivors and 316 with at least 5 years of follow-up. Early mortality was 9% (45 patients). Five- and 10-year mortality rates, excluding early mortality, were 13% and 18%, respectively. Deaths were sudden cardiac death in 29 patients, nonsudden cardiac death in 45, noncardiac death in 19, and deaths from unknown or other causes in 7. There were 74 patients (15%) with early SVTA. According to multivariate analysis, significant predictors of early-onset SVTA were atrioventricular valve regurgitation, preoperative SVTA, and abnormal atrioventricular valve anatomy. The frequency of late-onset SVTA was 6% at 1 year, 12% at 3 years, and 17% at 5 years. According to multivariate analysis, risk factors for late-onset SVTA were age older than 10 years or younger than 3 years, and valve replacement (Fig 3).

Conclusion.—The frequency of SVTA is not related to the type of Fontan modification used.

▶ Figure 3 indicates that clinically significant SVTAs continue to occur with increased follow-up after a Fontan procedure. Preoperative arrhythmia and patient age at operation were strong predictors of postoperative arrhythmia, as were atrioventricular valve regurgitation and an abnormal atrioventricular valve. The latter 2 variables are associated with a large atrium before and after repair. Thus, atrial size may have been a major determinant of atrial arrhythmia.

T.P. Graham, M.D.

Results of a Restrictive Use of Antiarrhythmic Drugs in the Chronic Treatment of Atrioventricular Reentrant Tachycardias in Infancy and Childhood
Pfammatter J-P, Stocker FP (Univ Children's Hosp, Berne, Switzerland)
Am J Cardiol 82:72-75, 1998   2–45

Objective.—Oral long-term prophylactic drug therapy is usually recommended for infants and children with supraventricular tachycardia (SVT). The value of digoxin and the value of β blockers in the oral long-term therapy of an unselected population of children with SVT were retrospectively reviewed.

Methods.—Between January 1988 and January 1996, 50 children (23 male), aged newborn to 13 years, who had SVT received either no drug therapy (n = 11), digoxin (n = 28), or a β blocker (n = 11). Children were studied for a minimum of 12 months; all children were examined and had Holter monitoring in 1996.

Results.—The average age at the first SVT episode was 2 years, with 33 patients (66%) experiencing the first episode before age 1. Underlying heart disease was diagnosed in 11 patients. SVT responded favorably to drug treatment in 29 (75%) of 39 patients, with both drug therapies being equally effective. Nine of 10 patients who failed first-line therapy required class I or II antiarrhythmic drugs. Six of 11 children without drug therapy had no SVT recurrences, and 5 had either frequent short attacks or rare attacks.

Conclusion.—Treatment of SVT in children with digoxin or β blockers is successful in approximately two thirds of patients, obviating the need for class I or II antiarrhythmic drugs.

▶ These authors recommend the use of digoxin and/or a β blocker for first-line therapy in pediatric patients with atrioventricular re-entry tachycardias. Digoxin was the drug of choice in infants less than 1 year old and a β blocker the drug of choice in older children. With this approach, the authors were 75% successful. They did not try to differentiate between atrioventricular nodal re-entry tachycardia and tachycardia using a concealed accessory atrioventricular bypass before initial treatment. An alternative is to attempt, with transesophageal pacing, to determine mechanism and effectiveness of initial treatment at diagnosis, before discharge on chronic therapy. There has been no direct comparison of these 2 approaches and such a comparison needs to be done.

T.P. Graham, M.D.

Miscellaneous

Reduced Penetrance, Variable Expressivity, and Genetic Heterogeneity of Familial Atrial Septal Defects

Benson DW, Sharkey A, Fatkin D, et al (Brigham and Women's Hosp, Boston; Children's Hosp, Boston; Washington Univ, St Louis)
Circulation 97:2043-2048, 1998

2–46

Introduction.—A secundum atrial septal defect (ASD) occurs in up to 10% of individuals with congenital heart disease. Some familial ASD kindreds have associated family histories of the defect or other congenital heart malformations and coexisting heart blockage. Three kindreds with ASD inherited as an autosomal dominant trait were clinically examined and genetically investigated to determine the genetic basis for familial ASD.

Methods.—A history, medical record review, physical examination, 12-lead ECG, and 2-dimensional transthoracic echocardigraphy with color flow Doppler interrogation in 4 standard and subcostal views were performed in family members from 3 unrelated ASD kindreds. Peripheral lymphocytes were used to analyze genomic DNA. Two-point linkage analyses, multipoint analysis, and genetic heterogeneity for familial ASD were conducted.

Results.—Secundum ASD was transmitted as an autosomal dominant trait in each of the 3 families. An atrial septal defect was the most frequently occurring anomaly; other heart defects occurred alone or in association with ASD in individuals from each kindred. Genome-wide linkage evaluation in 1 kindred localized a familial ASD disease gene to chromosome 5p. Of 20 family members with the disease haplotype, 9 had ASD, 8 were clinically unaffected, and 3 had other cardiac defects. Familial ASD did not map to chromosome 5p in 2 kindreds.

Conclusion.—Familial ASD may be caused by a gene mutation on chromosome 5p. This genetically heterogeneous disorder may be caused by defects in other undefined genes. The observance of ASD or other congenital heart defects in more than 1 family member should cause suspicion; clinical evaluation should be undertaken in all relatives.

▶ Although the familial secundum ASD is a relatively rare occurrence, there are families with clear evidence of this defect transmitted as an autosomal dominant trait. At least 1 chromosomal location is at 5p, although other cases do not map to this location. Investigating the etiology of congenital heart disease is an exciting frontier, and the next 10 to 20 years should involve major breakthroughs in understanding causation.

T.P. Graham, M.D.

compared these results with the 2 out of 7 survivors, or 29%, achieved before this unit was available. The numbers are small and more data are needed to determine whether this rapid deployment unit yields a significantly better outcome than conventional ECMO when a larger number of patients are subjected to analysis.

T.P. Graham, M.D.

Acute Changes in Preload, Afterload, and Systolic Function After Superior Cavopulmonary Connection
Donofrio MT, Jacobs ML, Spray TL, et al (Children's Hosp of Philadelphia)
Ann Thorac Surg 65:503-508, 1998
2–49

Introduction.—Previous studies have shown a change in ventricular geometry occurs with volume reduction after superior cavopulmonary connection (SCPC). Nine patients were studied before and after SCPC, and at hospital discharge, to determine the effects of the procedure on preload, wall stress (or afterload), and systolic ventricular function.

Methods.—Diagnoses in the patient group included hypoplastic left heart syndrome in 4, double-outlet right ventricle in 2, unbalanced atrioventricular canal in 1, and tricuspid atresia in 2. Echocardiography was performed to estimate preload, using the ventricular end-diastolic area (EDA); wall stress was calculated at end-systole and peak systole. Ventricular function was represented by rate-corrected velocity of circumferential fiber shortening and fractional area change divided by rate-corrected ejection time. All measurements were made 3 times, with the average used for calculations.

Results.—Mean heart rate, diastolic blood pressure, and mean blood pressure were unchanged after SCPC, but systolic pressure decreased significantly. Mean EDA decreased by 34% immediately after SCPC, a change that persisted until hospital discharge. Wall stress decreased, and ventricular wall thickness increased with a concomitant decrease in cavity area.

Conclusion.—In single ventricles, an immediate decrease in preload and afterload occurs after SCPC. Alterations in ventricular geometry are the main cause of the decrease in afterload. Systolic function did not improve, but the reduction in loading conditions may preserve myocardial performance in the long-term.

▶ These authors report quantitative data on the changes in volume work of the single ventricle after SCPC. There is a nicely documented decrease in ventricular size and afterload (estimated by wall stress) with a concomitant increase in wall thickness. Hopefully, these changes will translate into improved diastolic and systolic function that will prove beneficial over the long run in these patients who are destined for a Fontan repair.

T.P. Graham, M.D.

Evidence for Rejection of Homograft Cardiac Valves in Infants

Rajani B, Mee RB, Ratliff NB (Cleveland Clinic Found, Ohio)
J Thorac Cardiovasc Surg 115:111-117, 1998

2–50

Introduction.—There is concern about the durability of small homograft cardiac valves in younger pediatric patients. Because homografts can induce specific immune responses, early homograft failure in young children appears to be associated with immunologic factors. If this were confirmed, a short course of immunosuppression therapy might improve homograft valve durability. Homograft cardiac valves removed at reoperation (n = 11) or autopsy (n = 1) were examined for immunohistochemical findings.

Methods.—A search of files at the study institution yielded 12 explanted homograft valves, 6 from adults (all male), 5 from infants, and 1 from a 13-year-old child. The valves from infants had inflammatory infiltrates, and sections from these valves were prepared for immunohistochemical studies with antibodies against smooth muscle actin, CD20, CD43, CD34, and CD68.

Results.—Homografts from the 6 adults and the older child showed histologic findings characterized by fibrosis, degeneration of leaflet collagen, calcification, and leaflet. None had signs of inflammation. Median graft survival time in the adult patients was 6 years. Each of the valves from infants had failed in less than 8 months. Microscopic examination of valve leaflets and aortic sleeves revealed a markedly thickened cellular intimal layer, with numerous spindle cells positive for smooth muscle actin. All 5 homografts contained multiple foci of inflammation (5 with T lymphocytes and 3 with B lymphocytes). Gomori methenamine silver and Gram stains for organisms were negative.

Discussion.—Findings in the explanted aortic homograft valves of infants were consistent with cellular rejection. The hyperplastic intima in all 5 valves and thrombus formation in 1 are similar to findings of transplant-associated vascular disease seen in coronary arteries.

▶ The evidence for rejection of homograft cardiac valves in these 5 infants is strong. This phenomenon may explain some of the early homograft failures in infants and young children, which continue to plague the pediatric cardiologist and cardiac surgeon. The current literature linking homograft failure to rejection is not consistent. It would be useful to know the blood group and HLA type for all homografts that are now used, so that future studies might shed some light on whether these factors play a significant role in homograft failure.

T.P. Graham, M.D.

3   Cardiac Surgery

Introduction

In what looks like the greatest change in cardiac surgery since the heart-lung machine, the rush to "minimally invasive" operations now threatens to stampede the standard approaches to coronary surgery as well as render the median sternotomy obsolete. Most patients don't really understand what is meant by *minimally invasive*. As a matter of fact, many surgeons would differ among themselves if asked to supply a definition for this often-requested new surgical technique.

A year or two ago, the term was used to connote small—as in smaller incisions, smaller scars, and shorter hospital stays. Now it has been redefined by many surgeons to indicate a procedure that does not require use of the heart-lung machine with its whole-body inflammatory response. Thus, an operation that uses a standard median sternotomy may be advertised as minimally invasive because the heart-lung machine is avoided. Of course, there are operations that are minimally invasive because they use a small incision, even though the heart-lung machine is used. So, you can claim to provide minimally invasive cardiac surgical operations for nearly any purpose except, perhaps, transplantation and for nearly any number of small incisions or even big ones. Just about the only characteristic that unites the various minimally invasive procedures is often the greater hazard or lesser benefit to the patient than most standard approaches provide.

Some systems of instrumentation for cardiac surgery allow for harvest of internal mammary arteries, various anastomotic techniques, and various valve operations—all of which can be done without any incision longer than 2 or 3 inches. So much for the future and some of the present.

But for the past and most of the present, there are still a lot of operations to study. These abstracts illustrate new and useful procedures and present results as described by skilled surgeons from numerous countries including the United States.

John J. Collins, Jr., M.D.

Generic Topics in Cardiac Surgery

Atrial Fibrillation After Bypass Surgery: Does the Arrhythmia or the Characteristics of the Patients Prolong Hospital Stay?

Borzak S, Tisdale JE, Amin NB, et al (Wayne State Univ, Detroit)
Chest 113:1489-1491, 1998   3–1

Background.—Atrial fibrillation or flutter (AF) is common after coronary artery bypass graft (CABG) surgery and is associated with clinical instability and stroke. AF is also associated with prolonged hospital stay and increased hospital costs. Whether the prolonged hospitalization of these patients is caused by the characteristics of the patients or by the arrhythmia itself has not been documented. A prospective case series study was performed to define the relative contributions of AF and patient characteristics to hospitalization after CABG surgery.

Study Design.—All patients undergoing isolated CABG surgery at Henry Ford Hospital between December 1994 and May 1996 were prospectively screened for this study. Demographic, outcome, and length-of-stay data were obtained for all 436 participants. Stepwise linear regression analysis was performed to identify factors associated with length of stay.

Findings.—Of the 436 consecutive CABG surgery patients, 23% developed AF. The AF patients were older and more likely to have obstructive lung disease. AF was the strongest predictor of prolonged hospital stay; other predictors were age, sex, and race. When an analysis of covariance was performed to adjust length of stay for age, gender, and race, AF remained a significant predictor.

Conclusions.—Although AF is more common in older patients, it is an independent predictor of prolonged hospital stay. Aggressive strategies to restore sinus rhythm may be useful in these patients to reduce hospitalization costs and should be investigated in prospective clinical trials.

▶ This interesting article shows that advanced age as such is not the principal cause of postoperative atrial fibrillation. However, atrial fibrillation remains a significant problem associated with operating on elderly patients.

J.J. Collins, Jr., M.D.

Right-Sided Maze Procedure for Right Atrial Arrhythmias in Congenital Heart Disease

Theodoro DA, Danielson GK, Porter CJ, et al (Mayo Clinic and Mayo Found, Rochester, Minn)
Ann Thorac Surg 65:149-154, 1998   3–2

Introduction.—Congenital heart anomalies are commonly associated with atrial tachyarrhythmias, particularly atrial fibrillation and atrial flutter, which cause right atrial dilatation. Patients with a right-sided congenital heart disease had surgery with a concomitant right-sided maze procedure to correct atrial fibrillation.

Methods.—A concomitant right-sided maze procedure was performed to reduce the incidence of atrial tachyarrhythmias after repair of right-sided congenital heart disease. There were 22 patients in 2 years who had right-sided congenital heart disease associated with atrial fibrillation or flutter. The patients ranged in age from 11 to 68 years. The procedure was performed in association with Ebstein's anomaly, congenital tricuspid insufficiency, or isolated atrial septal defect. The procedure was a modification of the Cox maze II operation. Patients were studied from 3 to 17 months.

Results.—No early deaths, reoperations, or complete heart blocks were seen. There was sinus discharge rhythm for 16 patients and junctional discharge rhythm for 2 patients. At follow-up, all patients were in New York Heart Association class I. In 3 patients, early postoperative arrhythmias developed, and all were converted to sinus rhythm by antiarrhythmic drugs. No late deaths or reoperations were observed.

Conclusion.—In patients having congenital heart anomalies that cause right atrial dilatation and associated atrial tachyarrythmias, a right-sided maze procedure with cardiac repair is effective in eliminating or reducing the incidence of those arrhythmias. Early arrhythmias, those lasting less than 3 months, were common for the standard maze procedure. The experience has been encouraging, and more information is needed to determine further improvement of patients.

Preoperative Amiodarone as Prophylaxis Against Atrial Fibrillation After Heart Surgery

Daoud EG, Strickberger SA, Man KC, et al (Univ of Michigan Hosp, Ann Arbor; Wayne State Univ, Detroit)
N Engl J Med 337:1785-1791, 1997   3–3

Objective.—Postoperative atrial fibrillation can occur in as many as 40% of patients having cardiac surgery. Because amiodarone is effective against atrial fibrillation, its oral use as prophylaxis against that condition after heart surgery was investigated in a double-blind, randomized study.

Methods.—Between June 1995 and October 1996, 124 patients (84 men) undergoing cardiac surgery received either 600 mg oral amiodarone daily (n = 64) or placebo (n = 60) for an average of 13 days before surgery. Patients receiving amiodarone before surgery also received 200 mg amiodarone daily after surgery until discharge.

Results.—Significantly fewer amiodarone patients than placebo patients had atrial fibrillation postoperatively (25% vs. 53%) (Fig 1). During hospitalization, 23% of amiodarone patients and 42% of placebo patients had atrial fibrillation 2.5 and 2.7 days, respectively, after surgery. The maximal heart rate during atrial fibrillation was significantly lower in the

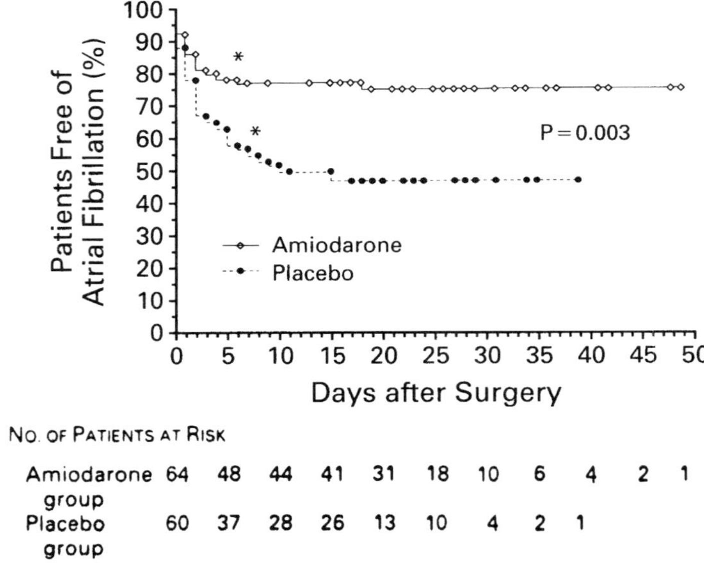

FIGURE 1.—Kaplan-Meier analysis of the percentages of patients remaining free of atrial fibrillation after surgery in the amiodarone and placebo groups. *Asterisks* indicate the mean days of hospital discharge. (Reprinted by permission of *The New England Journal of Medicine* from Daoud EG, Strickberger SA, Man KC, et al: Preoperative amiodarone as prophylaxis against atrial fibrillation after heart surgery. *N Engl J Med* 337:1785-1791, copyright 1997, Massachusetts Medical Society. All rights reserved.)

amiodarone group than in the placebo group (112 vs. 135 beats/min). The duration of atrial fibrillation was similar for the 2 groups. The use of β-blockers made no difference in the prevalence of atrial fibrillation. Patients with valvular surgery had a significantly higher incidence of atrial fibrillation than patients who had coronary bypass surgery (46% vs. 29%). Patients taking placebo were hospitalized significantly longer than patients taking amiodarone (7.9 vs. 6.5 days). The incidence of postoperative complications was similar for the 2 groups. There were postoperative complications in 8 placebo patients and 11 amiodarone patients. Morbidity occurred in 6 placebo patients and 8 amiodarone patients. Two placebo patients and 3 amiodarone patients died. Five placebo patients and 1 amiodarone patient had malignant ventricular arrhythmias. Amiodarone patients had significantly lower hospital costs than placebo patients did.

Conclusion.—Low-dose amiodarone, taken prophylactically, significantly and safely reduced both the incidence of atrial fibrillation and the cost of hospitalization in cardiac surgery patients.

▶ The papers by Theodoro and Daoud (Abstracts 3–2 and 3–3) and their associates allow some comparison of surgical vs. medical methods for prophylaxis against atrial fibrillation after cardiac surgery. In Dr. Theodoro's article, there was additional discussion because the paper was presented initially at the meeting of the Society of Thoracic Surgeons in February 1997.

It is surprising how enormous the impact of atrial fibrillation is on the care of postoperative cardiac surgical patients. Also, it is amazing that there is still considerable difficulty in controlling this common arrhythmia. The price paid for inability to control this condition is financial, functional, and serious.

J.J. Collins, Jr., M.D.

Early Results With Partial Left Ventriculectomy

McCarthy PM, Starling RC, Wong J, et al (Cleveland Clinic Found, Ohio)
J Thorac Cardiovasc Surg 114:755-765, 1997   3–4

Background.—An operation for patients with end-stage dilated cardiomyopathy was developed by Batista and coworkers. The procedure involves returning the enlarged heart to a normal diameter to reduce left ventricular wall tension.

Methods.—Partial left ventriculectomy was performed in 53 patients. The mean patient age was 53 years; 60% of patients were in class IV and 40% were in class III.

Results.—Two patients had mitral valve replacement. In 51 patients, the anterior and posterior mitral valve leaflets were approximated (Fig 3); ring posterior annuloplasty was also performed in 47 patients. In 51% of patients, one or both papillary muscles were divided, additional left ventricular wall was resected, and the papillary muscle heads were reimplanted. Significantly decreased left ventricular dimensions and reduced mitral regurgitation were seen, as well as increased forward ejection fraction. There was no significant increase in cardiac index. A perioperative left ventricular assist device was needed in 8 patients; 1 death in this group

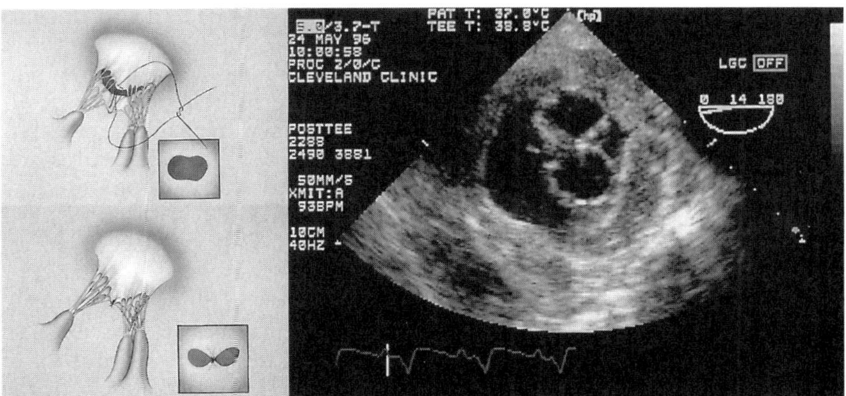

FIGURE 3.—To decrease mitral regurgitation and avoid prolapse from redundant mitral valve chordae, we sewed the free edge of the anterior and posterior mitral valve leaflets (**top left**) together with a 4-0 suture (Alfieri repair). After this suture is tied, the mitral valve has a double orifice (**bottom left**). Echocardiography revealed low gradients across the mitral valve, a "figure-of-eight" appearance, and good mitral valve area (**right**). (Courtesy of McCarthy PM, Starling RC, Wong J, et al: Early results with partial left ventriculectomy. *J Thorac Cardiovasc Surgery* 114:755-765, 1997.)

was the only perioperative death. At 11 months, survival was 87%, and 72% of patients did not relist for transplantation.

Discussion.—Better patient selection criteria may help avoid early failure. Longer follow-up and better data analysis are needed. This procedure may become a bridge or alternative to transplantation.

▶ McCarthy and associates at the Cleveland Clinic have reported this attempt at rigorous clinical evaluation of the partial left ventriculectomy operation introduced by Batista. This is a very useful report of the evolution of the operation in Cleveland. Every surgeon interested in performing this operation or knowing why the operation should or should not be performed in a particular patient would do well to become familiar with this publication. Additionally, because this presentation was originally read at the meeting of the American Association for Thoracic Surgery, expert commentary is provided that significantly adds to the value of the overall communication.

J.J. Collins, Jr., M.D.

Acute Hypovolemia May Cause Segmental Wall Motion Abnormalities in the Absence of Myocardial Ischemia

Seeberger MD, Cahalan MK, Rouine-Rapp K, et al (Univ of California, San Francisco)
Anesth Analg 85:1252-1257, 1997   3–5

Background.—New segmental wall motion abnormalities seen by echocardiography are regarded as sensitive and specific markers of myocardial ischemia. New segmental wall motion abnormalities were observed during pacing-induced reductions in left ventricular filling. These abnormalities resolved immediately after cessation of atrial pacing and restoration of filling.

Methods.—The ability of acute reduction in filling to induce new segmental wall motion abnormalities in the absence of ischemia was determined in 38 patients undergoing cardiopulmonary bypass surgery. The institution of cardiopulmonary bypass was used as a model of acute reduction in filling. When drainage of blood to the cardiopulmonary bypass machine emptied the heart, a beat-by-beat analysis of left ventricular contraction, filling, and blood pressures, as well as ECG was performed.

Results.—In 4 of the 38 patients, acute reduction in filling induced new segmental wall motion abnormalities. These 4 patients had preexisting abnormalities of left ventricular contraction, but neither translocation of these preexisting abnormalities nor myocardial ischemia accounted for the new segmental wall motion abnormalities.

Discussion.—Acute reduction in left ventricular filling can induce new segmental wall motion abnormalities in the absence of myocardial ischemia. The value of new segmental wall motion abnormalities as a marker of ischemia in the presence of acute reduction in filling is limited in the setting of acute hypovolemia.

▶ The observation that wall motion abnormalities may be a result of poor cardiac filling with no occurrence of ischemia is useful indeed. The more we understand about intraoperative echocardiography the more useful this procedure becomes.

J.J. Collins, Jr., M.D.

Activation of Coagulation and Fibrinolysis During Cardiothoracic Operations

Hunt BJ, Parratt RN, Segal HC, et al (Natl Heart and Lung Inst, Middlesex, England)
Ann Thorac Surg 65:712-718, 1998

3–6

Objective.—Open cardiac surgery with cardiopulmonary bypass (CPB) is associated with activation of hemostasis and fibrinolysis. However, it is unclear how much of this effect is directly attributable to CPB. Sequential blood samples from patients undergoing open cardiac vs. non-CPB thoracic surgery were compared to assess the separate effects of CPB and surgery on activation of coagulation and fibrinolysis.

Methods.—Eight patients were undergoing routine cardiac surgery with CPB and 7 patients were undergoing other thoracic surgical procedures without CPB. Sequential blood samples were obtained, preoperatively to 48 hours postoperatively, to assess activation of coagulation and the extent of fibrinolysis.

Results.—Duration of operation was shorter in the thoracic surgery group. These patients showed no significant increase in thrombin-antithrombin III complexes or D-dimers until 24 hours after surgery. The cardiac surgery group showed a sharp rise in both these measures during CPB. Fibrinolytic activity increased as a result of increased tissue plasminogen activator. At the time of the final blood sample, 48 hours after surgery, the cardiac surgery group were in a significantly more hypercoagulable state than the thoracic surgery group, and had higher levels of thrombin-antithrombin III complexes and of plasminogen activator inhibitor-1 activity.

Conclusions.—Cardiopulmonary bypass seems to be responsible for most of the activation of coagulation and fibrinolysis observed during and after cardiac surgery. In contrast, surgical cutting per se has little effect. Increased fibrinolysis, observed only with CPB, may result at least partly from thrombin generation. These findings underscore the need to make extracorporeal circuits more biocompatible, and to find ways of performing cardiac operations without CPB.

▶ This article presents more evidence that cardiopulmonary bypass is a major factor for activation of coagulation and fibrinolysis during open-heart operations.

J.J. Collins, Jr., M.D.

Impact of Minimum Hematocrit During Cardiopulmonary Bypass on Mortality in Patients Undergoing Coronary Artery Surgery

Fang WC, Helm RE, Krieger KH, et al (Univ of Massachusetts, Worcester; Cornell Univ, New York; North Shore Univ Hosp, Manhasset, NY; et al)
Circulation 96[suppl II]:II-194-II-199, 1997   3–7

Objective.—Over the years, a variety of measures have been used to reduce the need for blood transfusion during coronary artery bypass grafting (CABG). The hematocrit commonly falls to a low level in patients undergoing cardiopulmonary bypass (CPB), and there is debate over the minimum safe hematocrit level during this procedure. The mortality effect of the minimum hematocrit level achieved during CPB was investigated.

Methods.—The analysis included 1638 sequential patients undergoing CABG over 42 months. Patients requiring valve replacement or other concurrent surgical procedures were excluded. Minimum hematocrit level reached during CPB was analyzed, along with 31 preoperative risk factors, for effect on postoperative mortality.

Results.—The initial multiple logistic regression model identified 8 preoperative risk factors as independent predictors of postoperative mortality: shock, renal failure, ventricular arrhythmia, previous open heart surgery, IV nitroglycerin administration, congestive heart failure, aortoiliac disease, and older age. In a further model, minimum hematocrit during CPB was independently associated with mortality risk. With adjustment for other risk factors, patients with a minimum hematocrit of 14% or below had an increased probability of risk-adjusted mortality (odds ratio 2.70). For high-risk patients, a minimum hematocrit of 17% or lower significantly increased the risk of postoperative death (odds ratio 2.20). Factors independently associated with a minimum hematocrit value of 20% or less were low prebypass hematocrit, small body surface area, female sex, renal failure, and absence of chronic obstructive pulmonary disease.

Conclusions.—The extent to which hematocrit falls during CPB is an independent risk factor for post-CABG mortality. Risk of death is significantly increased for patients whose hematocrit drops to 14% or lower, or for high-risk patients whose hematocrit drops to 17% or lower. These data will help guide transfusion during CABG and improve overall cardiac surgical outcomes.

▶ These authors show that hematocrit levels that fall below about 14% during cardiopulmonary bypass are risk factors for increased mortality. Maintaining a hematocrit of around 18% to 20% appears to be safer.

J.J. Collins, Jr., M.D.

Platelet and Neutrophil Activation During Cardiac Surgical Procedures: Impact of Cardiopulmonary Bypass
Morse DS, Adams D, Magnani B (Harvard Med School, Boston)
Ann Thorac Surg 65:691-695, 1998   3–8

Purpose.—Reperfusion syndrome after acute coronary occlusion relies on platelet and neutrophil activation. By disrupting the balance between cellular activation and inhibition, ischemia and reperfusion may play a role in myocardial dysfunction occurring after blood flow is restored to hearts arrested by cardioplegia. Platelet and neutrophil activation in the coronary circulation after cold cardioplegic arrest and reperfusion was assessed.

Methods.—The study included 22 patients undergoing coronary artery bypass and/or valve surgery. Blood samples were taken from the coronary sinus and radial artery before bypass, immediately after cross-clamp release, and 5 minutes after cross-clamp release. These specimens were assessed for surface markers of platelet and neutrophil activation: CD62P and CD11b, respectively.

Results.—There was a significant increase in platelet activation during bypass. No difference was seen in the level of platelet activation between arterial and coronary sinus blood. Bypass was also associated with increased neutrophil activation, with no difference between arterial and coronary sinus samples. During the bypass, platelet count decreased, whereas granulocyte count increased.

Conclusions.—In patients undergoing cardiac surgery, cardioplegic arrest is not associated with the appearance of early indicators of reperfusion injury. However, there are still questions regarding the full extent of reperfusion injury associated with cardiac injury. Cardioplegia may protect against ischemia during cardiac arrest and cross-clamping. The cause of postoperative reperfusion syndrome remains to be determined.

▶ This very interesting article reports that cellular activation (often referred to as the sine qua non of maximal exposure open heart surgery) is no more significant after cold cardioplegic arrest with reperfusion than after other techniques of perfusion.

J.J. Collins, Jr., M.D.

Sternoplasty for Incomplete Sternum Separation
Robicsek F, Cook JW, Rizzoni W (Carolinas Med Ctr, Charlotte, NC)
J Thorac Cardiovasc Surg 116:361-362, 1998   3–9

Objective.—The authors have previously reported a technique for surgical repair of poststernotomy separation. In the sternal weaving technique, peristernal bilateral double-row wire sutures are placed, and transverse sutures are used to reunite the sternal halves, buttressed by the double axial suture lines. This technique is highly useful for patients with

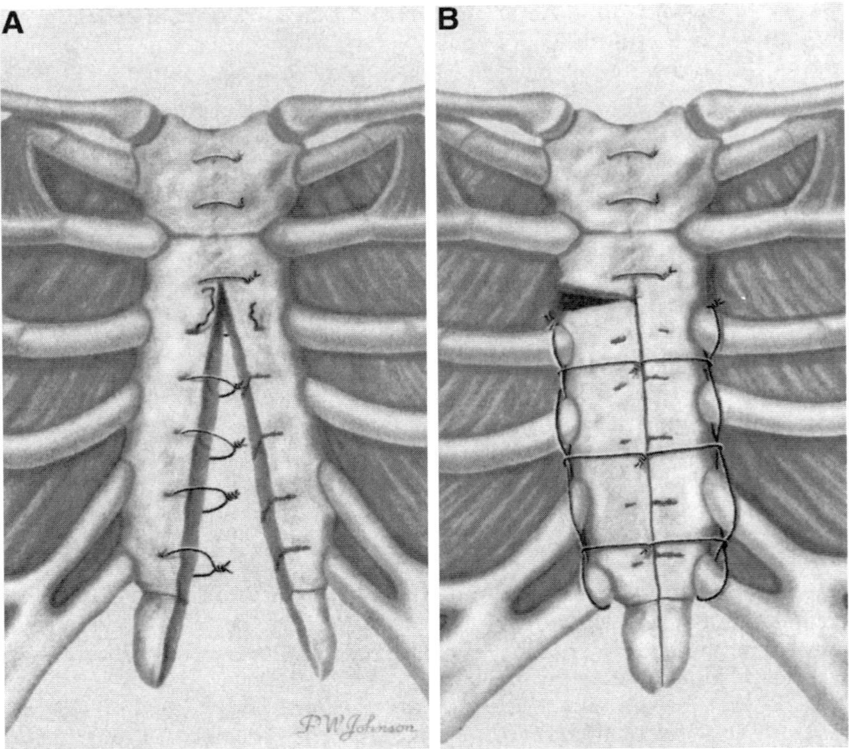

FIGURE 2.—Modified sternum weave applied in partial sternum separation. **A**, before repair. **B**, after repair. (Courtesy of Robicsek F, Cook JW, Rizzoni W: Sternoplasty for incomplete sternum separation. *J Thorac Cardiovasc Surg* 116:361-362, 1998.)

separation along the complete length of the sternum, but some patients have separation of only the lower portion of the sternal body. In the latter cases, the full sternum must sometimes be divided just to reapproximate the lower portion. A modified technique for reapproximation of the separated lower sternum is reported.

> *Technique.*—The lower sternum is exposed, and the pectoralis major muscles detached on both sides. Loose or broken wire sutures are removed, and the separated sternal edges are "freshened" to promote healing. A double row of wire sutures is placed on either side of the separated portion of the sternum, and carried to the upper edge of the separation. The right half of the sternum is mobilized by a transverse cut with an oscillating saw. The halves can now be easily approximated, and united by 3 or 4 transverse wire sutures (Fig 2). The detached pectoralis major muscles are then reattached.

Discussion.—This modified sternoplasty technique can be used in cases of partial postoperative sternal separation. This approach was successful in several patients with chronic, noninfected partial sternum separations. All patients showed good results, with early discharge from the hospital.

▶ These authors present a modification of the well-known Robicsek closure. The modification is likely to be useful not only in partial sternum separation but in prophylactic sternal closure in those patients having a small or particularly weakened sternum.

J.J. Collins, Jr., M.D.

An Experimental Model of Sudden Death Due to Low-Energy Chest-Wall Impact (Commotio Cordis)

Link MS, Wang PJ, Pandian NG, et al (Tufts-New England Med Ctr, Boston; Christ Hosp and Med Ctr, Oak Lawn, Ill; Minneapolis Heart Inst Found)
N Engl J Med 338:1805-1811, 1998   3–10

Introduction.—Commotio cordis, sudden death occurring in a young athlete who is struck in the precordium by a baseball or other object, usually occurs in youngsters aged 5 to 15 years who have no pre-existing heart disease, and it is associated with no structural damage to the chest or heart. The few reported survivors have shown precordial S-T segment elevation. To study the mechanism of commotio cordis, the authors developed an animal model of low-energy impact to the chest. The effects of using softer baseballs were assessed as well.

Methods.—The study used 4- to 8-week-old domesticated pigs weighing 2 to 12 kg. A wooden object the size and shape of a regulation baseball was used to strike the chest at a velocity of 30 mph, timed to the cardiac cycle. Some animals underwent multiple impacts, whereas some underwent single impacts. In a further experiment, the effects of using safety baseballs that were softer than regulation baseballs were examined.

Results.—In the initial experiment, 9 of 10 impacts occurring between 30 and 15 msec before peak T wave on ECG resulted in ventricular fibrillation. This was the only time during the cardiac cycle that ventricular fibrillation was produced. Transient complete heart block occurred with 4 of 10 impacts during the QRS complex. When safety baseballs were used during the T-wave window of vulnerability, the risk of ventricular fibrillation was lower, decreasing in proportion to the softness of the ball used. Only 2 of 26 impacts produced ventricular fibrillation with the softest ball, compared with 8 of 23 impacts with the regulation ball.

Conclusions.—This animal model of low-energy chest impact closely reflects the clinical circumstances of commotio cordis. The occurrence of ventricular fibrillation depends on the timing of the impact during the upstroke of the T wave. Using softer baseballs may reduce the risk of commotio cordis for young athletes. The animal model could be helpful in devising chest-wall protective measures and resuscitative techniques to reduce the risk of death caused by chest-wall impact.

▶ I have rarely selected animal studies for the YEAR BOOK, but this beautiful article presents an outstanding example of careful experimentation that establishes both the cause and the mechanism of a fatal injury in young athletes. The suggestion that safer baseballs may be available for use by children is reasonable. The likelihood is very great that deaths in some hockey players have probably been caused by a similar mechanism.

J.J. Collins, Jr., M.D.

Aortic Valve Surgery

Aortic Valve Replacement With Cryopreserved Aortic Allograft: Ten-Year Experience
Doty JR, Salazar JD, Liddicoat JR, et al (Johns Hopkins Hosp, Baltimore, Md; LDS Hosp, Salt Lake City, Utah)
J Thorac Cardiovasc Surg 115:371-380, 1998   3–11

Introduction.—Replacing the aortic valve with an aortic valve allograft has produced favorable long-term results in hemodynamic performance and freedom from reoperation. Since the initial procedures, operative techniques for aortic valve replacement with an aortic valve allograft have evolved, and include freehand valve replacement with intact noncoronary sinus and aortic root replacement by root inclusion or freestanding root techniques. Midterm studies of aortic valve replacement with cryopreserved aortic valve allografts have previously demonstrated encouraging results. The long-term results of cryopreserved aortic allograft valves in the aortic position were examined.

Methods.—There were 117 patients who had aortic valve replacement with cryopreserved aortic allografts in 1 year. The patients had a mean age of 45.6 and ranged in age from 15 to 83. Four operative techniques involving cryopreserved aortic allografts were used: freehand aortic valve replacement with 120-degree rotation, aortic root enlargement with intact noncoronary sinus, freehand aortic valve replacement with intact non-coronary sinus, and total aortic root replacement. During the operation in 78 patients (66%), echocardiography was used to assess valve function; and after operation, echocardiography was used for assessment in 77 patients (65%). The patients were studied for up to 11 years, with a mean of 4.6 years.

Results.—No significant aortic valve incompetence was seen with intra-operative echocardiography. There were 7 late deaths and 4 operative deaths (3%). At 10 years, freedom from valve-related mortality was 9:3% ± 4.55%. In 98 patients (94%), the New York Heart Association functional status at last follow-up was normal. There was no or trivial aortic valve incompetence seen in 90% of patients on postoperative echocardiography. There was 92% freedom from reoperation for valve-related causes requiring explantation (Fig 2). At 10 years, freedom from throm-

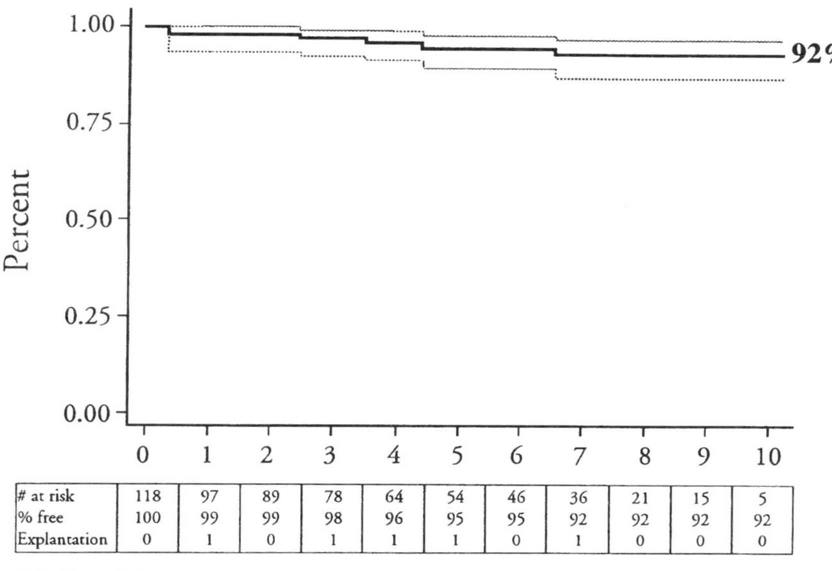

	0	1	2	3	4	5	6	7	8	9	10
# at risk	118	97	89	78	64	54	46	36	21	15	5
% free	100	99	99	98	96	95	95	92	92	92	92
Explantation	0	1	0	1	1	1	0	1	0	0	0

FIGURE 2.—Freedom from valve explantation for any cause at 10 years (Kaplan-Meier methods; 95% confidence interval, 82% to 97%). (Courtesy of Doty JR, Salazar JD, Liddicoat JR, et al: Aortic valve replacement with cryopreserved aortic allograft: Ten-year experience. *J Thorac Cardiovasc Surg* 115: 371-380, 1998.)

boembolism was 100% and freedom from endocarditis was 98% ± 2.47%.

Conclusion.—Low perioperative and long-term mortality can result with aortic valve replacement performed with cryopreserved aortic allografts. Reoperation for valve-related causes is unusual, and most patients have excellent functional status. Excellent freedom from thromboembolism, endocarditis, and progressive valve incompetence was demonstrated by aortic valve replacement with cryopreserved aortic allografts.

▶ These authors report excellent results with the use of cryopreserved aortic allografts. Unfortunately, studying patients for 10 years shows excellent freedom from reoperation for virtually all bioprosthetic valves, not only for the cryopreserved aortic allografts. It is only after 12 years or so that porcine bioprosthetic valves begin to show accelerated deterioration. The important question is whether improved durability will last through the second decade after implantation.

J.J. Collins, Jr., M.D.

Valve Replacement With a Stentless Bioprosthesis: Versatility of the Porcine Aortic Root

Westaby S, Jin XY, Katsumata T, et al (John Radcliffe Hosp, Oxford, England)
J Thorac Cardiovasc Surg 116:477-484, 1998   3–12

Introduction.—Calcific aortic stenosis dominates aortic valve disease in elderly patients. It is important to achieve rapid improvement in ventricular mechanics, functional class, and quality of life for worthwhile event-free survival in this population. Important hemodynamic benefits are conveyed by stentless aortic bioprostheses. The widespread use of stentless xenografts in this age group, however, has been restricted by perceived difficulties of implantation and prolonged myocardial ischemic and cardiopulmonary bypass times. Patients older than 70 received a stentless bioprosthesis in the aortic position.

Methods.—There were 200 patients who had the Freestyle valve implanted by the modified subcoronary method. The patients received a tissue valve in the aortic position and by root replacement. Patients ranged in age from 30 to 86; 43% of patients were older than 75. New York Heart Association class III or IV applied to 142 (70%) of patients. Coronary bypass was performed in 40% of patients. Follow-up continued for 3 years.

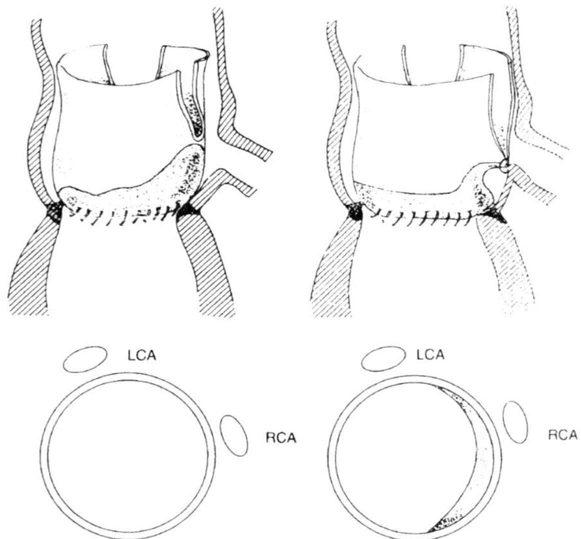

FIGURE 2.—Potential for a technical error, which produces an elevated transvalvular gradient after Freestyle valve implantation. If the distance between the valve anulus and right coronary ostium is less than the height of the inflow cloth beneath the porcine right coronary, the cloth may buckle. This can be avoided by rotating the porcine right coronary sinus to the human noncoronary sinus. *Abbreviations: RCA*, right coronary artery; *LCA*, left coronary artery. (Courtesy of Westaby S, Jin XY, Katsumata T, et al: Valve replacement with a stentless bioprosthesis: Versatility of the porcine aortic root. *J Thorac Cardiovasc Surg* 116:447-484, 1998.)

Results.—For isolated aortic valve replacement, mean ischemic time was 43 ± 6 minutes; and with concomitant procedures, it was 63 ± 14 minutes. There was 6% 30-day mortality, with no deaths related to the valve. Falling valve gradients and increased effective orifice areas were associated with improved hemodynamic function. Over 2 years, left ventricular mass fell within normal limits, but a non–valve-related upswing occurred at 3 years. There were no instances of hemolysis, valve thrombosis, or paravalvular leak. Distortion through bending of the Freestyle inflow could cause obstruction, prosthetic regurgitation, or contact of the xenograft cusp with the Dacron fabric; however, this problem can be avoided with the surgical learning curve (Fig 2).

Conclusion.—Virtually every patient with aortic valve disease is a candidate for the Freestyle valve, which provides superlative hemodynamic outcome. There are similar hospital morbidity and hospital mortality outcomes with the Freestyle valve and with the stented valves in an elderly population.

▶ The Medtronic Freestyle aortic valve bioprosthesis has demonstrated very satisfactory hemodynamic results. This article emphasizes the wide applicability of Freestyle valves and the authors' success, over the short term, with such valves in an elderly population. Even if valve size does not make much difference, the improved hemodynamics of the porcine aortic root should make the surgeon more comfortable.

J.J. Collins, Jr., M.D.

Aortic Valve Operations Under Deep Hypothermic Circulatory Arrest for the Porcelain Aorta: "No-Touch" Technique
Byrne JG, Aranki SF, Cohn LH (Harvard Med School, Boston)
Ann Thorac Surg 65:1313-1315, 1998   3–13

Introduction.—Aortic valve replacement or repair becomes a high-risk procedure in patients who have an ascending aorta that cannot be clamped because of extensive calcification and risk of cerebral embolus or because of extensive adhesions precluding safe dissection and clamping. This problem has been solved with several approaches, including replacement under deep hypothermic circulatory arrest. If accomplished relatively quickly and with minimal manipulation of the aorta, this method is preferred because of its simplicity, and because it minimizes aortic trauma and subsequent risk of cerebral embolus. Three patients had this technique performed.

Methods.—A 51-year-old woman had severe aortic regurgitation and heart failure with subaortic stenosis. A 69-year-old man with 2 previous cardiac operations, triple coronary artery bypass grafting and double coronary artery bypass grafting, had a massive dense adhesion precluding safe dissection of any mediastinal structures and aortic cannulation or clamping. An 84-year-old woman with unstable angina was the third patient, having moderate aortic stenosis that required an intra-aortic balloon pump before her operation.

Results.—Each of the operations for the 3 patients was performed in about 1 hour, with minimal manipulation of the aorta. Aortic trauma was minimized, as was subsequent risk of cerebral embolus. An unremarkable recovery without neurologic complications occurred in each patient. The results could be further improved by routinely using epiaortic and transesophageal echocardiography, by avoiding manipulation of the ascending aorta until the circulation is arrested, by avoiding antegrade cardioplegia, by routinely using retrograde cardioplegia and retrograde cerebral perfusion, when feasible, and by having minimal aortotomy or just enough to remove and replace or repair the valve.

Conclusion.—Aortic valve replacement or repair using the "no-touch" technique and deep hypothermic circulatory arrest is the preferred method when dealing with the porcelain or unclampable aorta.

▶ This article provides a recommendation for the management of aortic valve replacement in patients with severely calcified ascending aorta. There continues to be a significant hazard with these patients, but Dr. Byrne's suggestion that certain changes of technique be made for increased safety is well taken.

J.J. Collins, Jr., M.D.

Operation for Infective Endocarditis: Results After Implantation of Mechanical Valves
Bauernschmitt R, Jakob HG, Vahl C-F, et al (Univ of Heidelberg, Germany)
Ann Thorac Surg 65:359-364, 1998   3–14

Introduction.—Surgery is usually recommended before antibiotic therapy is completed in the treatment of infective endocarditis, resulting in a sick patient who is severely impaired by valve destruction and a systemic infectious process. Surgeons must grapple with the surgical rule not to implant prosthetic material into potentially infected tissue. Patients operated on for infective endocarditis were reviewed to determine factors influencing the perioperative risk and to establish strategies of perioperative management for more favorable outcomes.

Methods.—One hundred thirty-eight patients with infective endocarditis were operated on during 8 years. There was standardization of indication for operation, surgical approach, and postoperative antibiotic therapy during this period. Valve replacement was performed with mechanical prosthesis after radical débridement of all parts of infected tissue.

Results.—There was an overall early mortality of 11.5%. Significant risk factors for early mortality were New York Heart Association functional class, advanced age, and staphylococcal disease. Outcome was not affected by site of infection, multiple valve involvement, or prosthetic valve endocarditis. Early recurrent endocarditis was recorded in only 3 patients.

Complications included postoperative total atrioventricular block that required pacemaker implantation in 11 patients, re-exploration for bleeding in 7 patients, persistent septic symptoms in 6 patients, and transient postoperative psychological disorders in 12 patients.

Conclusion.—If radical operation and aggressive postoperative antibiotic therapy are performed, valve replacement with mechanical prosthesis is a safe procedure in cases of acute infective endocarditis. In patients with rapidly progressive cardiac deterioration or staphylococcal endocarditis, earlier operation will further improve results. The surgical approach may control infection and reduce the incidence of recurrent endocarditis.

▶ This article presents important data documenting that most patients with infected endocarditis do very well with wide débridement and long-term intravenous antibiotics, even when prosthetic valves are used. A great deal of attention has been paid to the use of tissue valves in these patients, and it is important to recognize that excellent results can be achieved with mechanical valves as well as with tissue valves.

J.J. Collins, Jr., M.D.

Aortic and Mitral Valve Replacement With Reconstruction of the Intervalvular Fibrous Body

David TE, Kuo J, Armstrong S (Univ of Toronto)
J Thorac Cardiovasc Surg 114:766-772, 1997   3–15

Introduction.—A fibrous body that extends from the lateral to the medial fibrous trigones connects the aortic and mitral valves. Combined aortic and mitral valve replacement can be difficult when this fibrous body is damaged by previous mitral valve replacement, infective endocarditis, or degenerative calcification. Experience with aortic and mitral valve replacement in patients who had reconstruction of the intervalvular fibrous body is described.

Methods.—Forty-three patients had reconstruction of the intervalvular fibrous body during aortic and mitral valve replacement. There were 25 women and 18 men, with a mean age of 58 ± 12. Fourteen patients had infective endocarditis with abscess; 9 had extensive calcification; 10 had lack of fibrous tissue because of multiple previous operations; and 10 needed to enlarge the aortic and mitral anuli. One or more previous heart valve replacements were performed in 32 patients. New York Heart Association functional classes III and IV included all the patients, and 9 patients were in shock before the operation. Patients were studied from 4 to 108 months, with a mean of 38 months. The operation involves approaching the aortic and mitral valves through the aortic root and the dome of the left atrium. The diseased fibrous body, aortic valve, and mitral valve are excised. To re-establish the aortic and mitral anuli, a patch of Dacron fabric or bovine pericardium is sutured to the lateral and medial fibrous trigones and to the aortic root (Fig 2) To close the left atriotomy

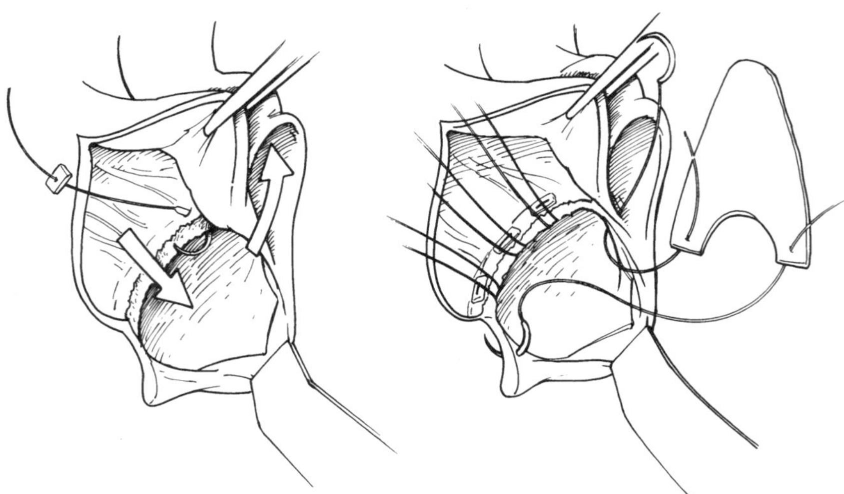

FIGURE 2.—A properly tailored patch is used to reconstruct the intervalvular fibrous body. (Courtesy of David TE, Kuo J, Armstrong S: Aortic and mitral valve replacement with reconstruction of the intervalvular fibrous body. *J Thorac Cardiovasc Surg* 114: 766-772, 1997.)

before implantation of a prosthetic aortic valve, a prosthetic mitral valve is implanted and a separate patch is used (Fig 3). The aortic anulus and patch is secured to the aortic valve prosthesis. The right side of the aortotomy is closed by the patch (Fig 4) (Fig 5).

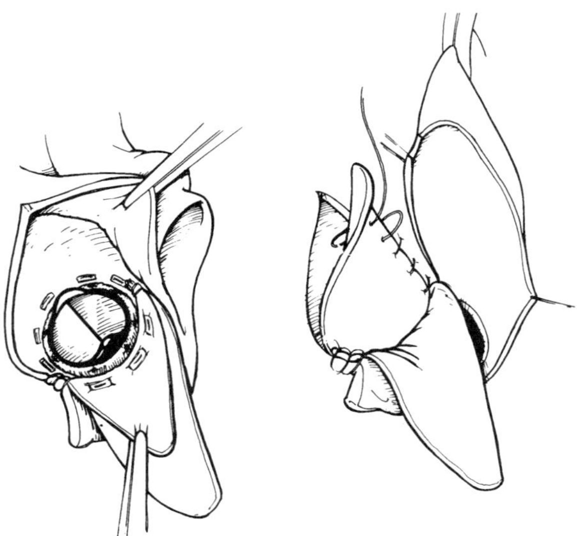

FIGURE 3.—A mitral valve prosthesis is secured to the mitral anulus posteriorly and to the patch superiorly. A separate patch is used to close the left atriotomy. (Courtesy of David TE, Kuo J, Armstrong S: Aortic and mitral valve replacement with reconstruction of the intervalvular fibrous body. *J Thorac Cardiovasc Surg* 114: 766-772, 1997.)

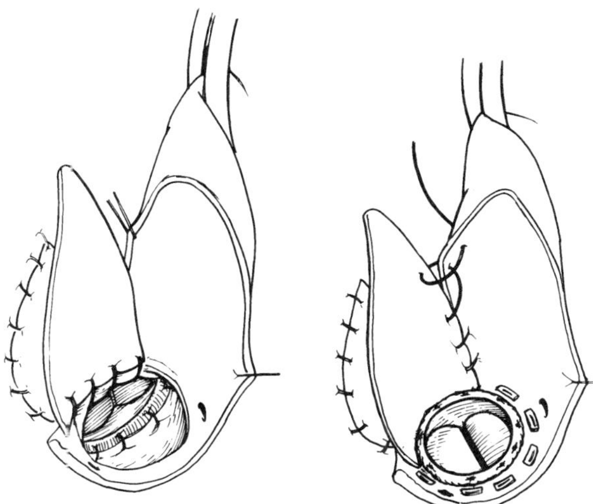

FIGURE 4.—An aortic valve prosthesis is secured to the aortic anulus and patch. The patch is used to close the right side of the aortotomy. (Courtesy of David TE, Kuo J, Armstrong S: Aortic and mitral valve replacement with reconstruction of the intervalvular fibrous body. *J Thorac Cardiovasc Surg* 114: 766-772, 1997.)

Results.—Seven operative deaths (16%) occurred. Two patients had early prosthetic valve endocarditis and needed reoperation. There were 6 late deaths. At 6 years, the actuarial survival was 56% ± 6%. Normal prosthetic valve function and anatomically intact anuli were found with Doppler echocardiograph in all 30 long-term survivors.

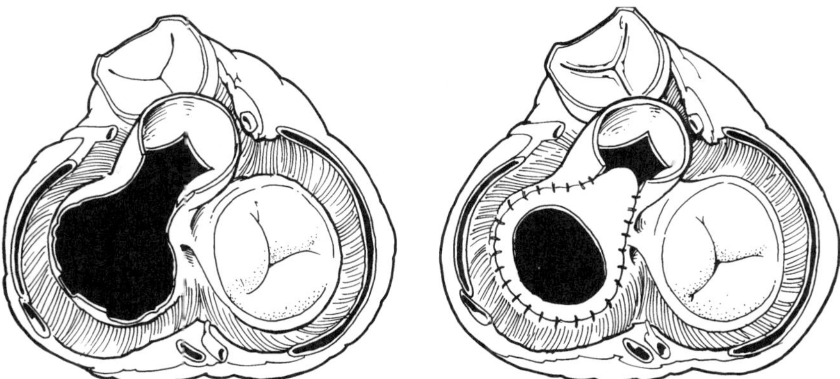

FIGURE 5.—Technique used to reconstruct the entire mitral anulus and the intervalvular fibrous body. (Courtesy of David TE, Kuo J, Armstrong S: Aortic and mitral valve replacement with reconstruction of the intervalvular fibrous body. *J Thorac Cardiovasc Surg* 114: 766-772, 1997.)

Conclusion.—In patients with complex valve anular pathology, reconstruction of the intervalvular fibrous body during aortic and mitral valve replacement is a satisfactory operative approach.

▶ This technique is really a radical undertaking. There certainly are patients with infective endocarditis who require wide débridement that can be accomplished only if an operation similar to this one is in the surgeon's toolbox. Dr. David is to be congratulated for his remarkable results with difficult patients such as these.

J.J. Collins, Jr., M.D.

Pregnancy in Patients With Pulmonary Autograft Valve Replacement

Dore A, Somerville J (Royal Brompton Hosp, London; Natl Heart and Lung Inst, London)
Eur Heart J 18:1659-1662, 1997   3–16

Background.—The ideal heart valve replacement for aortic valve disease in women of childbearing age is controversial. The pulmonary autograft operation is associated with low operative mortality, low incidence of late valve dysfunction, low risk of thromboembolism, and an absence of anticoagulants.

Methods.—The medical records of female patients who had pulmonary autograft valve replacement were reviewed.

Results.—From 1968 to 1993, 8 of 21 female survivors had 14 pregnancies. No patient received anticoagulants. There were no maternal deaths, thromboembolic or hemorrhagic events, or deterioration in valve function. One patient had dilated cardiomyopathy without aortic or pulmonary valve disease 6 months after delivery, but all others remained in Ability Index 1 after pregnancy. No significant progression of aortic regurgitation, pulmonary regurgitation, or right-sided obstruction occurred. In 2 patients, reoperation for right-sided obstruction was done 4 and 7 years after a second pregnancy.

Discussion.—In these patients, there were no valve-related complications during pregnancy, which did not seem to affect the function of the pulmonary valve autograft or right-sided homograft. The pulmonary autograft is an ideal procedure for young women who need aortic valve replacement.

▶ Early failure of porcine bioprostheses during or after pregnancy has been a poorly understood but readily recognized phenomenon for some time. This follow-up study in patients after pulmonary autograft transfer to the aortic position documents that these patients have done very well, and it is useful to know that no disadvantage from pregnancy was recognized in this small group.

J.J. Collins, Jr., M.D.

Thoracic Aortic Aneurysm

Composite Valve Graft Versus Separate Aortic Valve and Ascending Aortic Replacement: Is There Still a Role for the Separate Procedure?
Yun KL, Miller DC, Fann JI, et al (Stanford Univ, Calif)
Circulation 96[suppl II]:II-368-II-375, 1997   3–17

Introduction.—The surgical approach to aneurysm or dissection of the ascending aorta associated with aortic valve disease includes either conventional aortic valve replacement plus separate replacement of the ascending aorta or total replacement of the aortic root with a composite valve conduit. The rate of reoperation is not clearly defined. The survival rates and long-term results in a large number of patients who underwent either a composite valve graft (CVG) or separate graft and valve (GV) were assessed over 30 years to determine whether operative technique has any bearing on outcome.

Methods.—Medical records of 390 consecutive nonrandomized patients treated for aortic valve disease and ascending aortic aneurysm or type A dissection (278 and 112 patients, respectively) were reviewed. Of these patients, 135 underwent CVG and 255 had separate GV replacement. During surgery, 49 patients required profound hypothermic circulatory arrest. In earlier years, myocardial protection was accomplished using continuous topical 4°C saline with or without antegrade crystalloid cardioplegia.

Results.—Mean patient age was 52 years. Total patient-years of follow-up were 2,247 and extended to 27 years. Operative mortality rate was 10% and 15% for patients who underwent CVG and GV replacement, respectively (Fig 1). The 15-year actuarial survival estimate was higher for the CVG than GV group (53% vs. 36%). Reoperation on the aortic valve or ascending aorta was needed by 7 patients in the CVG group and 49 patients in the GV group. The probability of freedom from reoperation on the aortic root was 82% and 75% at 10 years, respectively, for patients in the CVG and GV groups. A multivariate model analyzed 30 variables. Pulmonary disease, higher New York Heart Association functional class, and longer cardiopulmonary bypass time were related to higher operative mortality risk. Older age, emergency operation, coronary artery disease, and liver dysfunction were independent predictors of late death. Younger age and use of a bioprosthesis were predictive of late reoperation. The type of surgical approach was not a significant determinant of any outcome variable.

Conclusion.—Long-term results after CVG and after GV did not differ, which indicated proper patient selection. The CVG theoretically offers more protection against recurrent aortic root aneurysm and is most appropriate in younger patients, patients with Marfan syndrome, and patients with marked pathological involvement of the sinuses. Use of GV also provides satisfactory results in carefully selected patients.

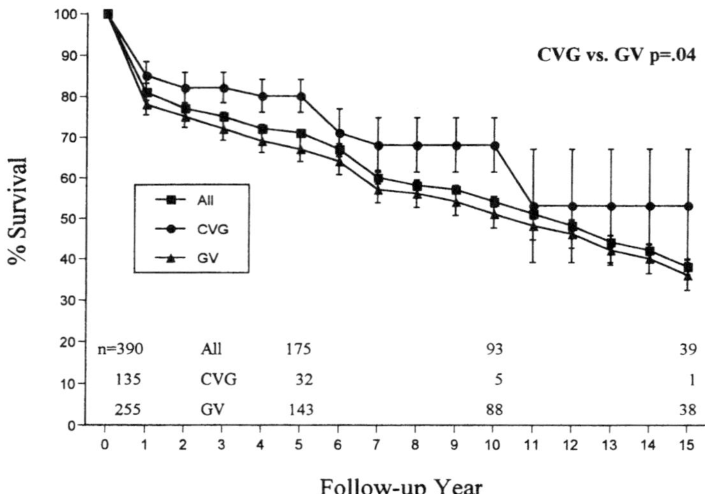

FIGURE 1.—Overall actuarial survival estimates for all patients, according to type of initial operative repair. (Courtesy of Yun KL, Miller DC, Fann JI, et al: Composite valve graft versus separate aortic valve and ascending aortic replacement: Is there still a role for the separate procedure? *Circulation* 96[suppl II]: II-368-II-375, 1997.)

▶ This article from Stanford confirms the authors' excellent results in dealing with the difficult problem of ascending aortic replacement with or without valved conduits. Carefully selected patients (those with a normal-sized aortic annulus) will do well with reconstructive surgery involving a separate aortic valve and ascending aortic graft.

J.J. Collins, Jr., M.D.

Replacing the Atherosclerotic Ascending Aorta Is a High-Risk Procedure

King RC, Kanithanon RC, Shockey KS, et al (Univ of Virginia, Charlottesville)
Ann Thorac Surg 66:396-401, 1998   3–18

Introduction.—New surgical techniques have been developed to minimize the risk of stroke in patients undergoing replacement of the chronically aneurysmal ascending thoracic aorta. Routine replacement of the severely atherosclerotic ascending thoracic aorta at the time of coronary artery bypass grafting (CABG) was assessed in 17 patients to determine whether hypothermic arrest and appropriate retrograde cerebral perfusion would significantly diminish the atherosclerotic morbidity and mortality rates associated with this patient population.

Methods.—Operative times for these patients were compared with those of a control group of 89 consecutive patients who underwent replacement of the ascending thoracic aorta for an ascending thoracic aortic aneurysm.

Results.—Hospital mortality was 23.5% (4 of 17) for patients undergoing replacement of the ascending thoracic aorta for severe atherosclerosis, compared to 2.25% (2 of 89) for patients in the control group. Deaths of 2 patients in the atherosclerotic group were caused by episodes of bleeding associated with coagulopathy and subsequent multisystem organ failure. The incidence of cerebrovascular accident was 17.6% (3 of 17) and 3.37% (3 of 89) for the atherosclerotic and control groups, respectively. Nine patients (52.9%) in the atherosclerotic group had operative morbidity. Control group patients had a nonfatal postoperative complication rate of 20.2% (18 patients).

Conclusion.—The severely atherosclerotic ascending aorta may be considered a marker of diffuse atherosclerosis. Patient outcome in this series is not as encouraging as in earlier series. The use of preoperative screening of the ascending aorta by chest CT may be appropriate in evaluating high-risk patients for potential surgery.

▶ The hazard of dealing with the atherosclerotic ascending aorta is emphasized by King and his associates from the University of Virginia. On the other hand, as they also point out, safety can probably be significantly improved by the use of hypothermic circulatoric arrest and retrograde cerebral perfusion.

J.J. Collins, Jr., M.D.

Experience With Antegrade Bihemispheric Cerebral Perfusion in Aortic Arch Operations

Veeragandham RS, Hamilton IN Jr, O'Connor C, et al (Rush Med College and Rush-Presbyterian-St Luke's Med Ctr, Chicago)
Ann Thorac Surg 66:493-499, 1998   3–19

Introduction.—Several techniques have been used for cerebral protection in aortic arch surgeries. Antegrade bihemispheric cerebral perfusion lost its first-line position to hypothermic circulatory arrest, which raises the problems of coagulopathy, time constraints, and prolongation of cardiopulmonary bypass time. Reported are clinical course, operative techniques, and results in a series of patients who underwent antegrade bihemispheric cerebral perfusion during aortic arch reconstruction over 10 years.

Methods.—Twenty consecutive patients with aortic arch disease underwent antegrade bihemispheric cerebral perfusion with moderate hypothermia. Of 20 patients, 12, 7, and 1, respectively, were treated for aneurysm, dissection, and traumatic tear. Five patients had undergone previous sternotomy for ascending aortic replacement. All patients underwent arch reconstruction; 7, 2, and 3 patients, respectively, also underwent aortic valve replacement or repair, Bentall procedure, and selective innominate reconstruction. Mean cerebral perfusion time was 51 minutes; 7 patients had cerebral perfusion times of 60 to 120 minutes.

Results.—In-hospital mortality and 30-day mortality were both 0%. Blood product requirements were significantly lower with moderate hypothermia. One patient (5%) had a cerebrovascular accident. There were no neurologic deficits in any of the 7 patients who had cerebral perfusion times of 60 to 120 minutes. These findings are superior to those reported for hypothermic circulatory arrest with or without retrograde perfusion.

Conclusion.—Antegrade bihemispheric cerebral perfusion with moderate hypothermia provides cerebral protection for patients undergoing aortic arch reconstruction. This approach significantly limits the need for blood products, extends the safe interruption of native brachiocephalic blood flow, and eliminates ischemic multiorgan injuries.

▶ This experience with antegrade bihemispheric cerebral perfusion, reported in this article by Veeragandham and associates, is a reminder that the older technique of antegrade cerebral perfusion still works pretty well for most patients. Retrograde cerebral perfusion is often easier and probably should be considered the procedure of choice for most patients who require cerebral protection in extensive aortic arch operations.

J.J. Collins, Jr., M.D.

Mitral Valve Surgery

Optimizing Mitral Valve Exposure With Conventional Left Atriotomy
McCarthy JF, Cosgrove DM III (Cleveland Clinic Found, Ohio)
Ann Thorac Surg 65:1161-1162, 1998   3–20

Purpose.—The mitral valve is most often approached through a longitudinal incision in the left atrium. However, this approach can result in poor valve exposure in certain situations. The authors report a method of obtaining better exposure of the mitral valve via left atriotomy.

Technique.—To provide maximal exposure, the heart is elevated out of the chest and rotated. As the apex is allowed to drop posteriorly, the right side of the heart is elevated, enhancing visualization of the valve and subvalvular structures. The pericardium to the right of midline is opened and sutured to the chest wall. After bypass and cardioplegia are initiated, any adhesions of the left side of the heart are separated, allowing the apex to rotate in a posterior direction. Mobility of the superior vena cava and right atrium are enhanced by incising the pericardium anterior to the superior vena cava. Greater elevation of the right side of the heart is achieved by placing a tourniquet around the inferior vena cava and applying traction (Fig 2).

A left atrial incision of adequate size is made at the junction with the right superior pulmonary vein. A self-retaining retractor is attached to the left side of the chest spreader, providing consistent exposure and reducing the need for assistance. One of 3 blades is placed at the cephalad extreme of the atriotomy, while the second exerts traction at the foot and the third is placed between them. Rotating the table away from the surgeon and elevating it provide

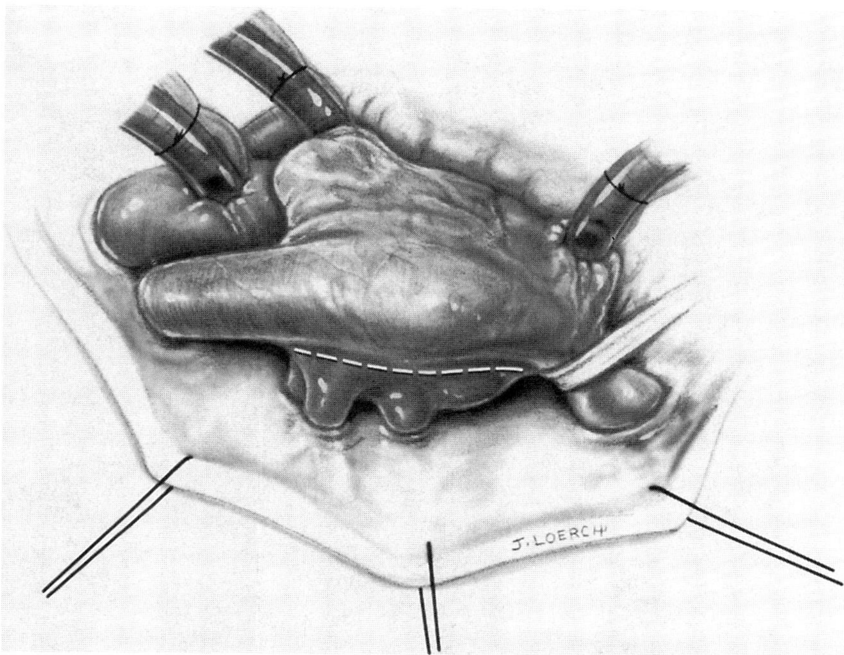

FIGURE 2.—A tourniquet is placed around the inferior vena cava, which is retracted inferiorly. This further elevates the right side of the heart. (Reprinted with permission from the Society of Thoracic Surgeons from McCarthy JF, Cosgrove DM III: Optimizing mitral valve exposure with conventional left atriotomy. *Ann Thorac Surg* 65:1161-1162, 1998.)

direct visualization (Fig 3). Additional maneuvers to enhance access to all aspects of the mitral valve are described.

Discussion.—Excellent and consistent visualization is the key to successful mitral valve surgery. The authors' technique of optimizing exposure facilitates all mitral valve procedures. With this technique, alternate approaches to the mitral valve are rarely needed.

▶ This article outlines Dr. Cosgrove's technique for improving visibility of the mitral valve, particularly when the left atrium is relatively small. This is an important description. Visualization of the mitral valve in patients with a small left atrium can be extremely difficult and all the tricks of the trade should be welcome, even to the experienced surgeon.

J.J. Collins, Jr., M.D.

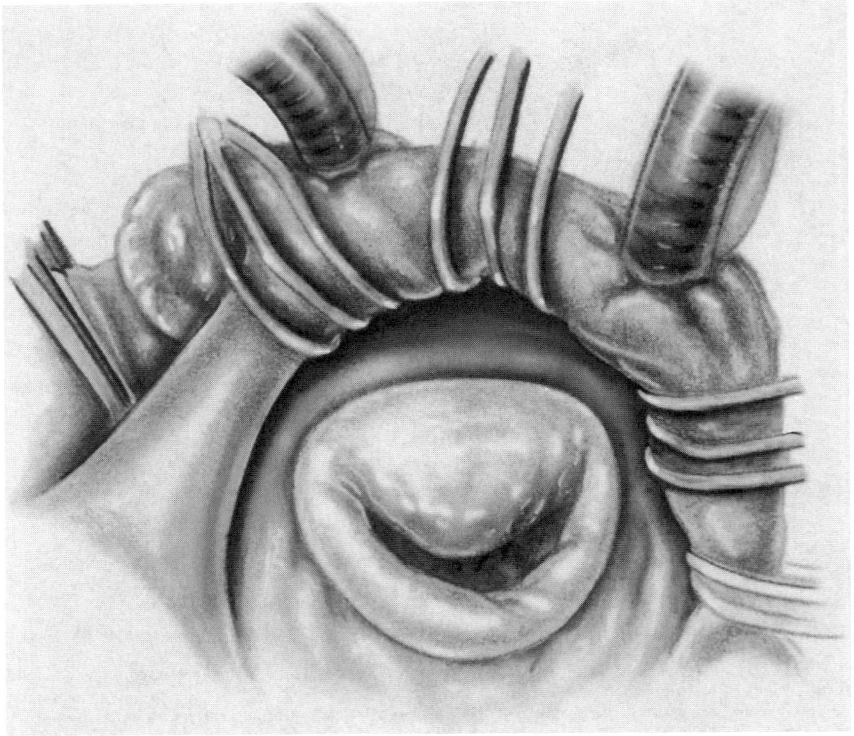

FIGURE 3.—The self-retaining retractor allows consistent and excellent exposure of the mitral valve. (Reprinted with permission from the Society of Thoracic Surgeons from McCarthy JF, Cosgrove DM III: Optimizing mitral valve exposure with conventional left atriotomy. *Ann Thorac Surg* 65:1161-1162, 1998.)

Video-Assisted Minimally Invasive Mitral Valve Surgery

Chitwood WR Jr, Wixon CL, Elbeery JR, et al (East Carolina Univ, Greenville, NC)

J Thorac Cardiovasc Surg 114:773-782, 1997   3–21

Background.—Several reports have described the use and potential benefits of minimally invasive cardiac surgery, including coronary grafting. Minimally invasive valve surgery may be even more promising, because it does not require complex vascular anastomoses. An experience with minimally invasive mitral valve surgery, performed with intraoperative video assistance, is reported.

Methods.—Over 10 months, the investigators used minithoracotomy with video assistance to perform mitral valve surgery in 31 consecutive patients, with a mean age of 59 (Fig 2). Mitral valve repair was performed in 20 patients and valve replacement in 11; the patients' ejection fractions ranged from 35% to 62%. The procedures were performed with the use of

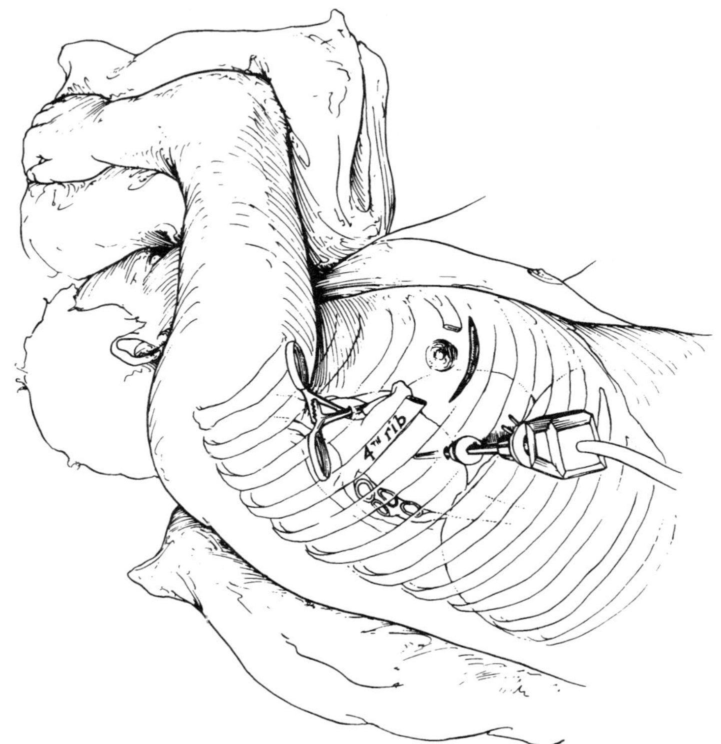

FIGURE 2.—A segment of the fourth rib anteriorly is removed. The transthoracic crossclamp is passed through the third intercostal space, in front of the superior vena cava, and through the transverse sinus to occlude the ascending aorta just caudal to the right pulmonary artery. Antegrade cardioplegia and aortic venting is provided by a videoscopically placed needle in the ascending aorta. The 5-mm telescope and thoracoscopic camera are inserted through a port in the fourth intercostal space. The camera port intercostal space is not selected until the superior pulmonary vein is identified. (Courtesy of Chitwood WR Jr, Wixon CL, Elbeery JR, et al: Video-assisted minimally invasive mitral valve surgery. *J Thorac Cardiovasc Surg* 114:773-782, 1997.)

antegrade/retrograde cold blood cardioplegia in 10 patients and antegrade cardioplegia in 19. The remaining 2 procedures were performed with a new transthoracic crossclamp or with ventricular fibrillation (Fig 3). Peripheral arterial cannulation was used in 28 patients and pump-assisted right atrial drainage in 26.

Results.—In-hospital mortality was zero, though 30-day mortality was 3%. There was 1 case of deep venous thrombosis and 1 of phrenic nerve palsy. There were no strokes, and no reoperations for bleeding. All patients but 1 had excellent valve function on postoperative echocardiography. Average cardiopulmonary bypass time was 183 minutes, and average cardiopulmonary arrest time 136 minutes. Mean hospitalization time was 5.1 days, compared with 8.6 days in a group of 100 patients undergoing conventional mitral valve surgery. In the latter part of the experience, most patients were discharged after 3 to 5 days. Minimally invasive surgery was

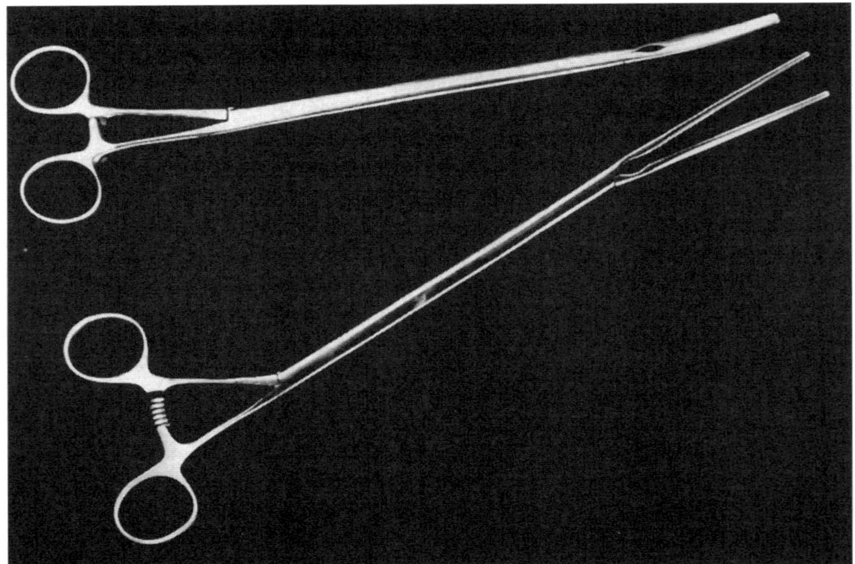

FIGURE 3.—The transthoracic crossclamp is shown in 2 pincer-tip lengths. The clamp mechanism works entirely within the thorax (Scanlan International, Minneapolis, Minn). (Courtesy of Chitwood WR Jr, Wixon CL, Elbeery JR, et al: Video-assisted minimally invasive mitral valve surgery. *J Thorac Cardiovasc Surg* 114:773-782, 1997.)

associated with a 27% reduction in hospital charges and a 34% reduction in hospital costs. The patients had minimal perioperative pain and quick recovery.

Conclusions.—The authors report good initial results with minimally invasive, video-assisted mitral valve surgery. This approach may reduce morbidity, shorten hospital stay, and reduce costs. Video assistance is always helpful in this application, and sometimes essential for achieving instrument access to intracardiac sites.

▶ Dr. Chitwood has written a very useful article about 31 patients who underwent operations of repair or replacement of the mitral valve using minimally invasive video-assisted techniques. The results certainly suggest that minimally invasive operations can be safely performed, and I'm sure the ease with which these operations can be accomplished will continue to increase.

J.J. Collins, Jr., M.D.

Robot-Assisted Minimally Invasive Solo Mitral Valve Operation

Falk V, Walther T, Autschbach R, et al (Univ of Leipzig, Germany)
J Thorac Cardiovasc Surg 115:470-471, 1998

3–22

Introduction.—Experience with minimally invasive mitral valve surgery is growing and points the way toward solo mitral valve operations. The authors report initial experience with minimally invasive solo mitral valve surgery, performed under videoscopic guidance provided by a voice-controlled robotic device.

Methods.—The investigators performed videoscopically guided mitral valve surgery in 8 consecutive patients with nonischemic mitral valve disease. The 3-dimensional videoscope was placed through a 10-mm port in the second right intercostal space and connected to the AESOP 2000 robotic arm (Fig 1). The robot was voice activated by the surgeon, who controlled its motion with 1- or 2-word commands.

Results.—All procedures were successfully completed without complications. The robot provided videoscopic guidance without the need for assistants other than a scrub nurse. The videoscopic picture was excellent

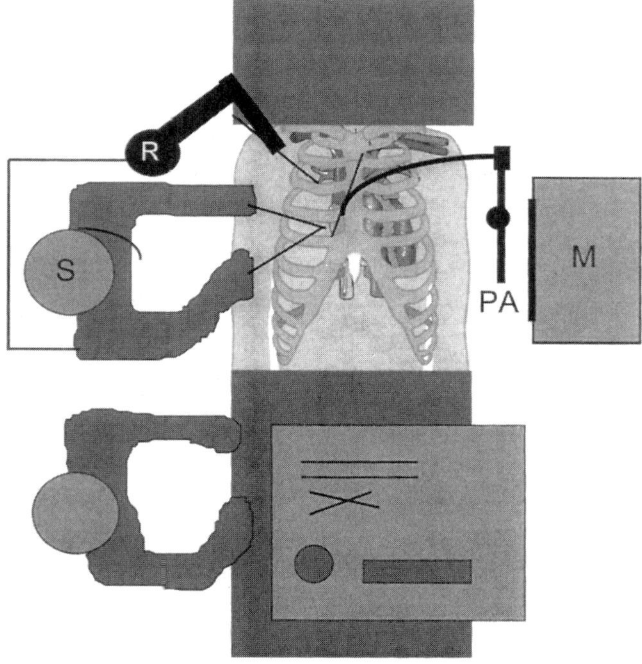

FIGURE 1.—Operative setting in minimally invasive solo mitral valve operation. The robotic arm (*R*) that holds the 3-dimensional videoscope is fixed at the operating table left of the surgeon (*S*) and operated by voice control. The left atrial retractor is fixed by a passive articulating arm that is mounted to the operating table opposite the surgeon. *Abbreviation: M,* video monitor. (Courtesy of Falk V, Walther T, Autschbach R, et al: Robot-assisted minimally invasive solo mitral valve operation. *J Thorac Cardiovasc Surg* 115:470-471, 1998.)

and steady. The robotic movements were smoother and more precise than possible with manually guided videoscopic assistance, producing superior exposure of all valvular and subvalvular structures. The robot was capable of memorizing positions and returning to them automatically. Using voice control, the surgeon could continue to operate without stopping to adjust the videoscope. Lens cleaning was rarely necessary, which led to reduced operating times. There were no technical complications.

Conclusions.—The authors report good initial experience with a robotic assistant to provide videoscopic guidance for minimally invasive mitral valve surgery. This technology opens the way to performance of solo cardiac surgery. Robotic guidance offers several potentially important advantages, but may raise the overall cost of the procedure.

▶ This article seems to speak to us from the next millennium. Even the illustration is a bit surreal. However, the message is quite clear.

J.J. Collins, Jr., M.D.

Mitral Valve Replacement: Randomized Trial of St Jude and Medtronic Hall Prostheses

Fiore AC, Barner HB, Swartz MT, et al (Saint Louis Univ)
Ann Thorac Surg 66:707-713, 1998

3–23

Background.—All the available heart valve prostheses have their own associated complications. Two commonly used devices—the bileaflet St. Jude and the tilting-disk Medtronic Hall prostheses—have attractive properties. A prospective, randomized trial was performed to compare the hemodynamic properties of these 2 heart valve prostheses.

Methods.—The study included 156 patients undergoing elective mitral valve replacement who were randomized to receive either the Medtronic Hall or the St. Jude replacement. The 2 groups were compared in terms of preoperative New York Heart Association class, left ventricular ejection fraction, incidence of mitral stenosis or mitral insufficiency, extent of coronary artery disease, completeness of revascularization, and cross-clamp or bypass time. Outcomes were assessed at a mean follow-up of about 5 years.

Results.—There were no significant differences in operative or late mortality. Operative mortality was 11% with the St. Jude valve vs. 13% with the Medtronic Hall valve; late mortality was 27% vs. 22%, respectively. Ten-year actuarial survival and freedom from valve-related events were also similar. Patients receiving the St. Jude valve did have a higher probability of freedom from reoperation. At follow-up, the 2 groups were similar in terms of patient functional status and echocardiographic hemodynamic parameters.

Conclusions.—This randomized trial finds no significant difference in the outcomes of patients receiving the St. Jude prosthesis and patients receiving the Medtronic Hall prosthesis. The late clinical and hemodynamic results are similar, providing no rationale to prefer 1 device over the other. The choice depends on the surgeon's experience and preference, which may be affected by factors such as ease of insertion, availability, and cost.

► This article should lay to rest any argument that there is a significant advantage in either the St. Jude or the Medtronic Hall prosthesis for mitral valve replacement. I think the design of the Medtronic Hall strut system makes the possibility of entanglement in the chordae greater but careful placement of the Medtronic Hall valves seems to obviate that disadvantage.

J.J. Collins, Jr., M.D.

Homograft Replacement of Mitral Valve in Children

Plunkett MD, Schneider DJ, Shah JJ, et al (Univ of Illinois, Peoria)
Ann Thorac Surg 66:849-852, 1998   3–24

Introduction.—Good results with cryopreserved mitral valve homografts have recently been seen in adult patients. These reports conclude that mitral valve homografts can significantly improve the limitations of mitral valve repair in selected adult patients. The results of homograft mitral valve replacement in 4 children with various valve complications are reported.

Methods.—Over 1 year, the investigators performed mitral valve replacement using cryopreserved mitral valve homografts in 4 pediatric patients. The children ranged in age from 5 to 15 years; 2 children had previous atrioventricular septal defects, 1 child with a history of previous prosthetic valve placement; and 2 children had rheumatic valvular disease. All patients had moderately severe to severe mitral valve regurgitation and/or stenosis, confirmed by preoperative echocardiography.

Results.—Homograft mitral valve replacements were successfully placed in all patients. At 10 months postoperatively, Doppler transesophageal and transthoracic echocardiograms showed reduced mitral regurgitation, with sharp decreases in pulmonary artery pressures. The valves were functioning well with normal hemodynamics, although all patients had mild residual gradients across the valves.

Conclusions.—Good initial results in homograft mitral valve replacement were seen in selected children. However, there is concern about the limited growth potential of the homografts and about the possibility of graft fibrosis and calcification over time. Long-term follow-up studies are needed to demonstrate the durability and function of mitral valve homografts in children.

► The research presented in this article should be followed with great interest. I cannot help but be concerned that the durability of these homograft valves will be limited. Avoidance of thrombosis and absence of the need for anticoagulation are certainly strong arguments for these valves, presuming they prove satisfactory over the medium or long term.

J.J. Collins, Jr., M.D.

Intermediate-term Outcome of Mitral Reconstruction in Cardiomyopathy

Bolling SF, Pagani FD, Deeb GM, et al (Univ of Michigan, Ann Arbor)
J Thorac Cardiovasc Surg 115:381-389, 1998   3–25

Introduction.—Heart transplantation is standard treatment for patients with severe congestive heart failure associated with end-stage heart disease. With the donor shortage, waiting times have increased and new strategies to manage end-stage heart disease are being sought. Mitral regurgitation is a significant complication of end-stage cardiomyopathy, and results from dilation of the annular-ventricular apparatus, altered ventricular geometry, or papillary muscle dysfunction. The intermediate outcome of mitral reconstruction in patients with dilated cardiomyopathy was assessed.

Methods.—Forty-eight patients who had cardiomyopathy with severe mitral regurgitation had mitral reconstruction in 4 years. The patients ranged in age from 33 to 79 and had left ventricular ejection fractions that ranged from 8% to 25%. Maximal drug therapy was being given to all patients who had New York Heart Association class III or IV with severe, refractory 4+ mitral regurgitation. Undersized flexible annuloplasty rings were inserted in all patients, coronary bypass grafts for incidental disease were performed for 7 patients, prior bypass grafts were performed for 11 patients, and tricuspid valve repair were performed in 11 patients.

Results.—Right ventricular failure caused 1 operative death. Seven patients had mild mitral regurgitation, according to postoperative transesophageal echocardiography, whereas 41 had no mitral regurgitation. Late deaths occurred in 10 patients at 2 to 47 months after mitral reconstruction. There was 82% survival at 1 year and 71% survival at 2 years. The number of hospitalizations for heart failure decreased at a mean follow-up of 22 months, with 1 patient having had a heart transplantation. Before the operation, the New York Heart Association class improved from 3.9 ± 0.3; after the operation, it improved to 2.0 ± 0.6. Left ventricular volume and sphericity decreased at 24 months after the operation, whereas ejection fraction and cardiac output increased.

Conclusion.—Whether this favorable modification of left ventricular function and geometry will persist is not known. New strategies for patients who have cardiomyopathy with mitral regurgitation are possible with mitral repair.

▶ This group of patients operated upon and studied by Dr. Bolling and his group show more improvement of left ventricular function then many of us would expect in patients with cardiomyopathy. If these results persist for a few more years, I think the point that repair of mitral regurgitation should be performed early in many patients with cardiomyopathy will have been made.

J.J. Collins, Jr., M.D.

Surgical Management of Mitral Regurgitation Associated With Marfan's Syndrome
Fuzellier J-FG, Chauvaud SM, Fornes P, et al (Broussais Hosp, Paris)
Ann Thorac Surg 66:68-72, 1998   3–26

Objective.—Eighty percent of patients with Marfan's syndrome have mitral valve dysfunction, the most frequent cause of morbidity and mortality in these infants. There is debate over the optimal surgical approach to this problem, particularly about whether the underlying connective tissue defect compromises the durability of mitral valve repair. The middle-term outcomes of surgery for mitral regurgitation in patients with Marfan's syndrome were assessed.

Methods.—Over 10 years, mitral valve surgery was performed in 30 patients with Marfan's syndrome. The patients were 18 females and 15 males, with a mean age of 30. Thirty patients had leaflet prolapse; other causes of mitral regurgitation were annulus dilation in 2 patients and restricted leaflet motion in 1. Mitral valve replacement was performed in 1 patient, and the other patients had mitral valve repair. Surgery was performed using standard hypothermic bypass with cold-blood cardioplegia. At surgery, 73% of patients were found to have chordal elongation. Twenty-four percent of these patients had chordal rupture of the posterior leaflet, 18% had chordal rupture of the anterior leaflet, 6% congenital malformation, and 24% annulus calcification. Mitral valve repair was most commonly carried out using Carpentier's techniques.

Results.—There were 2 perioperative deaths; the survivors were studied for a mean of 39 months. Three patients died in the late postoperative period, 2 because of aortic complications. Ten-year actuarial survival was 79%, with a freedom from mitral valve reoperation of 87%. Echocardiographic follow-up revealed absence of mild mitral regurgitation in 21 of 24 patients, and moderate regurgitation in the remaining 3.

Conclusions.—The results of mitral valve repair in patients with Marfan's syndrome are comparable to outcomes achieved in patients with other forms of degenerative mitral valve disease, with similar high rates of survival and freedom from reoperation. Valve repair can be successful in almost all patients, even when annulus calcification is present. The underlying connective tissue disorder of Marfan's syndrome does not appear to compromise the durability of mitral valve repair.

▶ This article by Fuzellier and associates presents results of mitral valve repair, which continue to indicate that mitral valve repair, even in patients with Marfan's syndrome, is safe and reasonably durable.

J.J. Collins, Jr., M.D.

Long-term Results of Mitral Valve Repair for Myxomatous Disease With and Without Chordal Replacement With Expanded Polytetrafluoroethylene Sutures

David TE, Omran A, Armstrong S, et al (Univ of Toronto)
J Thorac Cardiovasc Surg 115:1279-1286, 1998
3–27

Introduction.—Myxomatous disease is the most common cause of mitral regurgitation requiring surgical correction. Compared with mitral valve replacement, mitral valve repair has low operative mortality and beneficial effects on left ventricular function in patients with myxomatous mitral valve disease. The availability of expanded polytetrafluoroethylene (ePFTE) sutures for replacement of chordae tendineae has further increased the use of mitral valve repair. The long-term results of mitral valve repair—with and without chordal replacement with ePTFE sutures—are reported.

Methods.—From 1981 to 1995, 1 of the authors performed mitral valve repair in 324 patients who had mitral regurgitation caused by myxomatous disease. There were 241 men and 83 women, with a mean age of 58 years. Beginning in 1985, ePTFE sutures were used for chordal replacement in 165 patients. These patients were more likely to have prolapse of the anterior leaflet or of both leaflets, whereas patients not undergoing chordal replacement were more likely to have prolapse of the posterior leaflet. Annual follow-up included Doppler echocardiography. The patients were studied for a mean of 36 months.

Results.—There were 2 operative deaths and 21 late deaths; of the latter, 14 were of cardiac causes. Ten-year actuarial survival was 75%, freedom from stroke was 94%, freedom from transient ischemic attack 92%, freedom from endocarditis 99%, freedom from mitral valve operation 96%, and freedom from mitral regurgitation 93%. Outcomes were similar with and without chordal replacement.

Conclusions.—For patients with mitral regurgitation caused by myxomatous disease, mitral valve repair is highly successful. The rate of valve-related complications is low. Late outcomes are not affected by the use of ePTFE for chordal replacement. However, chordal replacement may increase the probability of successful repair. The reoperation rate is elevated for patients with advanced myxomatous disease of both leaflets.

▶ This article confirms the excellent results that this group of authors have seen with mitral valve repair. In particular, the results with chordal replacement are remarkably good, without evidence of substantial disadvantage at up to 10 years.

J.J. Collins, Jr., M.D.

Coronary Artery Surgery

Ulnar Artery as a Coronary Bypass Graft
Buxton BF, Chan AT, Dixit AS, et al (Univ of Melbourne, Australia)
Ann Thorac Surg 65:1020-1024, 1998   3–28

Background.—The ulnar artery (UA) has received relatively little attention as an alternative to the radial artery for coronary artery bypass grafting. This article describes the anatomy and use of the UA.

> *Technique.*—The incision starts 3 cm above the wrist and runs along the lateral border of the tendon flexor carpi ulnaris. Near the midpoint of the forearm, the incision curves anteriorly and stops 3 cm below the elbow. The UA is removed by initiating distal dissection. In the distal region of the forearm, the vascular pedicle containing the UA is close to the ulnar nerve. The upper end of the UA is dissected to the level of the median nerve and common interosseus artery. When a sufficient length is obtained, the UA is clipped, transected, and stored.

Results.—One UA was removed from each of 10 male patients, in whom removal of the radial artery was considered unsafe. In 2 patients the UA could not be used. In the remaining 8 patients, the UA was used for bypass grafting. There was no evidence of neurological dysfunction or hand ischemia. The arteries were grafted successfully.

Conclusions.—The ulnar artery was successfully used for coronary bypass grafting in 8 patients, when it was not safe to use the radial artery. Care must be taken in harvesting the ulnar artery, because it lies close to the ulnar nerve.

▶ This article reports the use of ulnar arteries as coronary bypass conduits. The increased risk of complications, caused by the proximity of the ulnar nerve to the ulnar artery, has only been postulated: no injury was observed in this small group. The authors' caution that there should be some significant indication for use of the ulnar artery is a reasonable one.

J.J. Collins, Jr., M.D.

Myocardial Damage After Minimally Invasive Coronary Artery Bypass Grafting on the Beating Heart
Bonatti J, Hangler H, Hörmann C, et al (Univ of Innsbruck, Austria)
Ann Thorac Surg 66:1093-1096, 1998   3–29

Introduction.—Previous studies have reported a 2% to 6% rate of perioperative myocardial infarction in patients undergoing conventional coronary artery bypass grafting. When troponins and other sensitive marker proteins are used, these rates rise even higher. There is little information about the rate of perioperative myocardial infarction or about myocardial marker protein release in patients undergoing minimally invasive direct coronary artery bypass grafting (MIDCABG) on the beating heart. Cardiac troponin I was used to determine the rate of myocardial damage in patients undergoing MIDCABG.

Methods.—The study included 15 consecutive patients undergoing MIDCABG via minithoracotomy. There were 11 men and 4 women, with a mean age of 60. Intraoperative and postoperative ischemic monitoring was carried out with ECG, transesophageal and transthoracic echocardiography, and measurement of creatine kinase-MB mass concentration and cardiac troponin I.

Results.—One patient had severe myocardial ischemia and ventricular fibrillation, and died despite mechanical cardiocirculatory support. Of the survivors, 44% had evidence of transient myocardial ischemia on ECG, echocardiography, or both. Another 21% had reversible signs of myocardial ischemia during and after surgery. Cardiac troponin I was elevated with 4 of 9 patients with ischemia. In 2 of these 4 patients, angiography showed pathology in the bypass graft or target vessel.

Conclusions.—Using a sensitive and specific marker of myocardial damage, these authors show that subclinical myocardial injury is common among patients undergoing MIDCABG on the beating heart. Serial measurements of cardiac troponin I are needed to determine whether this myocardial ischemia leads to necrosis. This marker could serve as the gold standard for diagnosis of perioperative myocardial infarction. Increased cardiac troponin I is an indication for repeat angiography.

▶ This interesting article presents data similar to those found by the group at Loma Linda (Abstract 3–30). Significant ischemic damage seems to be expected in nearly half the patients in whom careful postoperative examination is immediately available. This is another article confirming that great care is needed in selecting patients for coronary operations on the beating heart.

J.J. Collins, Jr., M.D.

Seven-Year Follow-up of Coronary Artery Bypasses Performed With and Without Cardiopulmonary Bypass
Gundry SR, Romano MA, Shattuck OH, et al (Loma Linda Univ, Calif)
J Thorac Cardiovasc Surg 115:1273-1278, 1998   3–30

Background.—To decrease the morbidity and hospitalization associated with coronary artery bypass grafting (CABG) by cardiopulmonary bypass (CPB), surgeons revascularize the beating heart (BH) without CPB. Patients treated, by the same surgeons, with either BHCABG or traditional CABG with CPB were compared. Long-term survival and intervention-free outcome in these 2 patient groups were assessed.

Study Design.—All patients seen by 3 attending surgeons at Loma Linda University Medical Center from June 1989 to July 1990 were offered revascularization without CPB. If the patient consented, the choice of operation was left to the operating surgeon. During that year, 107 patients had BHCABG and 112 patients had traditional CABG. The average age and risk factors for these 2 groups were identical. Patients undergoing BHCABG had an average of 2.4 grafts per patient, and patients undergoing traditional CABG had an average of 3.2 grafts per patient. All patients were studied for 7 years.

Findings.—At 7-year follow-up, 80% of BHCABG patients and 79% of traditional CABG patients were alive. Cardiac deaths occurred in 12% of BHCABG patients and 9% of traditional CABG patients. However, 30% of BHCABG patients required catheterization for their symptoms, whereas only 16% in the traditional CABG group required intervention. Angioplasty or a second coronary bypass was required by 20% in the BHCABG group, but by only 7% in the traditional CABG group. No patient in the traditional CABG group required reoperation. Percutaneous transluminal coronary angioplasty was required by 71% of the 21 patients in the BHCABG group who needed reoperation.

Conclusions.—CABG performed on a BH produced longevity and symptom status equivalent to those produced by traditional CABG, as measured at 7 years' follow-up. However, twice as many patients in the BHCABG group required catheterization and 3 times as many interventions were required in the BHCABG group to achieve this equivalence.

▶ These authors have found exactly what would be expected: twice as many patients in a beating heart surgical group required subsequent recatheterization and 20% required a second intervention. This is substantially different from what was observed in the cardioplegia group. This article suggests that safety and reliability of operations on the beating heart are not yet clear enough for them to entirely replace cardioplegia.

J.J. Collins, Jr., M.D.

Intraoperative MIDCABG Arteriography via the Left Radial Artery: A Comparison With Doppler Ultrasound for Assessment of Graft Patency

Elbeery JR, Brown PM, Chitwood WR Jr (East Carolina Univ, Greenville, NC)
Ann Thorac Surg 66:51-55, 1998   3–31

Background.—Minimally invasive direct coronary artery bypass grafting (MIDCABG) procedures generally involve anastomosis of the left internal mammary artery (LIMA) to the left anterior descending artery without cardiopulmonary bypass, using local occlusion and on the beating heart. Reported short-term MIDCABG results are favorable, but there are anecdotal reports of poor outcomes with this technically challenging procedure. The importance of early assessment of graft patency cannot be overemphasized. Intraoperative evaluation is possible with noninvasive techniques such as Doppler US, but coronary angiography remains the standard. These authors describe an intraoperative radial artery catheterization arteriography technique to assess early graft patency in MIDCABG patients.

> *Technique.*—A 4F introducer is exchanged for the arterial catheter and advanced into the aorta with fluoroscopic guidance. The catheter is withdrawn into the subclavian artery, with the tip positioned caudally. Small injections of contrast medium permit visualization and cannulation of the LIMA origin. A C-arm fluoroscopy unit is used to make arteriograms during forceful injection of contrast material. Total procedure time is less than 15 minutes. This procedure was used in 50 MIDCABG patients, the majority of whom were men, with an average age of 59 and an average ejection fraction of 55%. Hard copies of the intraoperative arteriographic image were made and judged by an independent observer.

Results.—There were no injuries detected in the LIMA. Anastomotic occlusions were identified by intraoperative MIDCABG arteriography in 4 patients. Two of these occlusions involved sequential diagonal and left anterior descending artery anastomoses. The anastomoses were corrected at surgery. Two corrections involved conversion to standard coronary artery bypass grafting. Qualitative evaluation of grafts with Doppler US did not definitively identify the 4 occlusions detected by arteriography. There were no deaths or perioperative infarctions in this series of 50 MIDCABG patients.

Conclusions.—Intraoperative catheterization and arteriography of the LIMA can be safely performed during MIDCABG to assess early graft patency, which should permit a 100% early graft patency rate. This technique should increase the safety and success rate of the MIDCABG procedure.

▶ LIMA angiography is very valuable during MIDCABG operations. The authors' experience with angiography via the left radial artery suggests that this is a significantly more accurate technique than Doppler US, and that it is reasonably safe.

J.J. Collins, Jr., M.D.

Results of 1,454 Free Right Internal Thoracic Artery-to-Coronary Artery Grafts

Tatoulis J, Buxton BF, Fuller JA (Univ of Melbourne, Australia)
Ann Thorac Surg 64:1263-1269, 1997
3–32

Background.—To overcome anatomic limitations of the pedicled right internal thoracic artery-to-coronary graft, its use was expanded electively as a free graft (FRITA). A 10-year experience in 1,454 consecutive patients who had a planned FRITA-to-coronary artery graft as part of coronary revascularization is described.

Study Group.—The 1,454 patients in the study group had an average age of 59. Eight percent had non–insulin-dependent diabetes and 0.5% had insulin-dependent diabetes. Decreased left ventricular ejection fraction was present in 12% and unstable angina was present in 9.9%. In 11 patients, the FRITA was the only graft. There were an average of 3.3 distal anastomoses per patient. The aortic clamp time was about 49 minutes and bypass time was about 69 minutes.

Findings.—Operative mortality was 0.9%; stroke occurred in 1% and myocardial infarction in 1.3% of these patients. Peak serum creatine kinase myocardial isoenzyme level averaged 20.6 IU/L. Complications included sternal infection in 1.2% of patients and reoperation for hemorrhage in 1.6%. Survival at 5 years was 96% and at 7 years was 94%. In 71 patients studied for an average of 42 months, 67 FRITAs were widely patent, 3 displayed a string sign, and 1 was occluded.

Conclusions.—The right internal thoracic artery can be safely and successfully used as a free graft as part of myocardial revascularization procedures. Short- and long-term results were similar to those of single thoracic artery grafting. Use of the FRITA permits greater flexibility in arterial coronary revascularization.

▶ The FRITA can be reliably used in most patients. Care must be taken to perform the aortic anastomosis with the largest possible portion of the graft. In the vast majority of people the graft can be taken directly from the base of the aorta. If there is any doubt about the size of the FRITA, a vein patch can be placed on the aorta first and the internal thoracic graft taken off the vein patch.

J.J. Collins, Jr., M.D.

Single Versus Bilateral Internal Mammary Artery Grafts: 10-Year Outcome Analysis

Pick AW, Orszulak TA, Anderson BJ, et al (Mayo Clinic and Mayo Found, Rochester, Minn)
Ann Thorac Surg 64:599-605, 1997   3–33

Background.—Because use of the left internal mammary artery (IMA) to bypass the left anterior descending coronary artery has been associated with superior graft patency, reduced cardiac events, and enhanced survival, some surgical groups have begun using both IMAs for revascularization. To determine whether bilateral use of both IMAs confers further advantage to patients at bypass surgery, a group of patients with bilateral IMA (BIMA) bypass procedures was compared to a group of patients with single IMA (SIMA) bypass procedures.

Study Design.—Beginning in January 1984 and continuing for 24 months, 160 patients with multivessel disease had coronary revasculariza-

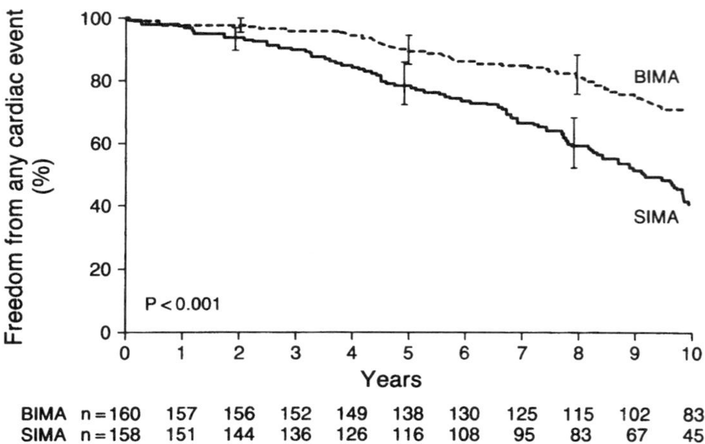

BIMA	n = 160	157	156	152	149	138	130	125	115	102	83
SIMA	n = 158	151	144	136	126	116	108	95	83	67	45

FIGURE 5.—Freedom from occurrence of any cardiac event for single (*SIMA*) vs. bilateral internal mammary artery (*BIMA*) grafts. (Reprinted with permission from the Society of Thoracic Surgeons from Pick AW, Orszulak TA, Anderson BJ, et al: Single versus bilateral internal mammary artery grafts: 10-year outcome analysis. *Ann Thorac Surg* 64:599-605, 1997.)

tion procedures with BIMA grafts plus saphenous vein grafts and 160 patients had saphenous grafts alone. During an expanded time to May 1986, a matched group of 161 patients with a SIMA and supplementary vein grafts operated on by the same surgeons were identified. These 3 groups of patients form the study group for this report. Clinical data were obtained from hospital records, physician notes, follow-up visits, patient surveys, and telephone interviews.

Findings.—The groups were matched for gender, preoperative angina class, priority status, coronary artery disease extent, left ventricular function, and distal anastomoses number. Diabetes was more common in the SIMA graft procedure group. Early outcome was similar for the single and bilateral IMA groups. Operative mortality was 0.6% in the SIMA group and 0% in the BIMA graft group. The average follow-up for the 320 hospital survivors was 10 years. Univariate analysis revealed significantly fewer overall deaths and lower late cardiac mortality in the BIMA graft group. Ten-year actuarial survival for patients who were dismissed from the hospital was 75% for the SIMA group and 85% for the BIMA group. Multivariate analysis found diabetes, age, and lower ejection fraction to be the only significant predictors of late cardiac death. Use of a SIMA graft was not significant, despite a risk ratio of 1.78. Use of a SIMA graft was associated with increased risk of angina recurrence, late myocardial infarction, and risk of any cardiac event (Fig 5).

Conclusions.—Bilateral internal mammary artery grafts are associated with reduced risk of angina recurrence, late myocardial infarction, and other late cardiac events after a bypass graft procedure. There was also a nonsignificant trend toward improvement in late survival in this study group. A larger study with longer follow-up will be necessary to clarify the long-term survival benefits of bilateral IMA grafting.

▶ This very useful article from the Mayo Clinic confirms that bilateral internal mammary artery grafting is an independent predictor of complications and late mortality after coronary surgery. Please note that this finding is not independent of diabetes mellitus.

J.J. Collins, Jr., M.D.

Minimally Invasive Coronary Artery Bypass: A Series With Early Qualitative Angiographic Follow-up

Gill IS, FitzGibbon GM, Higginson LAJ, et al (Univ of Ottawa, Ont, Canada)
Ann Thorac Surg 64:710-714, 1997

3–34

Background.—Minimally invasive direct coronary artery bypass grafting (MIDCABG) has advantages over conventional coronary operations involving cardiopulmonary bypass and cardioplegic arrest, but the technical accuracy of distal anastomosis made on a beating heart has been questioned. A consecutive series of selected patients undergoing MIDCABG were analyzed.

Study Design.—Between January and October 1996, 25 patients had MIDCABG operations at the University of Ottawa Heart Institute. All anastomoses were performed on a beating heart. Transit-time ultrasonic flows were monitored for the final 8 patients in this series after completion of the anastomosis. A postoperative angiogram was performed for all patients within 6 hours. Patients had follow-up visits at 2 weeks, 6 weeks, and 3 months. Follow-up was 100% complete and ranged from 15 days to 11 months.

Findings.—There were no anastomotic occlusions and graft patency was 97.5%. One internal thoracic artery was damaged. There was no mortality. There were no perioperative myocardial infarctions. All patients remain symptom free. Of the 26 anastomoses that could be evaluated, 81% were grade A and 19% were grade B. For comparison, 96% of the anastomoses created on an arrested heart by the same surgeon were grade A.

Conclusions.—In this small, select patient group, minimally invasive coronary bypass was performed effectively and safely. The development of sophisticated stabilizing devices and instrumentation should continue to improve the results of MIDCABG.

▶ This experience with only 25 patients is particularly significant. Surgeons in Ottawa are technically excellent and, as usual from this institution, follow-up is complete. The conclusion that minimally invasive coronary surgery is reasonable in select patients is entirely correct. The operative word is "select." And the operative consideration is surgical skill.

J.J. Collins, Jr., M.D.

Impact of Gender on Coronary Bypass Operative Mortality

Edwards FH, Carey JS, Grover FL, et al (Univ of Florida, Jacksonville; Torrance Mem Med Ctr, Calif; Univ of Colorado, Denver; et al)
Ann Thorac Surg 66:125-131, 1998
3–35

Introduction.—Women appear to have considerably higher risk of operative mortality after coronary artery bypass graft than men, with most studies reporting women's mortality as twice that of men. The reasons for this disparity are not clear, and include the possibility that a woman's smaller coronary arteries present a greater technical challenge or that women are seen for revascularization at a more advanced stage of disease. To determine whether a difference in operative mortality exists, surgical experience with coronary artery bypass graft was reviewed.

Methods.—The retrospective review included 344,913 patients who had coronary artery bypass graft operations. A variety of single risk factors and combinations of risk factors were examined and compared among men and women to determine the operative mortality rate. The risk factors studied included age, first operation, renal failure, morbid obesity, myocardial infarction, diabetes, triple-vessel disease, race, cardiomegaly, diuretic therapy, hypertension, and body surface area.

Results.—A significantly higher mortality for each of the risk factors was found among 97,153 women. Significantly higher mortality was found among the women when compared to equally matched men in the low- and medium-risk part of the spectrum. However, in the high-risk spectrum, no differences between men's and women's mortality were found.

Conclusion.—Except for patients in very high risk categories, gender was an independent predictor of operative mortality. The risk factors were virtually identical in men and women at presentation; however, the relative weight of some risk factors was very different. When the operative risk was near 30%, no significant differences in outcome were associated with gender.

▶ This article by Edwards and associates confirms the significant gender difference found in most studies of operative mortality risk. The disappearance of the gender factor in very high risk categories suggests that the quality of distal vessels has become a more powerful predictive factor than in less severely ill patients. It is our experience that women do very well as long as vessels beyond the obstructions are large enough and relatively free of severe disease. In patients with small or diffusely diseased vessels, the risk for surgery is higher.

J.J. Collins, Jr., M.D.

Reduction of the Inflammatory Response in Patients Undergoing Minimally Invasive Coronary Artery Bypass Grafting

Gu YJ, Mariani MA, van Oeveren W, et al (Univ Hosp, Groningen, The Netherlands)

Ann Thorac Surg 65:420-424, 1998

3–36

Introduction.—The induction of a systemic inflammatory response caused by cardiopulmonary bypass (CPB) is an important disadvantage of coronary artery bypass grafting (CABG). Minimally invasive CABG (MICABG)—performed through a small anterolateral thoracotomy without CPB—can reduce postoperative morbidity, though the mechanism of this benefit is unclear. The clinical and subclinical indicators of the inflammatory response in patients undergoing MICABG vs. conventional CABG were assessed.

Methods.—The study included 62 consecutive patients undergoing surgery for isolated stenosis of the left anterior descending artery. One group was randomized to undergo MICABG and the other to undergo conventional CABG with CPB. Inflammation-associated clinical morbidity was compared between groups. In 10 patients in each group, subclinical markers of the inflammatory response were measured: leukocyte elastase, platelet β-thromboglobulin, and complement C3a.

Results.—The MICABG group had a shorter duration of surgery, 104 vs. 140 minutes. The MICABG group also had less blood loss, 312 vs. 788 mL; a shorter duration of ventilatory support, 7.7 vs. 12.9 hours; and a shorter postoperative hospital stay, 4.4 vs. 7.7 days. The inflammatory markers were unchanged from baseline to the end of the bypass procedure in the MICABG group. In contrast, these markers increased significantly in patients undergoing conventional CABG with CPB.

Conclusions.—MICABG is associated with a significantly reduced inflammatory response, as indicated by subclinical inflammatory markers. The minimally invasive procedure also reduces postoperative morbidity and shortens hospital stay. These factors may overcome several of the important disadvantages associated with CABG.

▶ These authors make a good point that MICABG (operation without cardiopulmonary bypass) causes substantially less inflammatory response than operation using a heart-lung machine. Unfortunately, avoiding the use of the heart-lung machine also requires operating on a beating heart, which is difficult in all circumstances and impossible in some.

J.J. Collins, Jr., M.D.

Outcome of Coronary Bypass Surgery Versus Coronary Angioplasty in Diabetic Patients With Multivessel Coronary Artery Disease

Weintraub WS, Stein B, Kosinski A, et al (Emory Univ, Atlanta, Ga)
J Am Coll Cardiol 31:10-19, 1998

3–37

Background.—There is concern about revascularization in patients with diabetes mellitus and multivessel coronary disease because long-term event rates are higher than in patients without diabetes.

Methods.—Data were obtained retrospectively for 2,639 diabetic patients with multivessel coronary artery disease; 834 patients had percutaneous transluminal coronary angioplasty and 1,805 patients had coronary artery bypass graft surgery. The mean follow-up was 5.0 years.

Results.—Follow-up data were obtained for 96% of patients. There were more in-hospital deaths and a trend toward more Q wave myocardial infarctions after bypass surgery. After coronary angioplasty, 5-year survival was 78% and 10-year survival was 45%. After bypass surgery, 5-year survival was 76% and 10-year survival was 48%. For patients requiring insulin, 5-year survival was 72% and 10-year survival was 31% after coronary angioplasty; 5-year survival was 70% and 10-year survival was 48% after bypass surgery. Multivariate analysis showed that older age, low left ventricular ejection fraction, heart failure, and hypertension were associated with long-term mortality. In all patients, insulin requirement was associated with long-term mortality, and choice of therapy had a multivariate hazard ratio close to 1. In patients requiring insulin, the multivariate hazard ratio was 1.35 for coronary angioplasty vs. bypass surgery. In patients requiring insulin and after correcting for baseline differences, 5-year survival was 68% and 10-year survival was 36% after coronary angioplasty; 5-year survival was 75% and 10-year survival was 47% after bypass surgery. After coronary angioplasty, especially after additional revascularization, nonfatal events were more common than after bypass grafting.

Discussion.—In these patients with diabetes mellitus, there was a high rate of events, which raises additional questions about the use of angioplasty in such patients with multivessel disease.

▶ The observation that diabetes is a significant risk factor for early recurrence of obstruction in the coronary arteries after angioplasty is very useful.

J.J. Collins, Jr., M.D.

Lesions of the Target Vessel During Minimally Invasive Myocardial Revascularization

Alessandrini F, Gaudino M, Glieca F, et al (Catholic Univ, Rome; "R Calai" Hosp, Gualdo Tadino, Italy)
Ann Thorac Surg 64:1349-1353, 1997　　　　　　　　　　3–38

Background.—Minimally invasive coronary artery bypass grafting is a recent addition to cardiac surgery. The incidence of surgically induced distal target vessel stenosis in patients who undergo this procedure was studied.

Methods.—Postoperative Doppler evaluation of mammary artery flow was performed in 55 patients who had minimally invasive coronary artery bypass grafting. Angiography was performed in 37 patients.

Technique.—The left internal mammary artery (LIMA) was harvested skeletonized in 15 patients and pedicled in 40 patients. In most patients, the LIMA was harvested under direct vision, but a thoracoscopy was used in 3 patients. After administration of heparin, the LIMA was divided, injected with a papaverine solution, and evaluated for flow and quality.

Results.—In 32 of the first 35 patients, the anastomosis and the distal left anterior descending artery were normal. The other 3 patients had mammary artery occlusion, anastomotic stenosis, or stenosis of the anastomosis and the distal left anterior descending artery. In 2 patients who had late angiography, a distal left anterior descending artery stenosis was detected.

Discussion.—Surgically induced distal target vessel stenosis is a major disadvantage of minimally invasive coronary artery bypass grafting, a procedure that may soon transform surgical treatment of coronary artery disease. Improvements must be made in the means of achieving coronary artery occlusion, as well as in anticoagulant and antiplatelet therapy, before this procedure can be confidently used in clinical practice.

▶ Damage from suture encirclement of coronary arteries during coronary bypass surgery may be observed in operations done in a standard fashion as well as those occurring during minimally invasive surgery. In fact, the amount of tension necessary to establish total obstruction of antegrade blood flow by a suture ligature applied in a temporary fashion is much less in patients being operated on by a standard technique because it is done as a supplement to aortic clamping and not as the sole technique to resist blood pressure of the unclamped aorta.

J.J. Collins, Jr., M.D.

Thoracoscopic Transmyocardial Laser Revascularization

Horvath KA (Northwestern Univ, Chicago)
Ann Thorac Surg 65:1439-1440, 1998   3–39

Background.—Transmyocardial laser revascularization has been used for more than 6 years to treat patients with end-stage coronary artery disease who are not amenable to standard revascularization techniques and who suffer severe refractory angina. The operative approach for these patients has been through an 18- to 20-cm anterior thoracotomy. This author describes a minimally invasive technique for transmyocardial laser revascularization.

Case Report.—Woman, 67, with 2 previous myocardial infarctions, who had been treated with angioplasty and stenting, was seen with a third myocardial infarction. Repeat angiography revealed that stents were open and that there was little change in her diffusely diseased coronary arteries. She experienced significant substernal chest pressure that was refractory to medical treatment. Dual-isotope perfusion scanning revealed a large area of reversible ischemia. Under general anesthesia, a thoracoscopic port was placed in her fifth intercostal space along the midaxillary line. The pericardium was opened and retracted so that the carbon dioxide hand piece could be introduced through the fifth intercostal space incision. An additional 4-cm incision was made in the fourth intercostal space at the midclavicular line, under thoacoscopic guidance, to allow introduction of the laser through this incision and to create channels anteriorly and laterally close to the base of the heart. A single chest tube was placed through the fifth intercostal space incision. The procedure was completed in 65 minutes and the patient was extubated in the operating room. The postoperative course was unremarkable. The patient was discharged on postoperative day 3. She has been monitored for 8 months and has had no angina recurrences. Follow-up perfusion scans revealed improved perfusion in the laser-treated area. Incision discomfort was minimal.

Conclusion.—Thoracoscopic transmyocardial laser revascularization is a minimally invasive method for achieving transmural revascularization.

Electrical Stimulation Versus Coronary Artery Bypass Surgery in Severe Angina Pectoris: The ESBY Study
Mannheimer C, Eliasson T, Augustinsson L-E, et al (Östra Hosp, Gothenburg, Sweden; Sahlgren's Hosp, Gothenburg, Sweden)
Circulation 97:1157-1163, 1998

3–40

Background.—Since 1985, epidural spinal cord stimulation (SCS) has been used to treat intractable angina pectoris. This randomized, prospective trial compared the results of coronary artery bypass grafting (CABG) with those of SCS in patients accepted for CABG who had increased risk of surgical complications and a lack of prognostic benefit from CABG.

Methods.—The study group consisted of 51 patients who were randomized to CABG and 53 patients who were randomized to SCS from January 1992 to March 1995. CABG and SCS were compared with an "intention to treat" design. The primary end points were symptoms and myocardial ischemia. Secondary end points included total mortality and morbidity. Clinical outcome was recorded on a questionnaire after exercise testing.

Technique.—The stimulation equipment was implanted under local anesthesia, and the electrode positioned so that the patient felt a prickling sensation in the angina pain region. The electrode tip was placed at T1 to T2, and the pulse generator was placed subcutaneously in a pouch below the left costal arch. The pulse generator was telemetrically programmed with 2 stimulation strengths, the stronger for anginal pain and the weaker for prophylactic treatment. The prophylactic treatment was used for at least 2 hours 4 times daily.

Results.—Both SCS and CABG provided adequate symptom relief to this patient group. The CABG group had increased exercise capacity, less S-T segment depression, and an increase in the rate-pressure product. There were 7 deaths in the CABG group and 1 death in the SCS group during the follow-up. Mortality was lower in the SCS group, as was cerebrovascular morbidity.

Conclusions.—The limitations of this study included its small sample, short follow-up, and inability to blind either patients or physicians. In patients with an increased risk of surgical complications and no prognostic benefit from surgery, SCS may be a good therapeutic alternative to CABG. SCS provided symptomatic relief in patients with intractable angina pectoris.

▶ The rather short article by Horvath (Abstract 3–39) and the article by Mannheimer and associates (Abstract 3–40) both deal with controversial concepts in management of anginal pain. Horvath and Mannheimer report significant relief of angina with treatments that can only be described as alternative. Unfortunately, neither technique can be perfectly subjected to experimental conditions that would allow a definite conclusion. However, it may well be that no matter what the explanation for reduction of discomfort, the pain control alone may be very useful, especially for older patients or for those with severe comorbidities.

J.J. Collins, Jr., M.D.

Surgical Management of Spontaneous Left Main Coronary Artery Dissection

Thistlethwaite PA, Tarazi RY, Giordano FJ, et al (Univ of California, San Diego)
Ann Thorac Surg 66:258-260, 1998   3–41

Background.—Spontaneous coronary artery dissection is a rare cause of ischemic heart disease and sudden death. It occurs predominantly in healthy, young women in the third trimester of pregnancy or in the early postpartum period. Cardiac risk factors are usually absent. Early recognition is essential because coronary artery bypass grafting may be lifesaving.

> *Case Report.*—Woman, 34, 12 weeks postpartum, was first seen after 18 hours of chest pain, with acute anterior wall myocardial infarction. Cardiac catheterization revealed a dissection of the left main coronary artery extending into the left anterior descending artery. She underwent urgent bypass grafting, with bluish hemorrhage noted over the left main coronary artery and distal left anterior descending artery at operation. She was discharged on the sixth postoperative day. Transthoracic echocardiography after 2 months indicated improvement in both wall motion and ejection fraction.

Conclusions.—Most cases of primary coronary dissection occur in peripartum women without known cardiovascular risk factors. Young patients seen with acute ischemic symptoms should be considered for urgent angiography. If left main coronary artery dissection is detected, surgery with coronary artery bypass grafting is safe and effective. Rapid diagnosis and surgical intervention are lifesaving.

▶ Spontaneous dissection involving the left main coronary artery is certainly a management dilemma. As the authors point out, most surgeons would feel strongly that the safest management for these patients is open operation. I don't know of any reports (yet) of attempted stent placement in patients with left main coronary artery dissection. We have tended until now to treat these patients by prompt operation and I see no reason to change.

J.J. Collins, Jr., M.D.

Cardiac Transplantation

Implantable Left Ventricular Assist Devices Provide an Excellent Outpatient Bridge to Transplantation and Recovery

DeRose JJ Jr, Umana JP, Argenziano M, et al (Columbia Univ, New York)
J Am Coll Cardiol 30:1773-1777, 1997   3–42

Introduction.—The limited donor pool makes heart transplantation available for only 2,500 patients each year. Left ventricular assist devices (LVADs) have been successfully used as a bridge to transplantation for 10 years. Recent experience with outpatient LVAD support demonstrates the possibilities and limitations of long-term outpatient mechanical circulatory assistance.

Methods.—Thirty-two patients underwent implantation of the ThermoCardiosystems Heartmate vented electric LVAD during 1993 and 1994. This device is powered by batteries worn on shoulder holsters and is operated by a belt-mounted system controller that allows unrestricted patient ambulation and hospital discharge.

Results.—Mean duration of LVAD support was 122 days (range, 3-605 days). The survival rate to transplantation or explantation was 78%. Nineteen patients were discharged from the hospital at a mean postoperative time of 41 days (range, 17-68 days). Outpatient support time was a mean of 108 days (range, 2-466 days). Because of early transplantation, four patients were not available to participate in the discharge program. At final follow-up, three patients were awaiting discharge. The complication rate in this series was similar to that in an earlier series of 52 patients with a pneumatic LVAD.

Conclusion.—Outpatient LVAD support is safe and offers improved quality of life for patients awaiting transplantation. Wearable and totally implantable LVADs should be evaluated as permanent treatment options in patients who are not candidates for heart transplantation.

Clinical Outcomes, Quality of Life, and Cost Outcomes After Cardiac Transplantation

Hershberger RE (Oregon Health Sciences Univ, Portland, Ore)
Am J Med Sci 314:129-138, 1997   3–43

Introduction.—Improving survival is the most compelling reason to consider cardiac transplantation in patients with advanced heart failure, particularly those dependent on intravenous inotropic support or mechanical assistance. This procedure, however, is not curative; rather, it remains a treatment modality requiring indefinite immunosuppression and ongoing care. The cost of cardiac transplantation was also investigated.

Survival Analysis.—Primarily, cardiac transplantation should be considered because it improves survival. For populations of patients, mortality estimates of advanced heart failure have been assessed. For patients with advanced disease treated with the enalapril, the mortality rate was 40% at 1 year. Patients with class III or IV heart failure at initial evaluation had a 1-year mortality rate of 16%. Survival for cardiac transplants at 1 year was 81.8%.

Quality of Life.—An improved quality of life after cardiac transplantation has been found in most studies. At 1 year after transplantation, quality of life had improved because of less total symptom distress, better health perception, better overall functional status, and more overall satisfaction with life. The most common area of disability after transplantation was work-related. For patients with advanced heart failure who did not have cardiac transplantation, minimal changes were found in quality of life scores. Employment rates varied from 32% to 50% for patients with heart transplants.

Cost.—In 1988 dollars, the heart transplantation procedure charges from date of transplant to date of discharge were about $91,600, and in 1993 dollars, they were $209,100, with 5-year charges of $269,100. Although there are about 40,000 patients waiting for a heart transplantation, only about 2,500 donors are available, and this affects cost outcomes. The median waiting period for a new heart was 122 days in 1998 and was 215 days in 1992. As patients wait longer, they become sicker and then receive transplants in a more advanced state of disease, when costs are even higher. The implantable left ventricular assist device has become the most significant new technology development for cardiac transplantation, and is used as a bridge to cardiac transplantation, with a cost ranging from $30,000 to $60,000. Additional costs may accrue if these devices become part of the treatment paradigm.

▶ These articles by DeRose and associates (Abstract 3–42) and by Hershberger (Abstract 3–43) emphasize quality of life as well as cost and potential for rehabilitation related to cardiac transplantation surgery. Just getting the operation done is not enough. We must demonstrate that society can reasonably tolerate the admittedly enormous expense of improved technology in this area. With technology continuing to evolve, decisions may become more and more difficult. The introduction of simplicity into machinery for cardiac assist devices is paramount.

J.J. Collins, Jr., M.D.

Surgery for Congenital Heart Disease

Intermediate-term Results of Phase I Food and Drug Administration Trials of Buttoned Device Occlusion of Secundum Atrial Septal Defects
Zamora R, Rao PS, Lloyd TR, et al (Univ of Arizona, Tucson; Saint Louis Univ; Univ of Michigan, Ann Arbor; et al)
J Am Coll Cardiol 31:674-676, 1998   3–44

Introduction.—Only short-term follow-up studies have investigated the buttoned device used for transcatheter occlusion of secundum atrial septal defects, and the device has been shown to be safe, feasible, and effective.

The intermediate-term results of the multi-institutional trial of the buttoned device for transcatheter closure of secundum atrial septal defects were evaluated.

Methods.—Forty-six patients who had successful implantation of the device were prospectively studied and evaluated at 1, 6, and 12 months after device occlusion and yearly thereafter. They were studied from 51 to 68 months, with a mean of 60.8 months. The patients were evaluated by chest radiograph film, physical examination, history, electrocardiogram, and Doppler echocardiographic studies. The patients ranged in age from 1 to 62 years and had a median age of 4. They ranged in weight from 10 to 105 kg, with a median weight of 18 kg.

Results.—The patients had stretched atrial septal defects in which the sizes were 14 ± 4 mm (left to right shunts) and 10 ± 3 mm (right to left shunts.) Effective occlusion of their atrial septal defect occurred in 45 of the 46 patients (98%), and completed atrial septal defect closure occurred in 34 patients (74%). There was an incidence of residual shunts of 65% at 1 month after device placement and the incidence decreased to 27% at follow-up. All of the residual shunts were described as trivial. Reintervention for significant residual defects occurred in only 2 patients (4%). In the 224 patient-years of follow-up, there were no patients with endocarditis or thromboembolism.

Conclusion.—In 98% of patients in whom the buttoned device was successfully implanted, it provided effective closure for up to 5.5 years. During follow-up, the incidence of residual shunts decreased, and no instances of endocarditis or thromboembolism were observed.

▶ The placement of occlusion devices for treatment of secundum atrial septal defects will eventually be a sure and simple technique. It is interesting that conquering the interatrial septum has been more difficult technically than controlling apertures of the interventricular septum.

J.J. Collins, Jr., M.D.

Benefits of Early Surgical Repair in Fixed Subaortic Stenosis

Brauner R, Laks H, Drinkwater DC Jr, et al (Univ of California, Los Angeles)
J Am Coll Cardiol 30:1835-1842, 1997   3–45

Introduction.—It is a surgical challenge to fix subaortic stenosis. The disease is progressive, whether it is congenital or acquired. Subaortic lesions causing minimal or no obstruction are diagnosed increasingly in young, often asymptomatic patients. Because of diverging reports on outcomes of surgery for young patients, the subject is controversial. A retrospective review of young patients with subaortic stenosis who were treated with surgery was conducted to determine whether this strategy improved outcome by reducing recurrence, reoperation, and late aortic valve deterioration.

Methods.—There were 75 patients, ranging in age from 1 month to 44 years, with a mean age of 8.6 years and a median of 6 years with fixed subaortic stenosis, who had surgery and who were studied for a median of 6.7 years. At the time of referral, 49 patients (65.3%) were asymptomatic. In 68 patients, the lesion was discrete (91%), and of a tunnel type in 7 patients, with associated ventricular septal defect in 28 patients (37%). Transaortic resection was performed an all patients. Patients were divided into a low-gradient group and a high-gradient group.

Results.—No deaths occurred. In 15 patients (20%), there were 18 recurrences of subaortic stenosis. There were 17 reoperations in 13 patients (17%) for recurrence or aortic valve disease. There was an 8.9% cumulative hazard of recurrence at 2 years, 16.1% at 5 years, and 29.4% at 10 years. Recurrence of reoperation was 9.2% at 2 years, 18.4% at 5 years, and 35.1% at 10 years. After transaortic resection, a tunnel-type lesion was 5 times more likely to recur than a discrete lesion. There was a strong independent influence of the preoperative gradient on recurrence per patient-year of follow-up. Higher gradients in 35 patients were associated with a greater than seven-fold recurrence rate. The aortic valve required concomitant repair in 17 patients in the high-gradient group (48.6%), but in only 8 in the low-gradient group (20%). In the high-gradient group, progressive aortic regurgitation was noted at follow-up after 14 procedures (40%), and in the low gradient group, it was noted after 5 procedures (12.5%).

Conclusion.—Recurrence, reoperation, and secondary progressive aortic valve disease may be prevented by surgical resection of fixed subaortic stenosis before the development of a significant (greater than 40 mm Hg) outflow tract gradient.

▶ This article by Brauner and associates demonstrates that there is significant hazard in delaying repair of fixed subaortic stenosis and confirms the advice of other authors that promptness increases safety in these patients.

J.J. Collins, Jr., M.D.

Cardiac Surgery for Octogenarians

Cardiac Valve Surgery in Octogenarians: Improving Quality of Life and Functional Status

Khan JH, McElhinney DB, Hall TS, et al (Univ of California, San Francisco)
Arch Surg 133:887-893, 1998   3–46

Objective.—Open heart surgery can be performed on octogenarians with significant morbidity but acceptable mortality, but no studies have assessed the resulting quality of life and functional status of such patients. Factors that may predict survival, performance status, and medical resource use were retrospectively reviewed.

Methods.—Between June 1987 and May 1995, medical records of 61 patients (14 women), aged 80 to 89 years, who underwent cardiac valve surgery at a tertiary care hospital, were reviewed, and patients were interviewed by telephone. Patients were followed for a median of 30 months. They had a variety of co-morbid conditions, and all were symptomatic at the time of surgery. Functional status and Karnofsky performance status were assessed at discharge and at 3 months.

Results.—Patients underwent aortic valve replacement (n = 47), mitral valve replacement and/or repair (n = 14), and coronary artery bypass grafting with other procedures (n = 27). Seven patients (11.4%) died perioperatively, and 20 patients (37%) experienced significant postoperative complications. Hospital stays for patients with and without complications were 25.0 vs. 12.2 days, respectively. Of the 54 survivors, 15 were discharged to nursing homes, 9 of them for functional disabilities. There were 12 late deaths. The remaining 42 survivors had 18 hospital admissions. Actuarial survivals at 1 and 5 years were 85% and 66%, respectively. According to multivariable analysis, a preoperative stay in the ICU and New York Heart Association class 4 status were independent predictors of early mortality. Patients with postoperative complications had a longer hospital stay and decreased actuarial survival. One month after discharge, the New York Heart Association classification had improved a median of 2 classes; Karnofsky performance had improved to a median of 80% from a preoperative level of 30%. Results were similar at 3 months.

Conclusion.—Heart valve replacement in octogenarians is safe, improves symptoms and functional status, and enhances quality of life. More resources are used, and recovery is longer and more complicated.

Cardiac Operations in Octogenarians: Perioperative Risk Factors for Death and Impaired Autonomy
Kirsch M, Guesnier L, LeBesnerais P, et al (Hôpital Henri Mondor, Créteil, France)
Ann Thorac Surg 66:60-67, 1998   3–47

Objective.—With the aging of the population, cardiac surgeons are more frequently performing surgery on older, higher-risk patients. Records of 191 consecutive patients, aged 80 years or older, who underwent cardiac surgery were reviewed to identify risk factors for early and late postoperative mortality, impaired function, and reduced quality of life.

Methods.—Between January 1, 1991 and December 31, 1996, 191 patients (98 men), aged 80 to 91 years, in New York Heart Association class III or IV and a mean left ventricular ejection fraction of 0.55, underwent aortic valve replacement (n = 110), coronary artery bypass (n = 47), combined aortic valve replacement and coronary artery bypass grafting (n = 26), mitral valve replacement (n = 5), and other procedures (n = 3). Outcome measures were postoperative complications and 30-day hospital mortality rate. The patients, patients' relatives, or patients' physicians were interviewed by telephone.

Results.—The mean postoperative ICU stay was 6 days, and the mean postoperative hospital stay was 9.5 days. Complications occurring in 132 patients (91%) included cardiovascular in 82.6%, pulmonary in 32.5%, stroke in 9.4%, intra-abdominal complications requiring operative intervention in 2.1%, renal failure in 12.0%, and infection in 10%. The in-hospital mortality rate was 16.2%. Actuarial survivals at 1, 3, and 5 years were 79.2%, 74.9%, and 56.2%, respectively. The overall mortality rate was 31.0%. The most common causes of death were cardiac related. According to multivariate analysis, preoperative pulmonary hypertension and lower left ventricular ejection fraction were independent predictors of in-hospital mortality. Independent predictors of late mortality were combined aortic valve replacement, coronary artery bypass grafting, and female sex. At follow-up, 129 patients (63.6%) were completely autonomous. According to multivariate analysis, female sex was an independent risk factor for impaired autonomy. Subjective quality-of-life assessments revealed that 83% were satisfied, 8.55% were somewhat satisfied, and 7.8% were dissatisfied.

Conclusion.—The outcome after cardiac surgery in octogenarians is favorable, with the majority maintaining long-term autonomy and satisfactory quality of life.

Cost-Effectiveness of Coronary Artery Bypass Surgery in Octogenarians
Sollano JA, Rose EA, Williams DL, et al (Columbia Univ, New York)
Ann Surg 228:297-306, 1998   3–48

Objective.—Survival, quality of life, and economic outcomes are important issues to evaluate when considering the efficacy and cost effectiveness of coronary artery bypass graft (CABG) surgery in octogenarians. Results of a retrospective relative effectiveness, and cost-effectiveness analysis of CABG surgery vs. medical management in octogenarians was reported.

Methods.—Retrospectively, 2 cohorts were formed of patients with significant multivessel coronary artery disease treated with CABG (n = 176; 57% male; aged 80 to 90 years) or with medical management (n = 48; 75% male; aged 80 to 89 years) at Columbia Presbyterian Medical Center between 1992 and 1996. Medically managed patients were reasonable surgical candidates. End points were health outcomes, cost, and cost effectiveness.

Results.—Surgical and medically managed patients were followed for up to 38 and 31 months, respectively, and 3-year survivals were 80% and 64%, respectively. The perioperative mortality rate was 6.8%. A subgroup of medically managed patients who refused CABG had a 50% 10-month survival rate. EuroQol questionnaire scores were 64% for the surgical cohort and 73% for the medically managed cohort, with the surgical cohort scoring significantly better across all 5 dimensions. Average utility scores were 0.84 for the surgical cohort, 0.61 for the medically managed cohort, and 0.74 for a medically managed subgroup who refused CABG surgery. The costs of the index hospitalization for the surgery, medically managed, and medically managed subgroup patients were $41,348,

$12,467, and $15,232. The cost per quality-adjusted life years gained in comparing the surgical cohort with the medically managed cohort was $10,424, and in comparing the surgical cohort with the medically managed subgroup it was $9,423.

Conclusion.—CABG in octogenarians is cost effective and increases quality of life.

▶ These papers by Khan, Kirsch, and Sollano (Abstracts 3–46 to 3–48) demonstrate that the great interest in performing cardiac surgical operations in older patients continues. We, like many, are experiencing a gradual rise in the mean age of our patients. It is now not unusual to operate on patients over 80 years old on a daily basis. There can be no question that higher costs will be seen in older patients, although there is also no doubt that these patients will usually do well and are often totally rehabilitated for substantial lengths of time.

J.J. Collins, Jr., M.D.

Aortic Valve Replacement for Octogenarians: Are Small Valves Bad?
Medalion B, Lytle BW, McCarthy PM, et al (Cleveland Clinic Found, Ohio)
Ann Thorac Surg 66:699-706, 1998   3–49

Introduction.—Many octogenarians are candidates for aortic valve replacement, and many of the women have a small aortic annulus that causes uncertainty about optimal management. A residual gradient may result from small aortic prostheses, and the procedure can become more complicated with aortic root enlargement. The short- and long-term outcomes of aortic valve replacement in octogenarians were reviewed to determine whether small valve sizes were associated with a bad late clinical outcome.

Methods.—There were 248 octogenarians with a mean age of 82.6 ± 2.3 who had aortic valve replacement in 15 years. Of these patients, 99 had primary isolated aortic valve replacement and 149 had aortic valve replacement and coronary revascularization. In 26% of patients, 19-mm valves were used.

Results.—There was an 8.9% in-hospital mortality. Aortic valve replacement alone resulted in 5% mortality and aortic valve replacement and coronary revascularization resulted in 11.4% mortality. The 19-mm valves were associated with a 12.5% mortality, whereas the bigger valves were associated with a 7.7% mortality. At 1 year, survival was 85% and survival free from cardiovascular events was 80%. At 5 years, survival was 60% and survival free from cardiovascular events was 45%. At 10 years, survival was 30% and survival free from cardiovascular events was 21%. Triple-vessel disease and preoperative congestive heart failure were associated with increased risk for both in-hospital and late mortality, as identified with multivariate analysis. Late survival and event-free survival were not influenced by valve size, regardless of body surface area.

Conclusion.—The incidence of early or late mortality or of cardiac events is not adversely affected by the use of small aortic valve prostheses in octogenarians.

▶ This article fails to demonstrate a disadvantage in the use of small aortic valves in patients undergoing aortic valve replacement. Unfortunately, these authors do not consider any measurement of ventricular mass or whether survival may have been different in patients with large body surface area, in whom size mismatch would have been particularly severe.

J.J. Collins, Jr., M.D.

4 Coronary Heart Disease

Introduction

The last year has been exciting from a scientific standpoint and has been characterized by change as we grapple with the realities of providing optimum care in an environment of declining reimbursements. These constraints apply across the world, irrespective of the systems for health care delivery in different countries.

The sheer breadth of publications about coronary artery disease requires that the abstracts of the selected articles reflect the spectrum of new advances. Unfortunately, they cannot encompass more than a small segment.

The majority of the abstracts in the 1999 YEAR BOOK deal with the acute coronary syndromes and the role of thrombolytics vs. primary percutaneous transluminal coronary angioplasty. Another large section deals with the epidemiology of coronary disease and the emerging impact of the nontraditional risk factors on the incidence and prognosis of coronary artery disease. Advances in the secondary prevention of coronary artery disease and the explosion of new approaches to coronary revascularization by catheter-based techniques and bypass surgery are represented by selected papers. But even these do not do justice to all the advances made in these respective disciplines during the last year. Lastly, we should realize that the benefits of contemporary cardiovascular science and therapeutics have not been applied equally across nations and within countries or across all socioeconomic and racial groups. The relatively few papers addressing this topic in this YEAR BOOK should not belie the importance of the issue.

The year ends as it began. Advances in basic and clinical knowledge generate excitement and a continuation of opportunity for translational research and of the challenges involved in bringing these advances to the bedside. These challenges are compounded by the increasing role of fiscal realities on the practice of medicine in an environment of explosive growth, especially in the utilization of techniques based on scientific discovery. It is not the ideal situation, but one can envision many scenarios that are worse.

B.J. Gersh, M.B., Ch.B., D.Phil., F.R.C.P.

Myocardial Infarction: Acute and Long-term Prognosis

A Comparison of the Early Outcome of Acute Myocardial Infarction in Women and Men

Malacrida R, for the Third International Study of Infarct Survival Collaborative Group (Civic Hosp, Lugano, Switzerland; Mario Negri Inst, Milan, Italy; Univ of Oxford, England)

N Engl J Med 338:8-14, 1998   4–1

Background.—In previous gender-based studies of mortality and morbidity associated with myocardial infarctions, women have fared worse than men. However, these studies were not completely adjusted for coexisting conditions, including age. These studies also sampled a smaller test group than is needed to understand fully the gender implications of this condition. This larger study works to present a more accurate picture of the above by analyzing coexisting conditions.

Methods.—Researchers used data collected during the Third International Study of Infarct Survival (ISIS-3) which spanned days 0 to 35 of hospitalization and recorded major clinical events during this period. Women included in the study numbered 9,600 and men numbered 26,480. The women studied were older and more likely to have diabetes than the men. Test subjects were diagnosed with acute myocardial infarction, and physicians considered them candidates for fibrinolytic therapy. Researchers compiled data using the three following multiple logistic regression groups: (1) outcome in men and women without adjustment, (2) outcome in both sexes with adjustment for age, and (3) outcome with adjustment for other unfavorable prognostic factors recorded at baseline.

Results.—The odds ratios for each of the above groups (women versus men) are as follows. (1) Unadjusted was 1.73 (95% confidence interval, 1.61 to 1.86). (2) When adjusted for age (women were older than men), the ratio was 1.20 (95% confidence interval, 1.11 to 1.29). (3) When adjusted for other conditions (women were in worse condition than men), the ratio was 1.14 (95% confidence interval, 1.05 to 1.23) (Table 5).

Conclusion.—In a previous study that did not use adjustments, mortality was 40% higher for women than for men. In this same study, age adjustment dropped this figure to under 20%, making it unclear whether age and condition accounted for all of the difference between men and women. However, in this study, age adjustment reduced the unadjusted mortality figure by two thirds, and adjustment for other characteristics reduced this figure by another one third. The remaining 14% difference in men and women studied could well be the result of residual differences in characteristics of the test subjects.

TABLE 5.—Comparisons of Major Clinical Events During Hospitalization up to Day 35 Among the Women and Men, Before and After Adjustment for Age and Other Covariates*

Clinical Event	Women (N=9478) no. (%)	Men (N=26,147)	Unadjusted Odds Ratio (95% CI)	Odds Ratio Adjusted for Age (95% CI)	Odds Ratio Adjusted for Age and Other Covariates (95% CI)
Cardiogenic shock	979 (10.3)	1592 (6.1)	1.78 (1.63-1.93)	1.33 (1.22-1.45)	1.29 (1.17-1.42)
Heart failure	2050 (21.6)	4196 (16.0)	1.44 (1.36-1.53)	1.12 (1.05-1.19)	1.08 (1.02-1.16)
Cardiac rupture	229 (2.4)	266 (1.0)	2.41 (2.02-2.88)	1.70 (1.41-2.04)	1.62 (1.34-1.96)
Cardiac arrest	1137 (12.0)	2505 (9.6)	1.29 (1.19-1.39)	1.07 (0.99-1.16)	1.03 (0.95-1.11)
Reinfarction	433 (4.6)	777 (3.0)	1.56 (1.39-1.76)	1.34 (1.19-1.52)	1.35 (1.19-1.53)
Any stroke	157 (1.7)	263 (1.0)	1.66 (1.36-2.02)	1.21 (0.98-1.48)	1.16 (0.94-1.43)
Cerebral hemorrhage	57 (0.6)	101 (0.4)	1.56 (1.13-2.16)	1.19 (0.85-1.66)	1.12 (0.80-1.58)
Major bleeding	140 (1.5)	181 (0.7)	2.15 (1.72-2.69)	1.74 (1.38-2.19)	1.68 (1.33-2.12)

*Information on clinical events in the hospital was not available for all patients.

Abbreviations: CI, confidence interval.

(Reprinted by permission of *The New England Journal of Medicine* from Malacrida R, for the Third International Study of Infarct Survival Collaborative Group: A Comparison of the early outcome of acute myocardial infarction in women and men. *N Engl J Med* 338:8-14. Copyright 1998, Massachusetts Medical Society. All rights reserved.)

The adjusted ratios above suggest that women were not only older at the time of infarction but also were in much worse condition. Thus, female sex in itself cannot be considered more than a small independent associated risk in early mortality and morbidity in acute myocardial infarction.

▶ This very large substudy from a randomized trial database re-emphasizes the higher mortality of acute myocardial infarction in women in comparison with men.[1] The increased mortality can be accounted for almost completely by differences in age and in other baseline variables. Women in the study were not only older but also "sicker" in that they presented later after the onset of symptoms and were more likely to be diabetic. Virtually every other study has demonstrated a higher mortality in women and in those in which an adjustment could be made on the basis of baseline variables. The conclusions were that older age and other associated prognostic factors accounted for most of the difference in outcomes, although in some series, there appeared to be an independent adverse prognostic impact of female gender.[2]

What needs to be emphasized is that these data from the ISIS-3 trial apply to a large randomized population and, as such, relate to a very specific and carefully selected group of patients. Patients in randomized trials also have equal access to care. Whether the higher mortality in the community in women compared to men is related in part to different levels of access to care, a higher incidence of contra-indications to thrombolytic therapy and therefore less utilization of this procedure, or less exposure to invasive procedures, remains to be seen. Nonetheless, it would appear that the bulk of the difference in outcomes between men and women is readily understandable on the basis of the older age and greater incidence of other risk factors.

What was also of great interest in the study is the longer time between the onset of pain and randomization in women than in men. This has been shown in other trials, and the explanations are probably multifactorial. It may involve issues of access to care, the ability of single women to receive prompt therapy, and other patient-related factors, for example, denial of symptoms on the assumption that heart attacks are more likely to involve men than women. This is an area that needs further evaluation.

B.J. Gersh, M.B., Ch.B., D.Phil., F.R.C.P.

References

1. Vaccarino V, Krumholz HM, Berkman LF et al: Sex differences in mortality after myocardial infarction: Is there evidence for an increased risk for women? *Circulation*, 91:1861-1871, 1995.
2. Kostis JB, Wilson AC, O'Dowd K et al: Sex differences in the management and long-term outcome of acute myocardial infarction: A statewide study. *Circulation*, 90:1715-1730, 1994.

Coronary Angioscopic Findings in the Infarct-related Vessel Within 1 Month of Acute Myocardial Infarction: Natural History and the Effect of Thrombolysis

Van Belle E, Lablanche J-M, Bauters C, et al (Hôpital Cardiologique, Lille Cedex, France)
Circulation 97:26-33, 1998

4–2

Purpose.—Re-occlusion is a major risk in recent myocardial infarction (MI)-related lesions. Coronary angioscopy has provided a great deal of useful information on the characteristics of plaque and thrombi. However, it has been little used to study the natural history of infarct-related plaque after MI, or the effects of thrombolytic therapy. This study used angioscopy to study the morphology and natural history of infarct-related plaque, including the effects of thrombolysis.

Methods.—Coronary angioscopy of the infarct-related lesion was performed in 56 patients with recent MI (within 1 month). Forty patients received initial thrombolytic therapy; the rest were managed conservatively. The morphologic findings of the infarct-related lesion were ana-

TABLE 4.—Relation of Angioscopic Characteristics to the Time Elapsed Between Myocardial Infarction and Angioscopy

	≤8 Days (n=18)	8<≤10 Days (n=10)	10<≤15 Days (n=14)	>15 Days (n=14)	p
Plaque shape, n (%)					
Smooth*	6 (37)	7 (87)	3 (30)	4 (40)	.22
Complex	3 (19)	0 (0)	2 (20)	3 (30)	
Ulcerated	7 (44)	1 (13)	5 (50)	3 (30)	
Total	16 (100)	8 (100)	10 (100)	10 (100)	
Predominant plaque color, n (%)					
White	4 (23)	2 (22)	3 (23)	2 (15)	.95
Yellow	13 (76)	7 (78)	10 (77)	11 (85)	
Total	17 (100)	9 (100)	13 (100)	13 (100)	
Darkest color of the plaque, n (%)					
White	0 (0)	0 (0)	2 (15)	1 (8)	.27
Yellow	17 (100)	9 (100)	11 (85)	3 (93)	
Total	17 (100)	9 (100)	13 (100)	13 (100)	
Thrombus, n (%)					
Absence	3 (17)	3 (30)	4 (29)	3 (21)	.95
Presence	15 (83)	7 (70)	10 (71)	11 (79)	
Total	18 (100)	10 (100)	14 (100)	14 (100)	
Thrombus size, n (%)					
Lining	8 (53)	6 (86)	7 (70)	5 (45)	.31
Protruding	7 (47)	1 (14)	3 (30)	6 (55)	
Total	15 (100)	7 (100)	10 (100)	11 (100)	
Thrombus color, n (%)					
White	1 (7)	2 (29)	1 (10)	3 (28)	.54
Red	3 (20)	2 (42)	3 (30)	4 (36)	
Mixed	11 (73)	3 (29)	6 (60)	4 (36)	
Total	15 (100)	7 (100)	10 (100)	11 (100)	

Some angioscopic variables were not evaluable in individual patients (see Table 3).
*Smooth includes smooth concentric and smooth eccentric defined in Table 2.
(Courtesy of Van Belle E, Lablanche J-M, Baueters C, et al: Coronary angioscopic findings in the infarct-related vessel within 1 month of acute myocardial infarction: natural history and the effect of thrombolysis. *Circulation* 97:26-33, 1998.)

TABLE 5.—Relation Between Angioscopic Characteristics and the
Prior Administration of Thrombolytic Therapy

	Thrombolysis (n=40)	No Thrombolysis (n=16)	P
Plaque shape, n (%)			
Smooth	12 (39)	8 (61)	.17
Complex	5 (16)	3 (23)	
Ulcerated	14 (45)	2 (16)	
Total	31 (100)	13 (100)	
Predominant plaque color, n (%)			
White	7 (31)	4 (18)	.32
Yellow	32 (69)	9 (82)	
Total	39 (100)	13 (100)	
Darkest color of the plaque, n (%)			
White	0 (0)	3 (23)	.01
Yellow	39 (100)	10 (77)	
Total	39 (100)	13 (100)	
Thrombus, n (%)			
Absence	7 (18)	6 (37)	.12
Presence	33 (82)	10 (63)	
Total	40 (100)	16 (100)	
Thrombus size, n (%)			
Lining	23 (70)	3 (30)	.02
Protruding	10 (30)	7 (70)	
Total	33 (100)	10 (100)	
Thrombus color, n (%)			
White	4 (12)	3 (30)	.15
Red	8 (24)	3 (30)	
Mixed	21 (64)	4 (40)	
Total	33 (100)	10 (100)	

Some angioscopic variables were not evaluable in individual patients (see Table 3).
*Smooth includes smooth concentric and smooth eccentric defined in Table 2.
(Courtesy of Van Belle E, Lablanche J-M, Baueters C, et al: Coronary angioscopic findings in the infarct-related vessel within 1 month of acute myocardial infarction: natural history and the effect of thrombolysis. *Circulation* 97:26-33, 1998.)

lyzed, and the natural history was evaluated in terms of time since MI. The effects of thrombolytic therapy on the angioscopic findings were analyzed as well.

Results.—The angioscopic picture was a complex lesion with an ulcerated shape in 54% of patients. The plaque was mainly yellow in 79% of patients, purely white in just 6%. Seventy-seven percent of patients had angioscopically visible thrombus. Though just 7% of patients had angina after MI, angioscopy commonly showed signs of instability. The angioscopic findings did not change significantly within the month after MI, though there was a slight increase in white plaque (Table 4). Thrombolytic therapy was associated with reduced thrombus size and less protruding thrombi. However, the frequency of plaque containing thrombi was unchanged, and the incidence of ulcerated plaques was nonsignificantly increased from 16% to 45% (Table 5).

Conclusions.—The angioscopic appearance of recent MI-related plaque is described. Such lesions require longer than one month to heal, the results suggest. During that time, many lesions show "unstable" yellow plaque with adherent thrombus. This finding could partially account for the tendency of recent infarct-related lesions to reocclude. The effects of thrombolytic therapy on plaque stabilization are not as impressive as its clinical benefits.

▶ This elegant study using intracoronary angioscopy provides a pathophysiological explanation for the high incidence of re-occlusion in the month after thrombolysis and also for the higher rates of restenosis and re-occlusion after percutaneous transluminal coronary angioplasty (PTCA) of recent infarct-related lesions.[1]

This study suggests that the process of vascular healing requires at least one month. During that period of time, the milieu of an unstable complex plaque with persistent thrombus and ulcerated lesions is present in the majority of infarct-related vessels. It is interesting to note that thrombolytic therapy appears to reduce thrombus burden and the presence of "protruding thrombus," but it does *not* increase plaque stability. On the contrary, prior lytic therapy may enhance the frequency of unstable residual plaque, perhaps by exposing an underlying ulcerated lesion that is inherently unstable.

These data certainly imply that there is a great window of opportunity for the newer classes of platelet inhibitors and stents. Time will tell, but I suspect that the answers will be forthcoming, sooner rather than later.

B.J. Gersh, M.B., Ch.B., D.Phil., F.R.C.P.

Reference

1. Meijer A, Verheugt FWA, Werter CJPJ et al: Aspirin versus coumadin in the prevention of reocclusion and recurrent ischemia after successful thrombolysis and coronary prospective placebo-controlled angiographic study. *Circulation*, 87:1524-1530, 1993.

Non–Q-Wave Versus Q-Wave Myocardial Infarction After Thrombolytic Therapy: Angiographic and Prognostic Insights From the Global Utilization of Streptokinase and Tissue Plasminogen Activator for Occluded Coronary Arteries-I Angiographic Substudy
Goodman SG, for the GUSTO-I Angiographic Investigators (Univ of Toronto; Duke Univ, Durham, NC; George Washington Univ, Washington, DC; et al)
Circulation 97:444-450, 1998   4–3

Objective.—The appearance of abnormal new Q waves on ECG is a clinically and prognostically important factor in patients with acute myocardial infarction. However, there are few data on the effects of thrombolytic therapy and the subsequent development of Q waves or on the prognosis of non–Q-wave infarction. Using data from the Global Utilization of Streptokinase and Tissue Plasminogen Activator for Occluded Coronary Arteries-I (GUSTO-I) angiographic substudy, the investigators analyzed the impact of thrombolytic therapy on non–Q-wave and Q-wave myocardial infarction.

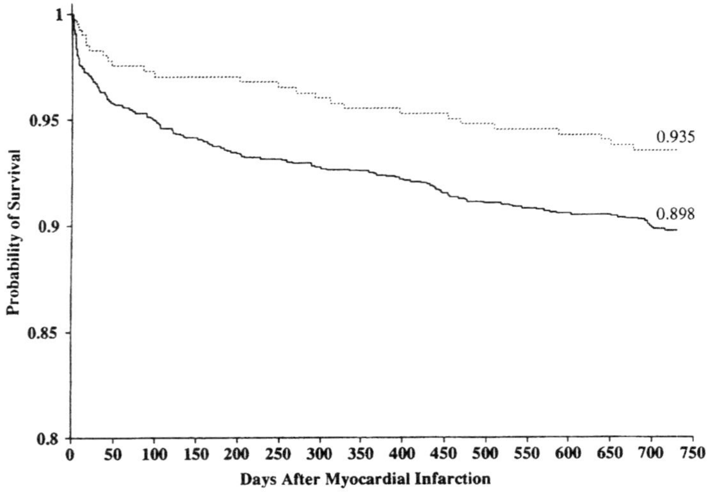

FIGURE 2.—Kaplan-Meier Plot of 2-Year Survival Among Patients Who Developed Non–Q-Wave (Dashed Line, n = 409) or Q wave (Solid Line, n = 1637) MI After Thrombolysis. (Courtesy of Goodman SG, for the GUSTO-I Angiographic Investigators: Non–Q-wave versus Q-wave myocardial infarction after thrombolytic therapy: angiographic and prognostic insights from the Global Utilization of Streptokinase and Tissue Plasminogen Activator for Occluded Coronary Arteries-I Angiographic Substudy. *Circulation* 97:440-450, 1998. Reproduced with permission, copyright 1998, American Heart Association.)

Methods.—The analysis included 2,046 patients with ST-segment elevation infarction. The presence of Q-wave myocardial infarction was assessed from a follow-up ECG performed 24 hours or longer after initiation of thrombolysis. The ECG, coronary anatomy, left ventricular function, and mortality data were analyzed to assess the pathophysiology and prognosis of Q-wave versus non–Q-wave infarction after thrombolytic therapy.

Results.—The rate of non–Q-wave myocardial infarction was 20%. Patients with non–Q-wave myocardial infarction had significantly lower maximal CK and CK-MB values than those with Q-wave infarction. The non–Q-wave patients also had lower ECG indicators of infarct severity than the Q-wave patients; that is, the median number of leads with ST-segment elevation was 3 in the non–Q-wave patients versus 4 in the Q-wave patients. In non–Q-wave infarctions, the infarct-related artery was more likely to be nonanterior and distally located. The non–Q-wave patients had greater early and complete infarct-related patency and better global and regional left ventricular function. In-hospital mortality tended to be lower in the non–Q-wave group (1.5% vs. 3.0%). After 2 years, the difference in mortality was significant (6.4% vs. 10.1%) (Fig 2). On multivariate analysis, non–Q-wave myocardial infarction was an independent predictor of reduced 2-year mortality. There was no significant difference in the use of in-hospital coronary revascularization between groups. Patients with non–Q-wave infarction were less likely to have cardiogenic shock and congestive heart failure, but there was no difference in the rate of reinfarction, recurrent ischemia, or stroke.

Conclusions.—Patients with non–Q-wave myocardial infarction have an excellent prognosis after thrombolytic therapy. This prognostic advantage is related to their high rate of early, complete, and sustained infarct-related patency, leading to limited left ventricular infarction and dysfunction. Among patients with non–Q-wave infarction, mortality is similar whether in-hospital revascularization is performed.

▶ Studies from the prethrombolytic era suggested that although non–Q-wave MI was associated with a lower in-hospital mortality rate, cardiac events after discharge, including re-infarction and late mortality were increased in comparison to patients with Q-wave myocardial infarctions. This was attributed to the lower rate of initial total coronary occlusion followed by thrombus progression, in addition to the presence of extensive collaterals to the infarct-related artery[1] and a greater prevalence of diffuse and multivessel disease.[2]

This study (the largest among a population treated with thrombolytic therapy) highlights the dramatic differences in a population of patients with non–Q-wave myocardial infarction undergoing thrombolysis (presenting primarily with ST-segment elevation) versus patients in the prethrombolytic era who presented primarily with ST-segment depression. Non–Q-Wave myocardial infarction in patients treated with lytics is a marker of early, complete, and sustained perfusion of the infarct-related artery; less disease of the left anterior descending coronary artery; a lower prevalence of multivessel disease; and an excellent prognosis with a lower hospital and 2-year mortality in comparison with thrombolytic-treated patients who develop Q waves.

This study has implications for predischarge risk stratification and treatment. Whereas a more aggressive approach is justified in patients presenting with ST-segment depression who evolve to a non–Q-wave myocardial infarction (without lytic therapy), in the subset of patients described in this study, 30-day and 1-year mortality rates are strikingly low, irrespective of whether patients underwent revascularization. This certainly would justify a conservative approach at the time of discharge.

B.J. Gersh, M.B., Ch.B., D.Phil, F.R.C.P.

References

1. DeWood, M.A., Stifter WF, Simpson CS, et al: Coronary arteriographic findings soon after non–Q-wave myocardial infarction. *N Engl J Med* 315:417-423, 1986.
2. Gibson RS, Beller GA, Gheorghiade M, et al: The prevalence and clinical significance of residual myocardial ischemia 2 weeks after uncomplicated non-Q wave infarction: A prospective natural history study. *Circulation* 73:1186-1198, 1986.

Gender Difference in Autonomic and Hemodynamic Reactions to Abrupt Coronary Occlusion

Airaksinen KEJ, Ikäheimo MJ, Linnaluoto M, et al (Univ of Oulu, Finland; Univ of Tampere, Finland)
J Am Coll Cardiol 31:301-306, 1998

4-4

Introduction.—The clinical presentation of acute ischemic events may be modified by changes in heart rate, blood pressure, and heart rate variability. In patients with coronary artery disease, a temporal relationship between changes in heart rate variability and life-threatening ventricular tachyarrhythmias has also been demonstrated. In the autonomic modulation of heart rate, recent research has shown that there are gender-related differences. In a prospective series of patients having clinically indicated coronary angioplasty, potential gender-related differences in autonomic responses to abrupt coronary occlusions were assessed.

Methods.—In 149 men and 65 women referred for single-vessel coronary angioplasty, the changes in heart rate, heart rate variability and blood pressure and the occurrence of ventricular ectopic beats during a 2-minute coronary occlusion were analyzed. By analyzing a control group of 19 patients with no ischemia during a 2-minute balloon inflation in a totally

TABLE 2.—Signs of Ischemia, Ventricular Ectopic Beats, and Abnormal Reactions in Heart Rate, Systolic Blood Pressure, and Heart Rate Variability During Balloon Occlusion of Coronary Artery Stenosis by Gender

	Women (n=65)	Men (n=140)	p Value
Chest pain	49 (75)	83 (59%)	< 0.05
Severity*	3.1 ±2.3	2.4 ± 2.1	< 0.05
ST seg changes	42 (65%)	59 (42%)	< 0.01
Bradycardia	20 (31%)	18 (13%)	< 0.01
Severe	14 (22%)	7 (5%)	< 0.001
B-J reaction†	10 (16%)	1 (0.7%)	< 0.0001
Tachycardia	12 (19%)	13 (9%)	NS
Severe	5 (8%)	2 (1%)	< 0.05
HR variability‡			
Increase	16 (25%)	16 (11%)	< 0.05
Decrease	5 (8%)	7 (5%)	NS
Hypotension†	18 (28%)	15 (11%)	< 0.01
Severe	10 (17%)	6 (4%)	< 0.01
VEBs§	5 (8%)	18 (13%)	NS

Note: Data presented are mean values ± standard deviation.

*Borg scale (Borg G, Holmgren A, Lindblad I: Quantitative evaluation of chest pain. *Acta Med Scand* 209 (suppl 644): 43-45, 1981) of severity of pain: 1 to 10.

†Data for only 134 men and 64 women because of technical failure in blood pressure recordings in 6 men and 1 woman, of whom 1 man and 1 woman had significant heart rate reactions.

‡Data for only 139 men and 64 women because of extrasystoles during the occlusion data, which made the analysis unreliable in 2 cases.

§Data for only 125 men and 60 women (15 men and 5 women with at least 1 ventricular ectopic beat in the baseline period were excluded).

Abbreviations: B-J, Bezold-Jarisch; *seg*, segment; *VEB*, ventricular ectopic beat; *HR*, heart rate.

(Reprinted with permission from the American College of Cardiology courtesy of Airaksinen KEJ, Ikaheimo MJ, Linnaluoto M, et al: Gender difference in autonomic and hemodynamic reactions to abrupt coronary occlusion. *J Am Coll Cardiol* 31:301-306, 1998.)

occluded coronary artery, the ranges of nonspecific responses were determined.

Results.—During the occlusion, women had ST segment changes and chest pain more often than men (Table 2). Women had significant bradycardia (31% vs. 13%) or increase in heart rate variability (25% vs. 11%) as a sign of vagal activation compared with men. A decrease in blood pressure was caused by coronary occlusion more often among women than men (28% vs. 11%). The incidence of Bezold-Jarisch–type reaction (simultaneous bradycardia and decrease in blood pressure) was the most pronounced female preponderance (16% vs. 0.7%). An independent predictor of bradycardiac reactions, hypotensive reactions, and Bezold-Jarisch–type response was female gender, according to logistic regression models developed to analyze the significance of gender while controlling for baseline variables and signs of ischemia. There was borderline significance of female gender as a protector against early coronary occlusion–induced ventricular ectopic beats.

Conclusion.—During abrupt coronary occlusion, vagal activation is more common and may have beneficial antiarrhythmic effects, modifying the outcome of acute coronary events.

▶ This study is fascinating and emphasizes, yet again, gender differences in cardiac physiology and pathophysiology. It has been previously shown that the risk of sudden cardiac death before hospital admission in patients with myocardial infarction is higher in women.[1] This clinical study suggests that women have a greater vagal or parasympathetic response to coronary occlusion, and it has previously been shown in animal models that enhanced parasympathetic activity has protective antifibrillatory effects during acute myocardial ischemia. On the other hand, the greater propensity for females to have hypotensive and severe bradycardiac reactions to coronary occlusion may also contribute to the higher incidence of shock and syncope in women during myocardial infarction and of complications after percutaneous transluminal coronary angioplasty.[2]

B.J. Gersh, M.B., Ch.B., D.Phil., F.R.C.P.

References

1. Tunstall-Pedoe H, Morrison C, Woodward M, et al: Sex differences in myocardial infarction and cardiac death in the Scottish MONICA population of Glasgow 1985-1991: Presentation, diagnosis, treatment, and 28-day case fatality of 3991 events in men and 1551 events in women. *Circulation* 93:1981-1992, 1996.
2. Malenka DJ, O'Connor GT, Quinton H, et al: Differences in outcomes between women and men associated with percutaneous transluminal coronary angioplasty: A regional prospective study of 13,061 procedures. *Circulation* 94 (suppl II) II99-II104, 1996.

Baroreflex Sensitivity and Heart-Rate Variability in Prediction of Total Cardiac Mortality After Myocardial Infarction

La Rovere MT, for the ATRAMI (Autonomic Tone and Reflexes After Myocardial Infarction) Investigators (Fondazione "Salvatore Maugeri" Pavia, Italy)

Lancet 351:478-484, 1998   4–5

Background.—In survivors of acute myocardial infarction, left ventricular dysfunction and presence of frequent ventricular premature complexes each double the risk of death. It has been shown that the autonomic nervous system is involved in the triggering of sudden death. There is evidence that changes in autonomic balance might help identify patients who are at high risk of life-threatening arrhythmias during acute myocardial ischemia after myocardial infarction. The 2 autonomic markers currently receiving much attention are heart-rate variability and baroreflex sensitivity. There are clinical data that support the value of heart-rate variability in predicting risk after myocardial infarction.

Methods.—The Autonomic Tone and Reflexes After Myocardial Infarction (ATRAMI) study is a prospective, international, multicenter study designed to evaluate the independent prognostic value of baroreflex sen-

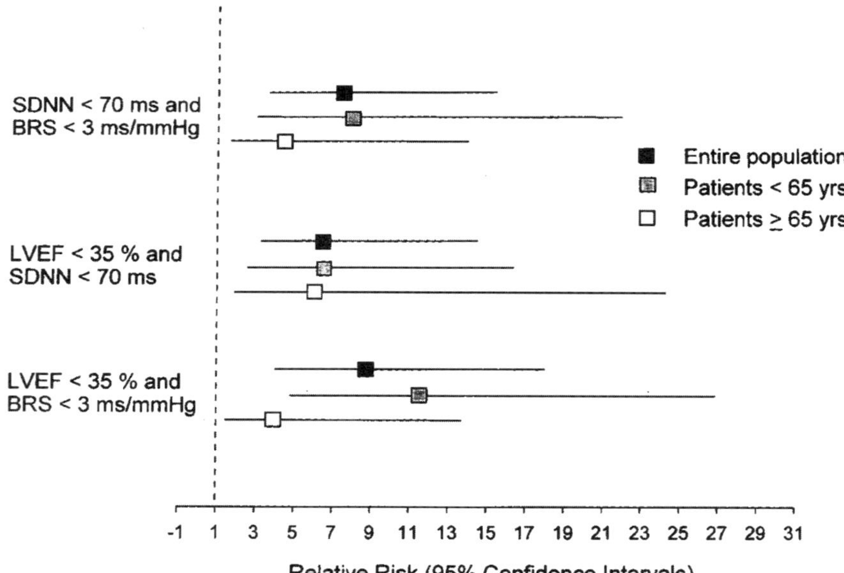

FIGURE 2.—Relative risks of total cardiac mortality for the combination of low standard deviation of all normal beats (*SDNN*) and baroreflex sensitivity (*BRS*) and for their association with low left ventricular ejection fraction (*LVEF*) in the whole study population and for patients younger than and older than 65 years. *Bars* indicate 95% confidence interval. (Courtesy of La Rovere MT, for the ATRAMI (Autonomic Tone and Reflexes After Myocardial Infarction) Investigators. Baroreflex sensitivity and heart rate variability in prediction of total cardiac mortality after myocardial infarction. *Lancet* 351:478-484, copyright 1998 by The Lancet Ltd.)

sitivity and to re-evaluate the value of heart-rate variability in predicting risk of cardiac mortality after myocardial infarction in patients with known left ventricular ejection fraction and ventricular arrhythmias. There were 1,284 patients enrolled who had had myocardial infarction within the previous 28 days. Heart-rate variability and ventricular arrhythmias were measured with 24-hour Holter recording; heart-rate variability was measured as the standard deviation of normal to normal reciprocal of heart rate intervals (SDNN). Baroreflex sensitivity was determined by measuring the rate-pressure response to IV phenylephrine. The main outcome measure was cardiac mortality. Follow-up was 21 months.

Results.—During follow-up, there were 44 cardiac deaths and 5 nonfatal cardiac arrests. A significant multivariate risk of cardiac mortality was seen with low values of either heart-rate variability or baroreflex sensitivity. A further increased risk was seen with an association of low SDNN and baroreflex sensitivity (Fig 2); the 2-year mortality rate was 2% when both were well-preserved and 17% when both were below the cutoff points. Compared with patients with a left ventricular ejection fraction higher than 35% and less compromised SDNN and baroreflex sensitivity, patients with low SDNN and a left ventricular ejection fraction of less than 35% had a relative risk of 6.7; patients with low baroreflex sensitivity and a left ventricular ejection fraction of less than 35% had a relative risk of 8.7.

Discussion.—These findings show that after myocardial infarction, analysis of vagal reflexes has significant independent predictive value independently of left ventricular ejection fraction and ventricular arrhythmias and significantly adds to the prognostic value of heart-rate variability. This study is limited by the protocol that required all patients to be eligible for an exercise stress test.

▶ The late prognosis of myocardial infarction in the reperfusion area is improving, and the lower incidence of late events is reflected in the declining positive predictive value of most of our standard tests that are used to risk stratify acute infarct survivors.[1] The strengths of the ATRAMI Study is that it is relatively recent (1991-1994) and, as such, documents a contemporary experience in 63% of the patients who receive thrombolytic therapy. Moreover, late cardiac mortality and nonfatal cardiac arrest rates were low.

Nonetheless, the 2 noninvasive indices of autonomic tone, namely, heart rate variability and baroreflex sensitivity, were independently predictive of cardiac mortality and nonfatal cardiac arrest. Moreover, these indices provided incremental information over and above that obtained by measurements of left ventricular ejection fraction and the frequency of ventricular premature extrasystoles.

Nonetheless, before we introduce these methods of risk stratification into clinical practice, additional studies need to be carried out. It appears that reduced heart rate variability and baroreflex sensitivity are associated with an absence of thrombolytic therapy and, presumably, a closed infarct-related artery. It would, therefore, be helpful to know whether the prognostic power of these indices holds up in the group who received reperfusion therapy and, presumably, had a patent infarct-related artery.

What is also unclear is the predictive value when one takes into account other clinical determinants of reduced autonomic sensitivity such as old age, female sex, and anterior myocardial infarction.[2] The editorial referenced here also questioned the impact of β-blockers and angiotensin-converting enzyme inhibitors on the findings of this study. These drugs were used in only 20% and 14% of patients, respectively, and it would be expected that more widespread use of these agents might have favorably altered mortality and affected the positive predictive value of the test. Despite these caveats, the ATRAMI study does point in a new direction for the identification of high-risk postinfarct survivors in the modern era. The next question to be answered is whether the prognosis can be improved by tailored therapy, including implantable defibrillators.

B.J. Gersh, M.B., Ch.B., D.Phil., F.R.C.P.

References

1. Shaw LJ, Peterson ED, Kesler K, et al: A metaanalysis of predischarge risk stratification after acute myocardial infarction with stress electrocardiographic, myocardial perfusion, and ventricular function imaging. *Am J Cardiol* 78:1327-1337, 1996.
2. Barron HV, Viskin S: Autonomic markers in prediction of cardiac death after myocardial infarction (editorial). *Lancet* 351:461-462, 1998.

Prospective Temporal Analysis of the Onset of Preinfarction Angina Versus Outcome: An Ancillary Study in TIMI-9B
Kloner RA, and the TIMI-9B Investigators (Good Samaritan Hosp, Los Angeles; Univ of Southern Calif, Los Angeles; Harvard Med School, Boston; et al)
Circulation 97:1042-1045, 1998   4–6

Objective.—Preinfarction angina pectoris has been shown in some studies to confer a protective effect on myocardial infarction (MI), possibly by initiating ischemic preconditioning. Few studies have examined the relationship between onset of angina and outcome after MI. The 30-day outcomes after MI were prospectively compared in patients with more than 24 hours or 24 hours or less between onset of angina and MI.

Methods.—Angina was reported before acute MI in 425 of 3,002 patients in the TIMI-9B study. Major cardiac events within 30 days of hospitalization were recorded. The 2 groups of patients were compared statistically.

Results.—Patients in the 24 hours or less group had significantly lower event rates than did patients in the more than 24 hours group (Table 1). Patients in the 24 hours or less group had nonsignificantly lower creatine kinase (CK) values than did patients in the more than 24 hours group (1,133 vs. 1,416). Patients in the 24 hours or less group had significantly

TABLE 1.—Time of Onset of Angina

	≤24 h	48 h	72 h	1 wk	1 mo	>1 mo	No Angina	>24 h	Any Time
No. of patients with events	2	8	4	19	9	23	309	63	65
Total No. of patients	45	41	34	99	93	113	2,577	380	425
%*	4%	20%	12%	19%	10%	20%	12%	17%	15%

*P=.03; 24 hours or less vs. more than 24 hours. (Courtesy of Kloner RA, and the TIMI-9B: Prospective temporal analysis of the onset of preinfarction angina versus outcome: An ancillary study in TIMI-9B. *Circulation* 97:1042-1045, 1998.)

lower maximum CK values than did patients without angina (1,133 vs. 1,570). A history of angina was not associated with a reduced rate of cardiac events. A reduced rate of cardiac events was not related to aspirin use, antianginal drugs, hypertension, or hypercholesterolemia.

Conclusion.—Patients with preinfarction angina had better outcomes than patients without preinfarction angina.

▶ Previous studies have demonstrated that preinfarction angina is associated with a better outcome and smaller infarcts in patients who go on to sustain an acute MI.[1] This prospective study takes the data one step further by demonstrating that the major benefit is in patients with angina onset within 24 hours of an MI, in whom 30-day cardiac events were significantly less than in patients without preceding angina or in those in whom the onset was more than 24 hours before infarction. This time frame is consistent with the concept of cardioprotection induced by ischemic preconditioning.[2, 3] The role of collaterals is less likely because they probably require more than 24 hours to develop. Alternative explanations lie in the possibility that patients with recent preinfarction angina have more complete thrombolysis because of an effect of antecedent ischemia on platelet-mediated thrombosis.[4] Whatever the mechanism, the data from this and many other studies all point in the same direction. Recent-onset angina within 24 hours of an MI is a marker of a more favorable early outcome. On the other hand, among patients with a long history of preceding angina, the opposite may be the case, as in many of these patients, because such a history is a marker of multivessel disease—an important determinant of an adverse late prognosis.

B.J. Gersh, M.B., Ch.B., D.Phil., F.R.C.P.

References

1. Anzi T, Yoshikawa T, Asakura Y, et al: Effect on short-term prognosis in left ventricular function of angina pectoris prior to first Q-wave anterior wall acute myocardial infarction. *Am J Cardiol* 74:755-759, 1994.
2. Ottani F, Galvani M, Ferrini D, et al: Prodromal angina limits infarct size: A role for ischemic preconditioning. *Circulation* 21:291-297, 1995.
3. Kloner RA, Yellon D: Does ischemic preconditioning occur in patients? *J Am Coll Cardiol* 24:1133-1142, 1994.
4. Hata K, Whittaker P, Kloner RA, et al: Brief antecedent ischemia attenuates platelet-mediated thrombosis in damaged and stenotic canine coronary arteries: Role of adenosine. *Circulation* 97:692-702, 1998.

Influence of Collateral Circulation on In-Hospital Death From Anterior Acute Myocardial Infarction

Pérez-Castellano N, García EJ, Abeytua M, et al ("Gregorio Marañón" Univ Gen Hosp, Madrid)
J Am Coll Cardiol 31:512-518, 1998

4–7

Introduction.—Nearly 40% of patients exhibit some degree of collateral circulation at the onset of acute myocardial infarction (AMI). Although some studies have shown a beneficial effect from the residual blood flow carried by collateral vessels, there is no evidence that collateral circulation improves prognosis after AMI. A study of 180 patients sought to determine whether the in-hospital prognosis of anterior AMI is influenced by pre-existent collateral circulation to the infarct-related artery.

Methods.—Eligible patients were admitted with suspected anterior wall AMI, showed complete occlusion of the left anterior descending coronary artery at diagnostic coronary angiography, and were treated by primary percutaneous transluminal coronary angioplasty within the first 6 hours of symptom onset. Angiographic assessment of collateral channels to the infarct-related artery before angioplasty established 2 patient groups: 115 patients without collateral vessels (group A), and 65 patients with collateral vessels (group B).

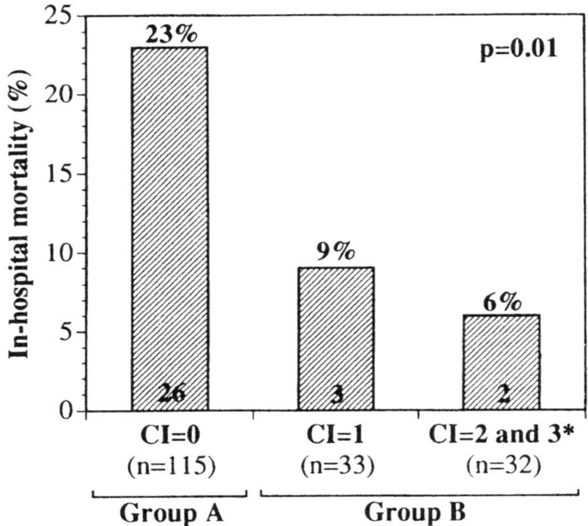

FIGURE 1.—Linear association between collateral index and in-hospital mortality rate (Mantel-Haenszel test, P = 0.01). *Abbreviation: CI,* collateral index. *Collateral indexes 2 and 3 were grouped because their expected values were less than 5. Collateral circulation was index 2 in 23 patients and index 3 in 9 patients; 1 patient from each of these subgroups died. (Reprinted with permission from the American College of Cardiology from Pérez-Castellano N, García EJ, Abeytua M, et al: Influence of collateral circulation on in-hospital death from anterior acute myocardial infarction. *J Am Coll Cardiol* 31:512-518, 1998.)

Results.—The 2 patient groups were similar in baseline characteristics, except that the prevalence of previous angina was greater in group B (34%) than in group A (15%). More hospital deaths occurred in group A (23%) than in group B (8%). Cardiogenic shock, which accounted for 74% of deaths, developed in 26% of group A patients vs. 6% of group B patients. A progressive decrease in the in-hospital mortality rate was noted (Fig 1) with increasing grades of collateral circulation.

Conclusion.—In this series of patients, the absence of collateral circulation appeared to be an independent predictor of both in-hospital death (odds ratio 3.4) and cardiogenic shock (odds ratio 5.6). By decreasing the occurrence of cardiogenic shock, the presence of operating collateral vessels to the left anterior descending coronary artery in the initial hours after anterior AMI reduced in-hospital mortality.

▶ This simple article provides quite striking clinical evidence of the benefits of the collateral circulation in patients with acute anterior myocardial infarction who are undergoing primary angioplasty. Some degree of collateral circulation is present in approximately 40% of patients with acute myocardial infarction, and prior studies have demonstrated a beneficial effect upon infarct size.[1] It is logical to assume that this might be translated into a reduced incidence of cardiogenic shock and improved survival, and this article suggests that this is indeed the case. It is of interest that patients with collaterals have an increased incidence of multivessel disease and preceding angina. The former might adversely affect prognosis, whereas the latter, if within the preceding 24 hours, might be beneficial via other mechanisms—for example, ischemic preconditioning.[2]

B.J. Gersh, M.B., Ch.B., D.Phil., F.R.C.P.

References

1. Christian TF, Schwartz RS, Gibbons RJ: Determinants of infarct size and reperfusion therapy for acute myocardial infarction. *Circulation* 86:81-90, 1992.
2. Yellon DM, Alkhulaifi AM, Pugsley WB: Preconditioning the human myocardium. *Lancet* 342:276-277, 1993.

Association Between Preinfarction Angina and a Lower Risk of Right Ventricular Infarction
Shiraki H, Yoshikawa T, Anzai T, et al (Yokohama Municipal Hosp, Japan; Keio Univ, Tokyo)
N Engl J Med 338:941-947, 1998   4–8

Introduction.—When inferior myocardial infarction caused by proximal occlusion of the right coronary artery occurs, the result is right ventricular infarction. Such infarctions are less common than would be expected from the frequency of proximal occlusion of the right coronary artery. The reasons for this are unclear. This study examined the possible

TABLE 6.—Association Between the Timing of Preinfarction Angina and the Short-term Outcome

Interval Between Angina and Onset of Infarction	Right Ventricular Infarction (N=53)		Complete Atrioventricular Block (N=24)		Hypotension and Shock (N=32)	
	Odds Ratio (95% CI)	P Value	Odds Ratio (95% CI)	P Value	Odds Ratio (95% CI)	P Value
24 Hr						
Univariate analysis	—	0.003	—	0.12	—	0.002
Multivariate analysis	0.7 (0.2-2.1)	0.47	0.5 (0.1-1.8)	0.30	0.4 (0.1-1.5)	0.18
24-72 Hr						
Univariate analysis	—	< 0.001	—	0.20	—	0.001
Multivariate analysis	0.2 (0-0.8)	0.02	0.4 (0.1-2.0)	0.32	0.1 (0-0.5)	0.02
72 Hr-1 wk						
Univariate analysis	—	0.002	—	0.54	—	0.02
Multivariate analysis	0.8 (0.2-3.8)	0.74	2.3 (0.4-18.3)	0.38	2.1 (0.2-26.2)	0.52

*P values were determined by logistic-regression analysis. Some patients had angina in more than 1 preinfarction interval. The odds ratios are for patients with angina during the interval in question, as compared with those patients without angina. Values are adjusted for age and sex and for the presence or absence of triple-vessel disease, proximal occlusion of the right coronary artery, hypertension, hypercholesterolemia, diabetes, and smoking.

Abbreviations: CI, confidence interval.

(Reprinted by permission of *The New England Journal of Medicine* from Shiraki H, Yoshikawa T, Anzai T, et al: Association between preinfarction angina and a lower risk of right ventricular infarction. *N Engl J Med* 338:941-947. Copyright 1998, Massachusetts Medical Society. All rights reserved.)

relationship between preinfarction angina and right ventricular infarction, including their short-term outcomes.

Methods.—The retrospective study included 113 patients with acute inferior myocardial infarction caused by right coronary artery occlusion. Of these patients, 62 had preinfarction angina—defined as at least 1 episode of typical chest pain, lasting less than 30 minutes, during the week before the infarction—and 51 did not. The investigators hypothesized that preinfarction angina was associated with a reduced incidence of right ventricular infarction, and thus with improved clinical outcome.

Results.—Patients without preinfarction angina were more likely to have right ventricular infarction (odds ratio 6.3, 95% confidence interval 2.7-15.1). They were also more likely to have complete atrioventricular block (odds ratio, 3.6; 95% confidence interval, 1.4-10.3) and combined hypotension and shock (odds ratio, 12.4; 95% confidence interval, 4.5-40.6). The strongest predictors of a reduced rate of right ventricular infarction were angina occurring 24 to 72 hours before infarction (adjusted odds ratio, 0.2; 95% confidence interval, 0-0.8) (Table 6) and combined hypotension and shock (adjusted odds ratio, 0.1; 95% confidence interval, 0-0.5). Patients with preinfarction angina had a lower incidence of ST-segment elevation in lead V_{4R}.

Conclusions.—Among patients with acute inferior myocardial infarction, preinfarction angina is independently associated with the absence of right ventricular infarction. The short-term outcomes of inferior infarctions are better when preinfarction angina occurs. The effects of delayed ischemic preconditioning may play a part in these favorable outcomes.

▶ What has been previously demonstrated in patients with anterior myocardial infarctions appears to apply to inferior and right ventricular myocardial infarctions.[1] Preinfarction angina is an independent predictor of the absence of right ventricular myocardial infarction in patients with acute inferior infarcts, and also a marker of better outcomes, characterized by a lower incidence of hypotension, shock, and complete atrio-ventricular block. The major impact of preinfarction angina was in patients in whom the interval between the last episode of angina and the onset of myocardial infarction was 24 to 72 hours. This finding is consistent with the effects of "delayed" ischemic preconditioning,[2] as opposed to the effect of "classic" preconditioning, in which the period of protection is brief. The mechanisms of protection by delayed preconditioning are unknown, but their eventual elucidation would open the window for the development of new pharmacologic approaches to myocardial protection.

B.J. Gersh, M.B., Ch.B., D.Phil., F.R.C.P.

References

1. Ottani F, Galvani M, Ferrini D, et al: Prodromal angina limits infarct size: A role for ischemic preconditioning. *Circulation* 91:291-297, 1995.
2. Yang XM, Baxter GF, Heads RJ, et al: Infarct limitation of the second window of protection in a conscious rabbit model. *Cardiovasc Res* 31:777-783, 1996.

Time to Therapy and Salvage in Myocardial Infarction
Milavetz JJ, Giebel DW, Christian TF, et al (Mayo Clinic and Mayo Found, Rochester, Minn)
J Am Coll Cardiol 31:1246-1251, 1998   4–9

Purpose.—Previous studies have suggested that earlier reperfusion is associated with improved outcome for patients with myocardial infarction (MI). However, even if perfusion is delayed, some patients have significant myocardial salvage. Time to reperfusion was evaluated as a determinant of myocardial salvage in patients undergoing reperfusion therapy.

Methods.—The study included 55 patients receiving successful angioplasty or thrombolysis after their first anterior MI. Reperfusion therapy was performed within 2 hours in 10 patients and after 2 hours in 45 patients. Before reperfusion therapy and at the time of hospital discharge, each patient underwent technetium-99m sestamibi studies to calculate the myocardial salvage index. The low point of the technetium-99m sestamibi curve was used to determine residual flow to the territory of the infarct.

Results.—The salvage index ranged from −0.4 to 1.0; 9% of patients had a salvage index of less than 0.10, while 25% had one of greater than 0.90. Patients undergoing reperfusion therapy within 2 hours or having good residual blood flow were likely to have a high salvage index. Residual blood flow was significantly correlated with salvage only in patients treated after 2 hours. Residual blood flow interacted significantly with time to therapy: each factor influenced the value of the other (Fig 3). None

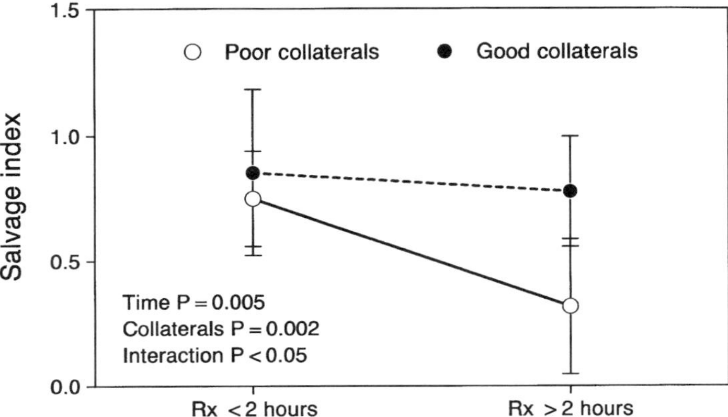

FIGURE 3.—Relation between time to reperfusion therapy (*Rx*) and residual blood flow on myocardial salvage index. Each variable, including interaction, was significant. (Reprinted with permission from the American College of Cardiology from Milavetz JJ, Giebel DW, Christian TF, et al: Time to therapy and salvage in myocardial infarction. *J Am Coll Cardiol* 31:1246-1251, 1998.)

of the historical or hemodynamic variables evaluated was significantly associated with residual flow or myocardial salvage.

Conclusions.—Reperfusion therapy provides the best results, in terms of myocardial salvage, if performed with 2 hours after acute MI. Thereafter, salvage rate appears to depend largely on the amount of residual blood flow to the infarct-related artery. These findings emphasize the importance of adequate collateral flow to the infarct territory in myocardial salvage.

▶ It is always reassuring when carefully collected clinical data support the animal models, and this article describes the relationships among infarct size, myocardium at risk, time to reperfusion, and the extent of the collateral circulation.[1] The implications for the preferred "routine" method of acute reperfusion therapy are quite provocative. Among patients first seen longer after the onset of symptoms, the time to reperfusion is less of a factor, and primary angioplasty is superior to thrombolytics in regard to the achievement of thrombolysis in MI Grade 3 flow—perhaps because with time, thrombi become more platelet-rich and more resistant to lytic agents. On the other hand, within the first 2 hours, time is of the essence, and at least during the first hour the key factor is speed, as opposed to the method of reperfusion (whether primary percutaneous transluminal coronary angioplasty or tissue-type plasminogen activator).

B.J. Gersh, M.B., Ch.B., D.Phil., F.R.C.P.

Reference

1. Reimer KA, Jennings RB, Cobb FR, et al: Animal models for protecting ischemic myocardium: Results of the NHLBI Cooperative Study. *Circ Res* 56:651-665, 1995.

Extended Mortality Benefit of Early Postinfarction Reperfusion

Ross AM, for the GUSTO-I Angiographic Investigators (George Washington Univ, Washington, DC; Thoraxcentrum, Rotterdam, The Netherlands; Duke Univ, Durham, NC; et al)
Circulation 97:1549-1556, 1998   4–10

Background.—Reperfusion therapy aims to restore flow to the infarct-related artery after acute myocardial infarction, thus preserving left ventricular function and survival. It was initially expected that successful reperfusion therapy would show increasing benefits over time. However, large clinical trials of thrombolytic therapy have shown maximum benefit

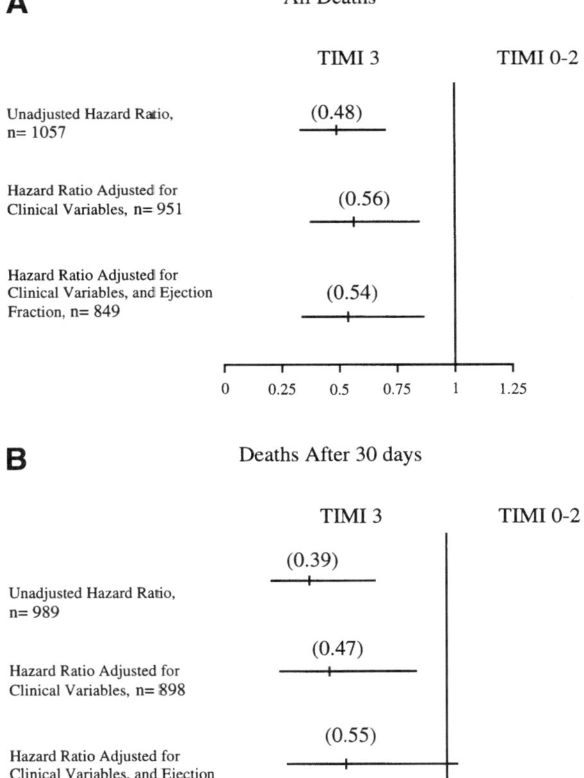

FIGURE 4.—Unadjusted and adjusted Thrombolysis in Myocardial Infarction (*TIMI*) flow hazard ratios and 95% confidence limits for 2-year mortality. **A**, hazard ratios calculated for all deaths; **B**, hazard ratios calculated for deaths that occurred after day 30. The number of patients entered into the model decreases after adjustment for clinical variables because of missing data and the absence of analyzable ventriculograms. (Courtesy of Ross AM, for the GUSTO-I Angiographic Investigators: Extended mortality benefit of early postinfarction reperfusion. *Circulation* 97:1549-1556, 1998.)

at 4 to 6 weeks, with no subsequent difference in survival. These studies compared the results in terms of assigned treatment, rather than treatment effectiveness. Data from the GUSTO-I study were analyzed to assess the impact of early, complete reperfusion on long-term survival.

Methods.—The analysis included data on 2,431 patients with myocardial infarction who were receiving 1 of 4 regimens of thrombolytic therapy. The patients were categorized as to whether or not they achieved early complete thrombolysis in myocardial infarction grade 3 (TIMI 3) flow in the infarct-related artery, and whether they achieved ejection fractions of 40% or less or of greater than 40%. The effects of these variables on 2-year survival were evaluated by Kaplan-Meier curves. Cox regression models were used to define hazard ratios for factors significantly affecting survival.

Results.—Survival beyond 30 days was significantly better for patients with early complete reperfusion and preserved ejection fraction. For patients with TIMI 3 flow, compared to those with lesser flow, unadjusted hazard ratio was 0.57 at 30 days and 0.39 at 30 to 688 days or beyond (Fig 4). Achieving early TIMI 3 flow reduced mortality by about 3 patients per 100 in the first month and 5 per 100 thereafter. Preserved ejection fraction was associated with an unadjusted hazard ratio of 0.25 at 30 days and of 0.20 thereafter. Lives saved by preserved ejection fraction at these intervals were 9 and 11 per 100, respectively.

Conclusions.—When reperfusion therapy provides early and complete restoration of flow to the infarct-related artery, with preservation of left ventricular function, the survival benefit continues to increase beyond the first postinfarction month. The findings emphasize the need for more effective reperfusion approaches. Cost-effectiveness analyses of reperfusion therapy should consider the additional late survival benefits.

▶ One of the more confusing aspects of the trials of thrombolytic therapy in studies to date has been the lack of any incremental late benefit in patients treated with thrombolytics. It appears that the maximum survival advantage was at 4 to 6 weeks, and thereafter the survival curves remained essentially parallel. One would have expected that the early effects of thrombolysis on myocardial salvage and left ventricular function would have translated into additional late benefits, with lower incidences of congestive heart failure and arrhythmia. This angiographic substudy, by documenting the presence or absence of normal flow (TIMI 3) is an important addition to the literature, because many prior studies used variables that were only indirectly related to perfusion. This GUSTO-1 article makes a case for the "open artery concept," by demonstrating a reduced late mortality in patients with TIMI 3 flow, *independent* of left ventricular ejection fraction—a surrogate for myocardial salvage. One needs to appreciate that this study antedates the use of stents, and the reocclusion rate in patients with initial TIMI 3 flow was probably quite high. One would expect even better long-term results in the current era.

B.J. Gersh, M.B., Ch.B., D.Phil., F.R.C.P.

Clinical Experience With Primary Percutaneous Transluminal Coronary Angioplasty Compared With Alteplase (Recombinant Tissue-type Plasminogen Activator) in Patients With Acute Myocardial Infarction: A Report From the Second National Registry of Myocardial Infarction (NRMI-2)

Tiefenbrunn AJ, Chandra NC, French WJ, et al (Washington Univ, St. Louis; Johns Hopkins Bayview Med Ctr, Baltimore, Md; Harbor Univ of California Los Angeles Med Ctr, Torrance; et al)

J Am Coll Cardiol 31:1240-1245, 1998   4–11

Introduction.—Results from a number of small studies comparing percutaneous transluminal coronary angioplasty (PTCA) with thrombolytic therapy in patients with acute myocardial infarction suggest a survival advantage for patients undergoing PTCA. Data from the Second National Registry of Myocardial Infarction were reviewed to describe the comparison of primary PTCA with alteplase (recombinant tissue-type plasminogen activator [rt-PA]) in a large number of patients.

Methods.—The phase IV study collected data from hospitals in 50 states. Eligible patients were transferred to participating hospitals and received treatment, either an IV thrombolytic agent or primary PTCA, within 12 hours of symptom onset. From June 1, 1994, through October 31, 1995, 4,939 patients underwent primary PTCA and 24,705 received rt-PA. Baseline characteristics of the 2 groups were similar after lytic-ineligible patients and those in cardiac shock at admission were excluded. Patients in the rt-PA group had thrombolytic therapy initiated at a median of 42 minutes after admission; the median time to first balloon inflation

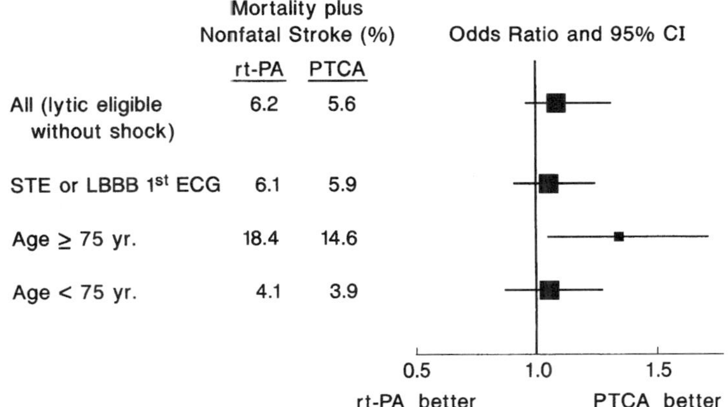

FIGURE 2.—Odds ratios and 95% confidence intervals for reduction in the combined end point of in-hospital mortality plus nonfatal stroke in patients treated with rt-PA compared with PTCA. *Abbreviations: rt-PA, recombinant tissue-type plasminogen activator; PTCA, percutaneous transluminal coronary angioplasty; CI, confidence interval.* (Reprinted with permission from the American College of Cardiology from Tiefenbrunn AJ, Chandra NC, French WJ, et al: Clinical experience with primary percutaneous transluminal coronary angioplasty compared with alteplase (recombinant tissue-type plasminogen activator) in patients with acute myocardial infarction: A report from the Second National Registry of Myocardial Infarction (NRMI-2). *J Am Coll Cardiol* 31:1240-1245, 1998.)

was 111 minutes after admission in the PTCA group, a significant difference.

Results.—In-hospital mortality was significantly higher in patients in shock after rt-PA (52%) than after PTCA (32%). Among lytic-eligible patients not in shock, the rate of in-hospital mortality was similar in the rt-PA (5.4%) and PTCA (5.2%) groups. Multiple logistic regression analysis was performed to determine variables predictive of increased mortality. Treatment modality was not an independent predictor of mortality, but increased mortality risk was independently predicted by Killip class 2 or 3, age 75 or greater, previous stroke, female gender, treatment interval greater than 4 hours from symptom onset, and anterior infarct location. Rate of reinfarction did not differ in the 2 groups (2.9% after rt-PA and 2.5% after PTCA), nor did the combined end point of death and nonfatal stroke (Fig 2).

Conclusion.—The Second National Registry of Myocardial Infarction data reflect recent clinical experience with a large number of patients treated at hospitals across the United States. For lytic-eligible patients not in shock after acute myocardial infarction, PTCA and rt-PA offer alternative means of reperfusion, yielding similar rates of in-hospital mortality, mortality plus nonfatal stroke, and reinfarction. Primary PTCA may be preferable for patients with a contraindication to lytic therapy, for those who are hemodynamically unstable, and for those at increased risk of intracranial bleeding.

▶ This is an observational study, subject to all the caveats that do not apply to randomized trials. This study has the advantage, however, of a more generalized applicability to the population at large. The total number of patients enrolled in this registry was 172,742. Although there was no difference overall in the rates of death and stroke, one has to bear in mind the possibility that "sicker" patients underwent PTCA as opposed to lytic therapy, despite the analyses being confined to patients who were "lytic-eligible," and patients with overt cardiogenic shock being excluded. Of interest, and supporting data from 2 large randomized trials, are the apparent (and I believe biologically plausible) benefits of primary PTCA in the elderly.[1, 2] One should appreciate that among the "universe" of patients presenting with acute myocardial infarction, PTCA was only employed in approximately 10%. The key to reperfusion therapy in the majority of patients presenting with acute myocardial infarction and S-T segment elevation remains the prompt administration of intravenous thrombolytic agents. I hope we will see the emergence of a new generation of more effective thrombolytic drugs in the immediate future.

B.J. Gersh, M.B., Ch.B., D.Phil., F.R.C.P.

References

1. Stone GW, Grimes CL, Browne KF, et al: Predictors of in-hospital and fixed-month outcome after acute myocardial infarction in the reperfusion era: The Primary Angioplasty in Myocardial Infarction [PAMI] Trial. *J Am Coll Cardiol* 5:370-377, 1995.
2. The Global Use of Strategies to Open Occluded Coronary Arteries in Acute Coronary Syndromes [GUSTO-IIb] Angioplasty Substudy Investigators: A clinical trial companying primary coronary angioplasty with tissue plasminogen activator for acute myocardial infarction. *N Engl J Med* 336:1621-1628, 1997.

Indications for ACE Inhibitors in the Early Treatment of Acute Myocardial Infarction: Systematic Overview of Individual Data From 100 000 Patients in Randomized Trials

Franzosi MG, for the ACE Inhibitor Collaborative Group (Istituto di Ricerche Farmacologiche "Mario Negri," Milan, Italy)
Circulation 97:2202-2212, 1998   4–12

Background.—Several trials have evaluated the use of angiotensin converting enzyme (ACE) inhibitors in acute myocardial infarction (MI). Although the utility of ACE inhibitors in MI is beyond question, some important questions remain. For example, do some patients benefit more from the therapy? Are some patients at greater risk? These authors examined individual data from 4 large trials to address these questions.

Methods.—The 4 large, randomized trials included were the Cooperative New Scandinavian Enalapril Survival Study II (CONSENSUS-II; n = 6,090), the Gruppo Italiano per lo Studio della Sopravvivenza nell'Infarto Miocardico (GISSI-3; n = 19,394), ISIS-4 (n = 58,050), and the Chinese Cardiac Study (CCS-1; n = 14,962). In these studies, the test group received ACE inhibitors within 0 to 36 hours of an acute MI and dosing continued for 4 to 6 weeks, whereas a placebo group received no ACE inhibitors. Data analyzed included baseline characteristics, survival at 30 days, and clinical events.

Findings.—Survival was significantly greater for the patients receiving ACE inhibitor therapy (3,501 deaths in 49,214 patients, or 7.11%) than in the controls (3,740 deaths in 49,269 patients, or 7.59%). Of the 239 fewer deaths in the patients receiving ACE inhibitors, 200 were avoided within the first week (Fig 3). Men and women benefited from treatment to a similar extent, as did patients between 55 and 74 years old. ACE inhibitors saved 22.7 lives/1000 for patients whose baseline heart rates were more than or equal to 100 beats/min and 8.7 lives/1,000 for those whose heart rates were between 80 to 99 beats/min. Absolute benefits of ACE inhibitors were significantly greater for patients with previous MI (8.9 lives saved/1,000), diabetes (17.3 lives saved/1,000), hypertension (9.0 lives saved/1,000), and Killip class more than 1 at baseline (14.1 lives saved/1,000). Of the patients receiving ACE inhibitors, those who had an anterior MI had significantly improved survival compared with those who had

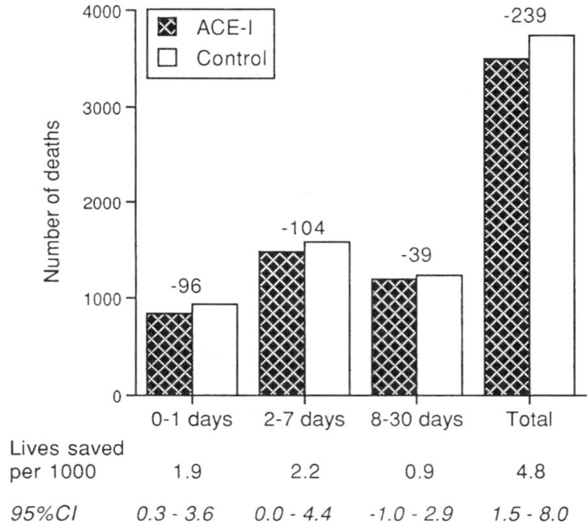

FIGURE 3.—Absolute effect of ACE inhibitor therapy on deaths for days 0 to 1, 2 to 7, and 8 to 30. (Courtesy of Franzosi MG, for the ACE Inhibitor Myocardial Infarction Collaborative Group: Indications for ACE inhibitors in the early treatment of acute myocardial infarction: Systematic overview of individual data from 100 000 patients in randomized trials. *Circulation* 97:2202-2212, 1998.)

MI at another site (10.6 lives saved/1,000). ACE inhibitor therapy saved 3.8 lives/1,000 low-risk patients and 13.6 lives/1,000 very high-risk patients. ACE inhibitor therapy also had a significant effect on nonfatal cardiac failure at 30 days compared with controls (14.6% vs. 15.2%, respectively). On the negative side, ACE inhibitor therapy was associated with significantly greater hypotension (84 cases/1,000 patients treated), cardiogenic shock (4.6 patients/1,000 treated), second- to third-degree atrioventricular block (5.4 cases/1,000 treated), and renal dysfunction (6.2 cases/1,000 treated). Patients 75 years old or greater had a significantly increased risk of renal dysfunction (17 cases/1,000 treated), and patients whose systolic blood pressure was less than 100 beats/min at baseline had a significantly increased risk of hypotension (132 cases/1,000 treated).

Conclusions.—ACE inhibitor therapy for 30 days saved about 5 lives/1,000 patients. The benefit was greatest in the first few days, and patients with a higher risk typically benefited to a greater absolute extent. Hypotension and renal dysfunction were the most common problems.

▶ Approximately 120,000 patients have been randomized in several large trials of ACE inhibitor therapy in acute MI. The trials can be broadly divided into those in which therapy was selective (patients with congestive heart failure or left ventricular dysfunction) as opposed to the 4 trials included in this analysis, in which the selection criteria were broad and inclusive of the majority of patients with acute myocardial infarction.[1] Virtually every trial demonstrated a benefit from an ACE inhibitor, but this was correspondingly greater in the "sickest" patients with left ventricular dysfunction in whom therapy was also continued for a longer period of time.

The 2 approaches to ACE inhibitor use in acute myocardial infarction are (1) to give the drugs to all patients and then reassess left ventricular function and the clinical status of the patient at 6 weeks, or (2) to use these drugs more selectively and to continue therapy indefinitely. The latter is my own preferred approach. An important conclusion from this meta-analysis, however, is to give the drugs orally and as early as possible once the patient is clinically stable because a significant proportion of lives saved were within the first 24 hours.

B.J. Gersh, M.B., Ch.B., D.Phil., F.R.C.P.

Reference

1. Latini R, Maggioni AP, Flather M, et al: ACE inhibitor use in patients with myocardial infarction: Summary of evidence from clinical trials. *Circulation* 92:3132-3137, 1995.

Transdermal Nitroglycerin Patch Therapy Improves Left Ventricular Function and Prevents Remodeling After Acute Myocardial Infarction: Results of a Multicenter Prospective Randomized, Double-blind, Placebo-controlled Trial
Mahmarian JJ, Moyé LA, Chinoy DA, et al (Baylor College of Medicine, Houston; Univ of Texas, Houston; Jacksonville Cardiovascular Clinic, Fla; et al)
Circulation 97:2017-2024, 1998   4–13

Introduction.—A multicenter trial examined the effects of transdermal nitroglycerin (NTG) patches on left ventricular (LV) remodeling in patients who survived acute Q-wave myocardial infarction. Prevention of LV dilation, which occurs more often in patients with LV dysfunction, might improve survival.

Methods.—The double-blind trial randomly assigned 77 patients to placebo and 214 to 3 different NTG patch dosages (0.4, 0.8, and 1.6 mg/h). Patients in the 4 groups were similar in mean age and other baseline characteristics; all underwent baseline gated radionuclide angiography. Dosages of NTG could be reduced, if necessary, to achieve a final tolerated dosage. Patients were evaluated monthly during the 6-month study period. Change in end-systolic volume index (ESVI) was the primary study end point.

Results.—Use of the 0.4-mg/h NTG patches significantly reduced both ESVI (mean −11.4 mL/m²) and end-diastolic volume index (mean −11.6 mL/m²). Patients who benefitted most from the treatment were those with a baseline LV ejection fraction less than or equal to 40%, and only at the 0.4-mg/h dose (Fig 3). Withdrawal of the NTG patch significantly increased ESVI, but values remained lower than those recorded before treatment.

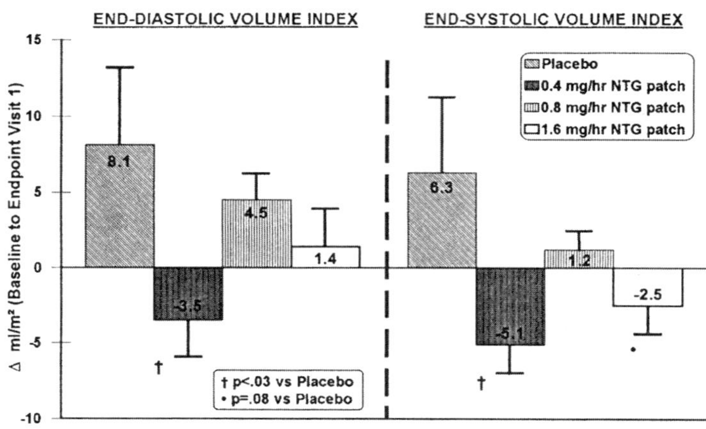

FIGURE 3.—Changes in LV end-diastolic volume diameter (EDVI) and ESVI (mL/m²) from baseline to end point visit 1 in the 4 randomized treatment groups. Only the 0.4-mg/h NTG patch dose significantly reduced cardiac volumes. Data are presented as mean ± SEM. (Courtesy of Mahmarian JJ, Moyé LA, Chinoy DA, et al: Transdermal nitroglycerin patch therapy improves left ventricular function and prevents remodeling after acute myocardial infarction: Results of a multi-center prospective randomized, double-blind, placebo-controlled trial. *Circulation* 97:2017-2024, 1998.)

Conclusion.—LV dilation was prevented by transdermal NTG patches when administered to patients who survived an acute myocardial infarction and had depressed LV function at baseline. Only the lowest dose (0.4 mg/h) was effective, and withdrawal of the patch after 6 months was followed by a significant increase in ESVI.

▶ In this small randomized trial, beneficial effects on left ventricular remodeling of 6 months were noted among patients receiving an intermittent 0.4-mg nitroglycerin patch. The benefits are likely to have been pharmacologic because ventricular volumes significantly increased within approximately 8 days after drug withdrawal. Among patients taking angiotensin-converting enzyme inhibitors, there was still a hemodynamic benefit from nitrate therapy, but only among patients with an ejection fraction of less than or equal to 0.40 (possibly a function of the small sample size). Two large megatrials failed to demonstrate any clinical benefit from nitrate therapy at 4 to 6 weeks, but the results were confounded by the large number of patients taking the placebo receiving nitrates in one trial and a limited or unknown number of patients with a depressed left ventricular ejection fraction.[1] The number was unknown in ISIS-4 and included only 5% of patients in the large Italian GISSI-3 trial.[2]

The crucial question is whether the hemodynamic benefits from nitrates will be translated into a clinical benefit, particularly in patients taking angiotensin-converting enzyme inhibitors. Remember also that long-term nitrate therapy means that sildenafil or Viagra is contraindicated; some may consider this a side effect of nitrate therapy.

B.J. Gersh, M.B., Ch.B., D.Phil., F.R.C.P.

References

1. ISIS-4: A randomized factorial trial assessing early oral captopril, oral mononitrate and intravenous magnesium sulfate in 58,050 patients with suspected acute myocardial infarction. *Lancet* 345:669-685, 1995.
2. GISSI-3: Effect of lisinopril and transdermal glycerol trinitrate singly and together on six-week mortality and ventricular function after acute myocardial infarction. *Lancet* 343:1115-1122, 1994.

Randomized Comparison of Direct Thrombin Inhibition Versus Heparin in Conjunction With Fibrinolytic Therapy for Acute Myocardial Infarction: Results From the GUSTO-IIb Trial

Topol EJ, for the Globa Use of Strategies to Open Occluded Coronary Arteries in Acute Coronary Syndromes (GUSTO-IIb) Investigators (Cleveland Clinic Found, Ohio; Green Lane Hosp, Auckland, New Zealand; Duke Clinical Research Inst, Durham, NC; et al)

J Am Coll Cardiol 31:1493-1498, 1998   4–14

Introduction.—Compared with streptokinase (SK) and either IV or subcutaneous heparin, the combination of SK and tissue-type plasminogen activator (t-PA) with IV heparin has provided a 15% relative reduction in 30-day mortality rate among patients with myocardial infarction (MI). A

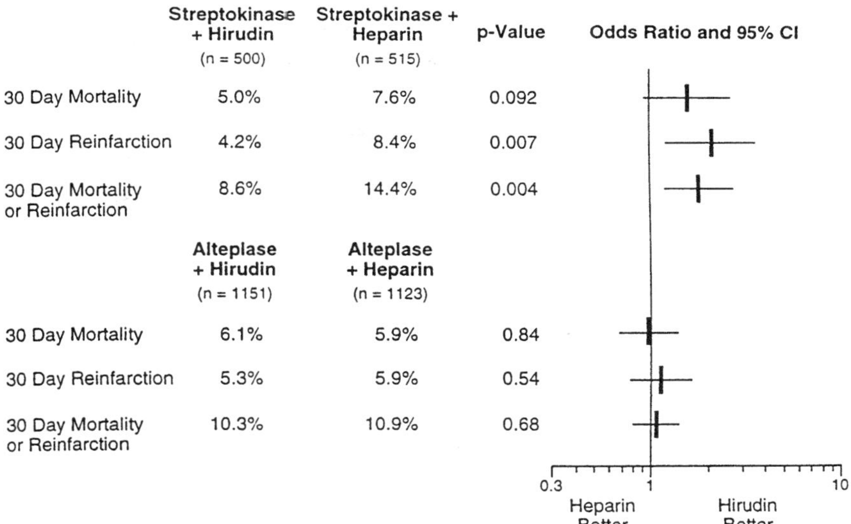

FIGURE 1.—Odds ratios and 95% confidence intervals for the unadjusted risk of death, reinfarction or death, or reinfarction at 30 days with hirudin versus heparin treatment with SK (*top*) or accelerated t-PA (*bottom*). (Reprinted with permission from the American College of Cardiology from Topol EJ, for the Global Use of Strategies to Open Occluded Coronary Arteries in the Acute Coronary Syndromes (GUSTO-IIb) Investigators: Randomized comparison of direct thrombin inhibition versus heparin in conjunction with fibrinolytic therapy for acute myocardial infarction: Results from the GUSTO-IIb trial. *J Am Coll Cardiol* 31:1493-1498, 1998.)

randomized study of patients with symptoms of acute MI and ST-segment elevation compared the effects of hirudin versus heparin in regimen of t-PA or SK.

Methods.—The study medication was to be infused for 3 to 5 days. All patients took chewable aspirin (160 mg) at admission, followed by up to 325 mg oral aspirin daily. The trial's primary end point was the composite incidence of death or nonfatal reinfarction within 30 days of enrollment. Of the patients treated with t-PA, 1,151 were randomly assigned to hirudin and 1,123 to heparin. Of those treated with SK, 500 were randomly assigned to hirudin and 515 to heparin.

Results.—In the SK group, death or reinfarction at 30 days occurred more often in those treated with heparin (14.4%) than in those who received hirudin (8.6%). Rates for t-PA–treated patients were 10.9% and 10.3%, respectively. Adjustment for baseline differences between groups yielded rates of 9.1% for SK with hirudin, 10.3% for t-PA with hirudin, 10.5% for t-PA with heparin, and 14.9% for SK with heparin, indicating that hirudin acts favorably with SK but not t-PA (Fig 1).

Conclusion.—Findings support the combination of hirudin and SK as an alternative to the current standard of t-PA with heparin. The use of SK and hirudin would also result in cost savings.

▶ The limitations of heparin and the theoretical advantages of the direct antithrombins created widespread expectations that were somewhat dashed by the results of 3 large randomized trials, demonstrating a modest benefit at best from hirudin in comparison with heparin.[1]

Many believe that the waning interest in the direct antithrombins is premature and that there are unanswered questions in regard to the optimal dose and its timing in relation to the administration of the thrombolytic agents. One always has to be wary of post hoc subset analyses, but the differential effects of hirudin in patients treated with streptokinase versus t-PA are consistent with 2 other trials, suggesting a higher patency rate in patients treated with streptokinase and hirulog givalirudin.[2]

Could the combination of acute thrombolytic agents such as streptokinase (in comparison with t-PA) plus hirulog produce patency rates and clinical results similar to those achieved with accelerated t-PA and intravenous heparin? This important question is currently the subject of ongoing trials. Stay tuned, since I do not believe that we have heard the end of the direct antithrombin story.

B.J. Gersh, M.B., Ch.B., D.Phil., F.R.C.P.

References

1. The GUSTO-IIb Investigators: A comparison of recombinant hirudin with heparin for the treatment of acute coronary syndrome. *N Engl J Med* 335:775-782, 1996.
2. White HD, Aylward PE, Frey M, et al: A randomized double blind comparison of hirulog versus heparin in patients receiving streptokinase and aspirin for acute myocardial infarction. *Circulation* 96:2155-2161, 1997.

Dangers of Delay of Initiation of Either Thrombolysis or Primary Angioplasty in Acute Myocardial Infarction With Increasing Use of Primary Angioplasty

Doorey A, Patel S, Reese C, et al (Med Ctr of Delaware, Newark; St Francis Hosp, Wilmington, Del)
Am J Cardiol 81:1173-1177, 1998

4–15

Introduction.—Early trials of primary angioplasty in the treatment of patients with acute myocardial infarction (AMI) yielded excellent results, but the therapy has been less successful in clinical practice. Patients treated with primary angioplasty or thrombolysis were examined.

Methods.—Three hospitals in Northern Delaware adopted primary angioplasty in 1995, after the release of favorable meta-analyses. When early results were unsatisfactory, factors contributing to these poor outcomes were evaluated. Treatment time intervals and outcomes for consecutive patients who received thrombolysis or angioplasty for AMI over 1 year were assessed. Reperfusion times were of interest because of the delays experienced with primary angioplasty.

Results.—In 1994, the hospitals had average thrombolysis time intervals of 20 to 30 minutes (Fig 1). Time intervals to thrombolysis increased at 1 of the hospitals after the new angioplasty protocol was announced in March 1995. Uncertainty about the use of thrombolysis vs. primary angioplasty was common, and often caused delays. Of 37 patients treated with primary angioplasty, 12 (32%) required emergency bypass surgery or died. With the increasing use of angioplasty, time intervals to thrombolysis

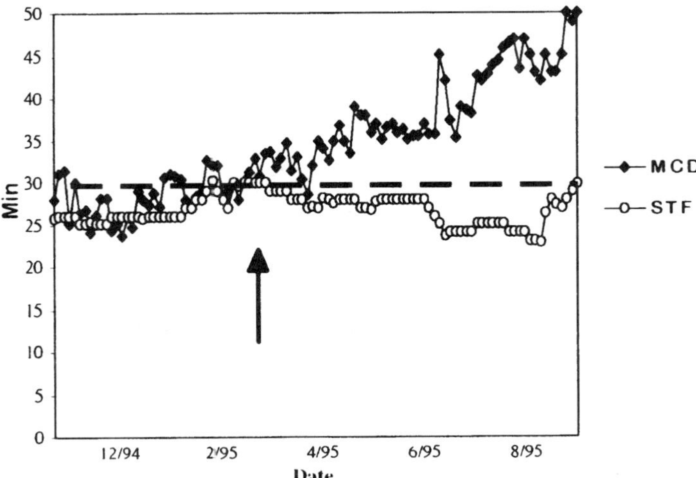

FIGURE 1.—Thrombolytic times from November 1994 to August 1995. The presentation of the new angioplasty protocol occurred in March *(arrow). Heavy dashed line,* the recommended maximum time interval of 30 minutes. A 10-point moving average is plotted. (Reprinted with permission from the American College of Cardiology from Doorey A, Patel S, Reese C, et al: Dangers of delay of initiation of either thrombolysis or primary angioplasty in acute myocardial infarction with increasing use of primary angioplasty. *Am J Cardiol* 81:1173-1177, 1998).

in patients not treated with angioplasty increased from an average of 29 to 39 minutes.

Conclusion.—The consideration of primary angioplasty can impair the timeliness of thrombolysis in patients with AMI. An algorithm should be established to minimize treatment delays.

▶ The role of "routine" primary angioplasty vs. thrombolysis is still the subject of some controversy, although I believe that the randomized trials have demonstrated the superiority of primary angioplasty with regard to the hard end points of death, recurrent infarction, and stroke. What needs to be emphasized is that "primary angioplasty may be great for some, but not for everyone," and that there is great variability in outcomes among institutions and operators. This frank account of events and outcomes in 2 community hospitals in the United States is fascinating and demonstrates what can happen when local circumstances and logistics create confusion among emergency room physicians. Not only were the results of primary angioplasty in this study poor, but the efficiency of the delivery of thrombolytic therapy deteriorated during the 12 months in which primary angioplasty was introduced for the first time to one of the hospitals. This is a "must read" for anyone planning to introduce primary angioplasty into an institution. This article emphasizes the importance of continuing to audit one's *own* results as opposed to relying on data published in the literature.

B.J. Gersh, M.B., Ch.B., D.Phil., F.R.C.P.

Influence of Treatment Delay on Infarct Size and Clinical Outcome in Patients With Acute Myocardial Infarction Treated With Primary Angioplasty

Liem AL, van 't Hof AWJ, Hoorntje JCA, et al (Hosp de Weezenlanden, Zwolle, The Netherlands)
J Am Coll Cardiol 32:629-633, 1998
4–16

Introduction.—There is a clear relationship between time to treatment and patency rate among patients given thrombolytic therapy for acute myocardial infarction, but this relationship is less evident in patients treated with primary angioplasty. The effect of delay caused by transfer to an angioplasty center was examined in a study of 207 patients.

Methods.—Outcome was compared for patients transferred from a community hospital to the study institution for primary angioplasty and patients admitted directly to the study institution. Each transferred patient was matched to a nontransferred patient. Primary angioplasty was considered successful if the residual stenosis in the infarct-related vessel was less than 50% and if thrombolysis in myocardial infarction grade 3 flow was present after the procedure.

Results.—The median additional delay for transfer patients was 43 minutes. Transferred and nontransferred groups were similar in baseline characteristics and in-hospital clinical outcome. At 6 months, 7% of patients in the transfer group and 6% in the nontransfer group had died. Reinfarction had occurred in 4% of transfer and 3% of nontransfer patients. Left ventricular ejection fraction at 6 months was 47% in nontransfer patients and 43% in transfer patients. Transferred patients also had a more extensive enzymatic infarct size.

Conclusion.—Although transferred acute myocardial infarction patients had a larger infarct size and lower left ventricular function than patients admitted directly to hospital for primary angioplasty, the patency rate and 6-month clinical outcome were not adversely affected by the delay.

▶ In patients treated with thrombolytic drugs, there is an inverse relationship between time to treatment and patency rate. This may be related to changes in the constituents of the thrombus which evolves from a clot composed primarily of erythrocytes to one that is platelet-rich. The latter, which manufactures plasminogen activator inhibitor - 1, PAI-1, is relatively resistant to fibrinolytic drugs, in contrast to primary angioplasty, which is equally effective against new or old clots.[1] One can therefore make a strong case for primary angioplasty in any setting in which there have been significant delays between the onset of symptoms and the time to treatment. This is particularly relevant because time becomes a less critical factor once the first 2 to 3 hours after the onset of symptoms have elapsed.[2] Nonetheless, the goal is to achieve reperfusion within 6 hours of symptoms and in this study, the delay incurred by transport was only 43 minutes. Is this the situation in your own institution?

B.J. Gersh, M.B., Ch.B., D.Phil., F.R.C.P.

References

1. Topol EJ: Toward a new frontier in myocardial perfusion therapy: Emerging platelet pre-eminence. *Circulation* 97:211-218, 1998.
2. Gersh BJ, Anderson JL: Thrombolysis and myocardial salvage: Results of clinical trials in the animal paradigm. *Circulation* 88:296-306, 1993.

Unstable Angina

Randomized Trial of an Oral Platelet Glycoprotein IIb/IIIa Antagonist, Sibrafiban, in Patients After an Acute Coronary Syndrome: Results of the TIMI 12 Trial

Cannon CP, McCabe CH, Eorzak S, et al (Harvard Med School, Boston; Henry Ford Hosp, Detroit; Hennepin County Med Ctr, Minneapolis, Minn; et al)
Circulation 97:340-349, 1998   4–17

Introduction.—Previous studies have showed that intravenous infusion of platelet glycoprotein IIb/IIIa receptor inhibitors can reduce the rate of ischemic complications in patients who have undergone coronary angioplasty or who have unstable angina. This benefit is lost after the infusion is stopped, however. Oral agents might be useful in the treatment and prevention of ischemic events in patients with acute coronary syndromes.

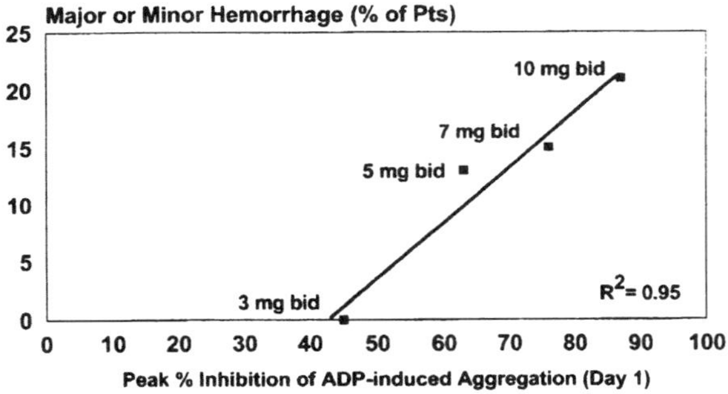

FIGURE 6.—Correlation of the median degree of platelet inhibition achieved in the twice-daily doses as measured in the PK/PD cohort plotted against the rate of total (major and minor) hemorrhage in both the PK/PD and safety cohorts. Pts indicates patients. (Courtesy of Cannon CP, McCabe CH, Borzak S, et al: Randomized trial of an oral platelet glycoprotein IIb/IIIa antagonist, sibrafiban, in patients after an acute coronary syndrome: Results of the TIMI 12 Trial. *Circulation* 97:340-349, 1998. Reproduced with permission, copyright 1998, American Heart Association.)

The Thrombolysis in Myocardial Infarction (TIMI) 12 trial assessed the pharmacokinetics, pharmacodynamics, safety, and tolerability of si-brafiban, an oral, peptidomimetic, selective antagonist of the glycoprotein IIb/IIIa receptor. In addition to this broad assessment, the study sought to define the doses achieving 2 different target ranges of inhibition of platelet aggregation and the effects of the rate of ischemic events.

Methods.—The phase II, double-blind, dose-ranging trial included 329 patients with acute coronary syndromes. A pharmacokinetics/pharmaco-dynamics cohort included 106 patients; a safety cohort included 223 patients. In the pharmacokinetics/pharmacodynamics cohort, patients were randomized to receive 28 days of treatment with sibrafiban in 1 of 7 dosages, ranging from 5 mg/day to 10 mg twice daily. In the safety cohort, patients were randomized to receive 28 days of treatment with sibrafiban in 1 of 4 doses, ranging from 5 mg/day to 10 mg twice daily, or with aspirin.

Results.—Sibrafiban produced high levels of platelet inhibition. All 7 doses in the pharmacokinetics/pharmacodynamics study achieved mean peak values of 47% to 97% inhibition of 20-µmol/L ADP-induced platelet aggregation after 28 days of treatment. Platelet inhibition was longer lasting with twice-daily dosing, which achieved a mean inhibition of 36% to 86% on day 28. With once-daily dosing, platelet inhibition returned to normal within 24 hours. Rates of major hemorrhage was 1.5% in the sibrafiban groups versus 1.9% in the aspirin group. Depending on dosage, 0% to 32% of sibrafiban-treated patients had mucocutaneous or other "minor" bleeding; none of the aspirin-treated patients had such minor bleeding. Factors associated with minor bleeding included total daily dose, once-daily versus twice-daily dosing, renal function, and diagnosis of unstable angina (Fig 6). In the safety cohort, all cardiovascular end-points were more frequent in the sibrafiban group, although the difference from the aspirin group was not significant.

Conclusions.—In patients who have had acute coronary syndromes, treatment with the oral glycoprotein IIb/IIIa antagonist sibrafiban produces effective, long-term platelet inhibition with a clear dose-response pattern. Sibrafiban produces a relatively high rate of minor bleeding. This study provides important information as to the best potential uses of oral IIb/IIIa inhibitors to reduce recurrent cardiac events after acute coronary syndromes.

▶ Despite the demonstrable benefits of aspirin in reducing clinical events in the acute ischemic syndromes, it is well accepted that aspirin is a relatively weak platelet inhibitor. The platelet surface glycoprotein IIb/IIIa receptor is the final common pathway of processes leading to platelet aggregation. Antagonists to this receptor have fulfilled their potential as more effective antiplatelet agents by demonstrating a reduction in ischemic complications after PTCA and in unstable angina.[1] Nonetheless, there are compelling reasons to prolong the period of IIb/IIIa inhibition, thus allowing time for plaque "passivation," anc the oral administration of IIb/IIIa receptor antagonists is a dynamic component of the "new frontier" of antithrombotic therapy.

The long-acting use of these agents is an enormously exciting prospect, and I expect that they will become a mainstay of therapy for acute ischemic syndromes in the future. Nonetheless, there are formidable issues which remain unresolved. First, as this study (the TIMI 12 trial) shows, a narrow window clearly exists between efficacy on one side and bleeding on the other. Second, additional questions which are crucial to resolving these issues include the relationship between drug dose, platelet count, body weight, and renal function. Third, how does one best assess the degree of platelet inhibition necessary to ensure optimal dosing and once this has been established, will they be reliable bedside assays?[2] Fourth, should one use a fixed dose and modify this according to the degree of bleeding, or is this a relatively crude approach? And finally, what is the role of aspirin in conjunction with IIb/IIIa inhibition and if so, is it because of its anti-inflammatory action or anti-platelet activity?

There are many questions and, to date, relatively few answers, but they will not be long in forthcoming. This really is an extraordinarily exciting area of investigation, and I suspect that this class of drugs will play a pivotal role in the posthospital management of patients with acute ischemic syndrome. What also remains to be determined would be the role of oral IIb/IIIa inhibitors in patients with chronic coronary artery disease.

B.J. Gersh, M.B., Ch.B., D.Phil., F.R.C.P.

References

1. The EPIC Investigators. Use of a monoclonal antibody directed against the platelet glycoprotein IIb/IIIa receptor in high risk angioplasty. *N Engl J Med* 330:956-961, 1994.
2. Collar BS, Land D, Scudder LE: Rapid and simple platelet function assay to assess glycoprotein IIb/IIIa receptor blockade. *Circulation* 95:860-867, 1997.

Platelet Activation With Unfractionated Heparin at Therapeutic Concentrations and Comparisons With a Low-Molecular-Weight Heparin and With a Direct Thrombin Inhibitor

Xiao Z, Théroux P (Univ of Montreal)
Circulation 97:251-256, 1998

4–18

Introduction.—Anticoagulant therapy is now used in the acute phase of coronary symptoms, leading to increased clinical use of heparin. This, along with the development of new antithrombotic agents, underscores the need to characterize the platelet effects of various anticoagulants. The platelet effects of heparin are unclear. In high doses, it causes enhanced platelet activation in vitro; however, in therapeutic doses in vivo, this effect

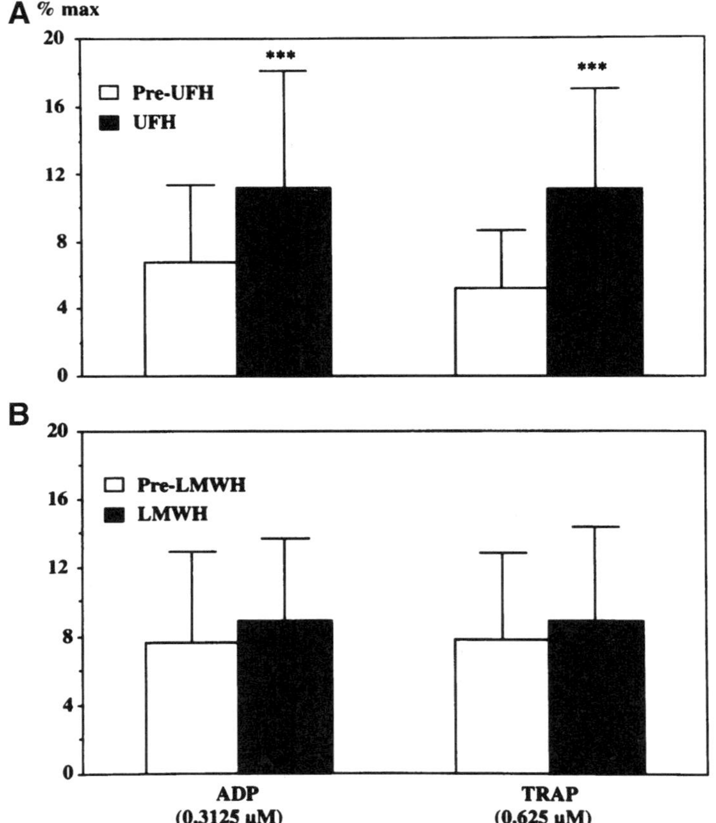

FIGURE 2.—Platelet aggregation (% maximum [max]) to ADP and to TRAP in the patients with unstable angina before and during the infusion of unfractionated heparin (**top**) and low-molecular-weight heparin enoxaparin (**bottom**). *$P < .001$ vs UFH. (Courtesy of Xiao Z, Théroux P: Platelet activation with unfractionated heparin at therapeutic concentrations and comparisons with a low-molecular-weight heparin and with a direct thrombin indicator. *Circulation* 97:251-256, 1998. Reproduced with permission, copyright 1998, American Heart Association.)

is not seen. The effects of 3 anticoagulant agents at therapeutic concentrations, namely, unfractionated heparin (UFH), the low-molecular-weight heparin enoxaparin, and the direct thrombin inhibitor argatroban, on platelet receptor activation and platelet aggregation were assessed.

Methods.—Forty-three patients with unstable angina were assessed before and during treatment with UFH or enoxaprin. Studies included measurement of platelet P-selectin (CD62) and activated GP IIb/IIIa (PAC-1) expression on the platelet membrane in whole blood, and measurement of platelet aggregation. Blood from 7 normal control subjects was studied ex vivo after addition of UFH, 0.25 U/mL; enoxaparin, 0.25 U/mL; argatroban, 1 ng/mL; or normal saline.

Results.—In the patients with unstable angina, UFH treatment increased the percentage of platelets positive to PAC-1 from 2.7% to 4.4%. The percentage of platelets positive to CD62 increased from 1.6% to 2.7%. The platelets also became hyperresponsive to stimulation with ADP and thrombin-receptor agonist peptide. During UFH treatment, aggregation to adenosine diphosphate (ADP) increased from 6.8% to 11.2%, while aggregation to thrombin receptor agonist peptide (TRAP) increased from 5.2% to 11.1% (Fig 2). When added to normal blood specimens, UFH caused activation of GP IIb/IIIa receptors, expression of P-selectin, and enhancement of platelet aggregation. Both in vivo and ex vivo, enoxaparin had little effect on platelets. Ex vivo argatroban had no detectable platelet effects.

Conclusions.—In therapeutic concentrations, UFH has platelet-activating effects both in vivo and ex vivo. These effects are modest, and of unknown clinical significance. They are reproducible, however, and could play a role at the site of thrombus formation.

▶ This study demonstrated (both in vivo and in vitro) the proaggregatory effect of unfractionated heparin on platelets. This was not seen with low-molecular-weight heparin or argatroban, a direct-thrombin inhibitor. The clinical relevance of these findings are unclear, but the much greater response in the presence of ADP and TRAP suggests that the interaction may be amplified at the site of thrombus formation. Prior studies have demonstrated in vivo that low doses of heparin are more apt to reduce the incidence of platelet aggregation and high doses are likely to increase it.[1]

There is increasing clinical evidence arising from studies in patients with acute myocardial infarction or those undergoing interventional procedures, to suggest that in regard to unfractionated heparin, less may be better. This study provides a theoretical basis for these observations. There is certainly much to learn about the interactions between unfractionated heparin, low-molecular-weight heparin, platelet function, aspirin and the IIb/IIIa inhibitors. This is one of the most dynamic areas of current investigation in coronary artery disease.

B.J. Gersh, M.B., Ch.B., D.Phil, F.R.C.P.

Reference

1. Westrick J, Scully M, Poll C, et al: Comparison of low molecular weight heparin and unfractionated heparin on activation in human platelets in vitro. *Thromb Res* 42:435-447, 1986.

Inhibition of the Platelet Glycoprotein IIb/IIIa Receptor With Tirofiban in Unstable Angina and Non–Q-Wave Myocardial Infarction

Théroux P, for the Platelet Receptor Inhibition in Ischemic Syndrome Management in Patients Limited by Unstable Signs and Symptoms (PRISM-PLUS) Study Investigators (Montreal Heart Inst)
N Engl J Med 338:1488-1497, 1998   4–19

Introduction.—New drugs that specifically inhibit the platelet glycoprotein IIb/IIIa inhibitor provide a new option for the treatment of thrombotic disorders. These drugs appear to prevent acute ischemic complications in patients undergoing angioplasty and in patients with unstable angina, whether or not they are undergoing interventional procedures. The platelet glycoprotein IIb/IIIa receptor tirofiban was evaluated for its ability to prevent acute ischemic events in patients with unstable angina and non–Q-wave myocardial infarction.

Methods.—The multicenter, randomized, double-blind trial included 1,915 patients with unstable angina or non–Q-wave myocardial infarction. The patients were assigned to receive either tirofiban 0.6 µg/kg/min IV for 30 min followed by an infusion of 0.15 µg/kg/min plus heparin placebo; adjusted-dose heparin plus tirofiban placebo; or tirofiban 0.4 µg/kg/min for 30 minutes followed by an infusion of 0.1 µg/kg/min plus adjusted-dose heparin. All patients received aspirin unless contraindicated. Treatment continued for a mean of 71 hours. After 48 hours, coronary angiography and angioplasty were performed as indicated. At 7 days after randomization, the 3 treatments were compared on a composite primary end point comprising death, myocardial infarction, or refractory ischemia.

Results.—Seven-day mortality rate was significantly increased for patients receiving tirofiban only—4.6% vs. 1.1% for patients receiving heparin only—leading to early stoppage of the trial. At 7 days, the composite primary end point was reached by 12.9% of patients receiving tirofiban plus heparin vs. 17.9% of those receiving heparin alone (risk ratio 0.68). At 30 days, 18.5% of the tirofiban plus heparin group had reached the composite end point compared with 22.3% of the heparin-only group; at 6 months the figures were 27.7% and 32.1%, respectively (Fig 1). The 7-day frequency of death or myocardial infarction was 4.9% with tirofiban plus heparin vs. 8.3% with heparin only. These figures rose to 8.7% vs. 11.9% at 20 days and 12.3% vs. 15.3% at 6 months, respectively. All patient subgroups received consistent benefit from tirofiban plus heparin, including those receiving medical treatment and those receiving angioplasty. The rate of major bleeding complications was 4.0% with tirofiban plus heparin and 3.0% with heparin only.

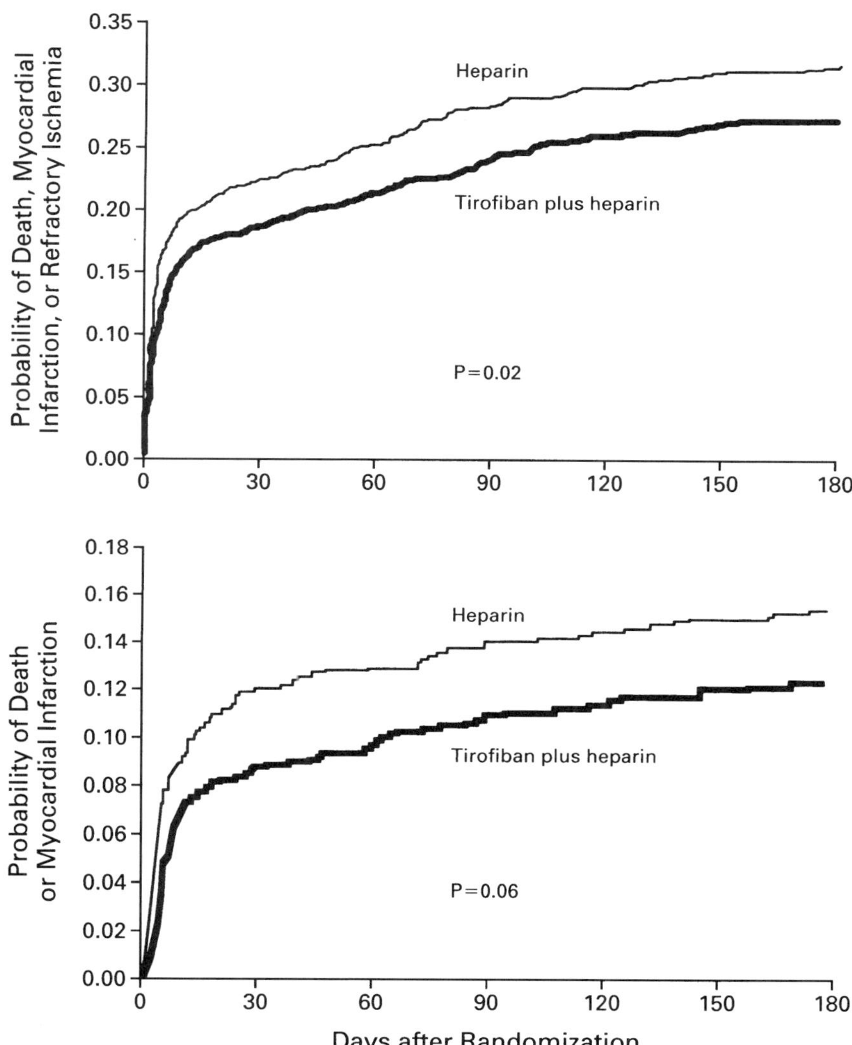

FIGURE 1.—Kaplan-Meier curves showing cumulative incidence of events among patients randomly assigned to receive tirofiban plus heparin or heparin alone. *P* values were computed by Cox regression analysis. *Top panel* shows composite end point of death, myocardial infarction, refractory ischemia, or rehospitalization for unstable angina; *bottom panel* shows the composite end point of death or myocardial infarction. (Courtesy of Pierre Théroux, for the Platelet Receptor Inhibition in Ischemic Syndrome Management in Patients Limited by Unstable Signs and Symptoms [PRISM-PLUS] Study Investigators: Inhibition of the platelet glycoprotein IIb/IIIa recptor with tirofiban in unstable angina and non–Q-wave myocardial infarction. *N Engl J Med* 338:1488-1497, 1998. Reprinted by permission of the New England Journal of Medicine, Copyright 1998 by the Massachusetss Medical Society. All rights reserved.)

Conclusions.—In patients with acute ischemic coronary syndromes, the combination of tirofiban, heparin, and aspirin reduces the incidence of ischemic events compared with heparin and aspirin only. The use of a platelet glycoprotein IIb/IIIa receptor inhibitor as part of a multitarget approach appears to offer an important new management strategy for these patients. Treatment with tirofiban alone carries an excess mortality rate at 7 days.

▶ One of the most dynamic and exciting topics in coronary artery disease is the concept of platelet receptor blockade with IIb/IIIa agents. Much of our knowledge to date is based on the role of these drugs in high-risk individuals undergoing interventional procedures.[1] This paper on the PRISM-PLUS study and its companion paper on the PRISM study compared aspirin plus tirofiban with aspirin plus heparin for unstable angina.[2] This paper extends these observations to an important group of patients with unstable angina and non–Q-wave myocardial infarction. In the PRISM-PLUS study, tirofiban plus heparin was associated with a lower risk of myocardial infarction and recurrent ischemia than heparin alone, although mortality rate was no different. In contrast to the PRISM trial, tirofiban alone was not effective in this study, which may relate to the fact that patients in PRISM-PLUS were at higher risk, although the difference between the 2 trials could be from chance alone.[3] In the PRISM-PLUS study, the differences diminish with time, and at 6 months the frequency of death and myocardial infarction was 12.3% in the tirofiban-heparin arm and 15.3% with heparin alone ($P = 0.06$). This raises the question whether a longer duration of infusion may be beneficial, and of course everyone is interested in the concept of oral platelet receptor blockade, which is currently the subject of several randomized trials.

B.J. Gersh, M.B., Ch.B., D.Phil., F.R.C.P.

References

1. The EPIC Investigators. Use of a monoclonal antibody directed against the platelet glycoprotein IIb/IIIa receptor in high-risk coronary angioplasty. *N Engl J Med* 330:956-961, 1994.
2. The platelet receptor inhibition in ischemic syndrome management. *N Engl J Med* 338:1498-1505, 1998.
3. Chesebro JH, Badimon JJ: Platelet glycoprotein IIb/IIIa receptor blockage in unstable coronary disease. *N Engl J Med* 338:1539-1541, 1998.

Epidemiology and Risk Factors

Fish Consumption and Risk of Sudden Cardiac Death

Albert CM, Hennekens CH, O'Donnell CJ, et al (Brigham and Women's Hosp, Boston; Massachusetts Gen Hosp, Boston; Harvard School of Public Health, Boston; et al)
JAMA 279:23-28, 1998   4–20

Background.—Fish consumption has been thought to reduce risk of sudden cardiac death through a selective benefit on fatal arrhythmias. This study investigates the relationship between eating fish and sudden cardiac death.

Methods.—As part of the U.S. Physicians' Health Study, male U.S. physicians ages 40 to 84 years were monitored up to 11 years after completing in 1982 a semiquantitative questionnaire on the frequency of fish consumption. Test subjects had no history of cancer, transient ischemic attack, or myocardial infarction at baseline. The physicians were also randomly assigned to take aspirin, beta-carotene, or placebos. Follow-up questionnaires on food consumption were administered at 12 and 18 months and at five years. Sudden cardiac death was determined through patient medical records and reports from relatives of test subjects.

Results.—During the study period, 133 sudden deaths occurred. Researchers controlled for coronary risk factors, age, and assignments for aspirin and beta-carotene and determined that the intake of dietary fish was associated with a decreased risk of sudden death. The threshold for this effect was one fish eaten per week (P for trend = 0.03). In comparison with test subjects who ate fish less than once a month, men who ate fish at least once a week had a multivariate relative risk of 0.48 (0.24-0.96; P = 0.04, 95% confidence interval) for sudden death. However, increasing intake beyond one serving per week did not further decrease the risk of sudden death. The n-3 fatty acid is suspected to provide these preventive effects. However, the effects were not consistent when dark meat fish was consumed. And yet, dark meat fish have a higher n-3 fatty acid content. Thus, some other unidentified nutrient may actually play a role. Eating fish was not correlated with decreased risk of nonsudden cardiac death, myocardial infarction, or total cardiovascular mortality. However, reduced risks of total mortality were found with threshold fish consumption.

Conclusion.—This cohort study has several possible flaws and is not clear-cut. For example, people with a family or personal history of hypertension, hypercholesterolemia, or coronary heart disease are more likely to eat fish. This complicates the relationship examined in this study. Nevertheless, the study shows that men who eat fish at least once per week have a reduced risk for sudden cardiac death.

▶ Good news all around? If you like fish, this study reinforces that it is good for you. If you dislike the stuff, the data suggest that you only have to eat it once a week.

This study does not provide clear-cut answers but does provide increasing support for other studies, suggesting a beneficial effect of fish oils upon sudden cardiac or arrhythmic deaths, but not on the incidence of myocardial infarction.[1,2] Discrepancies with other studies are addressed by the authors in their discussion and in the accompanying editorial.[3] In this respect, the lack of a dose-response relationship is somewhat puzzling.

What needs to be borne in mind is that only 9% of men in this study (the Physicians' Health Study), consumed fish less than once per week, and these men also had a higher prevalence of other coronary risk factors. Statistical adjustment for these differences cannot exclude a residual confounding inference.

This is a fascinating subject, but is there a "clinical" bottom line? It would certainly appear that the existing evidence suggests that 1-to-2 helpings of fish per week should be part of the "healthy heart diet."

B.J. Gersh, M.B., Ch.B., D. Phil., F.R.C.P.

References

1. Kromhout D, Bosschieter EB, DeLezenne Coulander C: The inverse relation between fish consumption and 20-year mortality from coronary heart disease. *N Engl J Med* 312:1205-1209, 1998.
2. Ascherio A, Rimm EB, Stampfer MJ, et al: Dietary intake of marine n-3 fatty acids, fish intake, and the risk of coronary disease among men. *N Engl J Med* 332:978-982, 1995.
3. Kromhout D: Fish consumption and sudden cardiac death. *JAMA* 279:65, 1998.

Polymorphisms in the Coagulation Factor VII Gene and the Risk of Myocardial Infarction

Iacoviello L, Di Castelnuovo A, De Knijff P, et al (Istituto di Ricerche Farmacologiche Mario Negri, Santa Maria Imbaro, Italy; Leiden Univ, The Netherlands)
N Engl J Med 338:79-85, 1998

4–21

Objective.—A growing body of evidence suggests that patients with high blood levels of coagulation factor VII are associated with an elevated risk of ischemic vascular disease. Environmental and genetic factors may affect the level of factor VII in the blood. However, the relationships among genetic polymorphisms of factor VII, blood levels of factor VII, and myocardial infarction risk are unknown. These associations were investigated in a case-control study.

Methods.—The cases were 165 patients (mean age, 55 years) with familial myocardial infarction. The controls were 225 individuals, (mean age, 56 years) with no personal or family history of cardiovascular disease. Each individual underwent DNA studies for polymorphisms involving R353Q and the hypervariable region 4 of the factor VII gene. Measurements of factor VII clotting activity and antigen levels were obtained as well. The effects of factor VII gene polymorphisms on myocardial infarction risk and on factor VII levels were analyzed.

Results.—The risk of myocardial infarction was reduced for patients with the *QQ* genotype (odds ratio, 0.08; 95% confidence interval, 0.01-0.9) and the *H7H7* genotype (odds ratio, 0.22; 95% confidence interval, 0.08-0.63). Analysis of the R353Q polymorphism suggested that risk was highest with the *RR* genotype, intermediate with the *RQ* genotype, and lowest for the *QQ* genotype. When the hypervariable region 4 polymorphism was considered, patients with the *H7H5* or *H6H5* genotype were at highest risk, followed by the *H6H6*, *H6H7*, and *H7H7* genotypes. Factor VII antigen level and factor VII clotting activity were reduced for patients with the *QQ* or *H7H7* genotype vs. the *RR* or *H6H6* genotype. Myocardial infarction risk was reduced for patients at the lowest vs. highest level of factor VII clotting activity (odds ratio, 0.13; 95% confidence interval, 0.05-0.34).

Conclusions.—Factor VII gene polymorphisms appear to influence myocardial infarction risk, perhaps acting through differences in factor VII levels. The mechanism by which the polymorphism influences factor VII levels is unknown. The clinical ramifications of these findings must be evaluated in prospective clinical trials.

▶ It is well documented that elevated plasma levels of factor VIIa is a strong risk factor for fatal myocardial infarction, and associations with other abnormalities of the coagulation system and coronary artery disease have been documented.[1] Moreover, other risk factors for myocardial infarction and coronary heart disease, such as a high-fat diet and diabetes, also raise plasma levels of factor VIIa.[2] This study suggests that certain polymorphisms of the factor VII gene may increase the risk of myocardial infarction, and one has to postulate that this may be mediated by alterations in factor VII levels.

This is a complex subject, in that polymorphisms are common and usually benign. But in some cases a polymorphism may be perverse, in which it is considered as a mutation. The correlation between a particular genetic polymorphism and a disease is of much less concern than whether the knowledge of such a polymorphism will lead to the means for diagnosis, prognosis, and treatment. For a useful discussion of these issues, the accompanying editorial is worth reading.[3]

B.J. Gersh, M.B., Ch.B., D.Phil., F.R.C.P.

References

1. Meade TW, Mellows S, Brozovic M, et al: Hemostatic function and ischaemic heart disease: Principal results of the Northwick Park Heart Study. *Lancet* 2:533-537, 1986.
2. Miller GJ, Cruickshank JK, Ellis LJ, et al: Fat consumption and factor VII coagulant activity in middle-aged men: An association between dietary and thrombogenic coronary risk factor. *Atherosclerosis* 78:19-24, 1989.
3. Rosenthal N, Schwarz RS: In search of perverse polymorphisms. *N Engl J Med*, 122-124, 1998.

Plasma Concentration of Soluble Intercellular Adhesion Molecule 1 and Risks of Future Myocardial Infarction in Apparently Healthy Men

Ridker PM, Hennekens CH, Roitman-Johnson B, et al (Brigham and Women's Hosp, Boston; Harvard Med School, Cambridge, Mass; Harvard School of Public Health, Boston; et al)
Lancet 351:88-92, 1998   4–22

Objective.—Leukocyte adhesion and transmigration to the vascular endothelial wall is thought to be a key step in the atherosclerotic process. This step is mediated by intercellular adhesion molecule (ICAM-1). It is unknown whether otherwise healthy people who go on to have acute myocardial infarction have elevated concentrations of soluble ICAM-1 (sICAM-1). This question was addressed using data from the Physicians' Health Study.

Methods.—The study was based on prospectively collected baseline plasma samples from nearly 15,000 healthy U.S. male physicians. Concentrations of sICAM-1 were measured in the samples of 474 research subjects with their first myocardial infarction and 474 controls who remained healthy during a 9-year follow-up period. The cases and controls were matched in terms of age and smoking status at the time of myocardial infarction. The effects of baseline sICAM-1 concentration on myocardial infarction risk were analyzed, including the influence of other lipid and nonlipid cardiovascular risk factors.

Results.—A high sICAM-1 concentration was associated with an increased risk of myocardial infarction. For men in the highest quartile of sICAM-1 concentration—greater than 260 ng/mL—the relative risk was 1.6, with a 95% confidence interval of 1.1 to 2.4. This relationship was present even in nonsmokers and after adjustment for other risk factors. Multivariate analysis suggested a 1.8 relative risk (95% confidence interval, 1.1 to 2.8) for subjects in the highest quartile of sICAM-1 concentration. Although sICAM-1 level was significantly correlated with fibrinogen, high-density lipoprotein cholesterol, homocysteine, triglycerides, tissue-type plasminogen-activator antigen, and C-reactive protein, adjusting for these factors had little impact on risk. The effects of sICAM-1 level of myocardial infarction risk appeared to increase with longer follow-up.

Conclusions.—An elevated baseline concentration of sICAM-1 is associated with an increased risk of later acute myocardial infarction. The findings strengthen the suggestion that ICAM-1 and other cellular mediators of inflammation are involved in the atherogenic process. They also suggest that anti-adhesion treatments could offer a new approach to the prevention of cardiovascular disease.

▶ The link between nontraditional risk factors and coronary artery disease continues to unfold, and the Physicians' Health Study has provided a fertile database in the past and continues to do so. The role of inflammation in the pathophysiology of atherosclerosis is extended by this study, which identifies a direct mediator of the inflammatory process (the intercellular adhesion molecule I) and the risk of myocardial infarction, as opposed to other studies involving C-reactive protein, which is simply a systemic marker.[1] The hypothesis that endothelial activation and inflammation are integral steps in the atherosclerotic process is substantiated by these data which document the association between concentrations of ICAM-I and the risk of a future myocardial infarction. Cellular adhesion molecules like ICAM-I are mediators of leukocyte-vascular wall interactions, which include the adhesion and transmigration of leukocytes from the vascular endothelial wall.[2]

B.J. Gersh, M.B., Ch.B., D. Phil., F.R.C.P.

References

1. Ridker PM, Cushman M, Stampfer MJ et al: Inflammation, aspirin and the risk of cardiovascular disease in apparently healthy men. *N Engl J Med*, 336:973-979, 1997.
2. Adams DH, Shaw S: Leucocyte-endothelial interactions and regulation of leucocyte migration. *Lancet*, 343:831-836, 1994.

Preventing Coronary Heart Disease: B Vitamins and Homocysteine

Omenn GS, Beresford SAA, Motulsky AG (Univ of Washington, Seattle)
Circulation 97:421-424, 1998   4–23

Background.—A new study from the European Concerted Action Projects suggests that homocysteine, plasma folate, and vitamin B6 have significant effects on the risk of atherosclerotic cardiovascular disease. Total homocysteine level had a striking dose-response relationship with risk of peripheral vascular and coronary heart disease. However, the study leaves many questions about the relationship between folate, vitamin B12, vitamin B6, and total homocysteine (tHey); the effect of homocysteine on cardiovascular risk; and the recommended risk reductions for individuals and patients. These questions are addressed in an editorial.

Homocysteine, B Vitamins, and Coronary Heart Disease Risk.—The available evidence suggests that a total homocysteine level of greater than 15 µmol/L is associated with a 1.4 relative risk of coronary heart disease mortality, compared with levels of less than 10 µmol/L. For disease prevention, total homocysteine levels should be reduced to a range of 9 to 10 µmol/L. This reduction and an accompanying increase in circulating folate levels is unlikely to be achieved by diet alone. The bioavailability of folic acid from dietary conjugated folates is about one half of that from supplements. Folic acid supplementation of 400 µg/day or greater is already recommended to prevent birth defects. The addition of vitamin B12, 200 to 1,000 µg, would prevent adverse outcomes even for subjects who lack intrinsic factor for B12 absorption. However, prevention trials are still needed to prove a cause-and-effect relationship and to rule out adverse effects.

Recommendations.—The available evidence strongly suggests that folic acid supplementation may reduce mortality from coronary heart disease. Everyone in the population should take at least 400 µg of folic acid per day. Manufacturers should include sufficient vitamin B12 in folic acid capsules to ensure adequate passive absorption even in the absence of intrinsic factor. If vitamin B12 is not also included in fortified grains, it should be prescribed to confer protection to older patients with vitamin B12 deficiency.

▶ This is an editorial in response to a multicenter European study which demonstrated a striking dose-response relationship between low homocysteine levels and the risk of peripheral vascular and coronary heart disease.[1]

An association between low folate and B6 levels in cardiovascular disease was present, but less striking, and this was even less so in regard to vitamin B12.

This superb editorial by Omenn et al. addressed a number of important and unresolved questions regarding the relationship of folate, vitamin B12, and vitamin B6 to levels of homocysteine and related moieties, in addition to the relationship between homocysteine and cardiovascular risk. Subjects addressed include the desired or optimum homocysteine blood levels, the amount of supplementation with folate and other B vitamins, the safety of this approach, genetic variability in folate and homocysteine levels, and the design and feasibility of randomized trials.

I agree with their statement that "statistical associations do not prove cause-and-effect relationships and do not rule out adverse effects." Associations should not be described as "effects." Nonetheless, the evidence is sufficiently strong to suggest that the daily intake of folic acid should be greater than or equal to 400 µg/day. Are higher doses needed in patients with increased homocysteine levels? It remains to be seen. I would also emphasize the recommendation to mandate inclusion of sufficient B12 in folic acid capsules (200 to 1,000 µg) to ensure adequate absorption by passive mechanisms, even in the absence of intrinsic factors.

B.J. Gersh, M.B., Ch.B., D.Phil, F.R.C.P.

Reference

1. Robinson K and the European Comac Group: Low circulating folate and vitamin B6 concentrations: Risk factors for stroke, peripheral vascular disease, and coronary artery disease. *Circulation* 97:437-443, 1998.

Folate and Vitamin B$_6$ From Diet and Supplements in Relation to Risk of Coronary Heart Disease Among Women
Rimm EB, Willett WC, Hu FB, et al (Harvard Med School, Boston)
JAMA 278:359-364, 1998   4–24

Background.—The relationship between intake of folate and vitamin B$_6$ and coronary heart disease (CHD) in women is being investigated. Low intake of these vitamins has been linked with hyperhomocysteinemia, but has yet to be linked with fatal CHD and nonfatal myocardial infarction (MI).

Methods.—In a prospective cohort study, information was gathered on food consumption from 80,082 women who were then followed up for 14 years and cases of nonfatal MI and fatal CD were documented. The women who completed the original survey had no history of diabetes, hypercholesterolemia, cardiovascular disease, or cancer. Test subjects were classified into quintiles for intake of folate and vitamin B$_6$. Adjustment was made for age.

Results.—A total of 658 cases of nonfatal MI and 281 of fatal CHD was documented within the test group. Data were controlled for smoking, hypertension, alcohol, fiber and vitamin E consumption, and the various fats (saturated, polyunsaturated, and *trans*). Comparing quintiles 1 (lowest intake) and 5 (highest intake), the relative risk (RR) was 0.69 (95% confidence interval [CI], 0.55-0.87) for folate and 0.67 (95% CI, 0.53-0.85) for vitamin B_6. The median intakes were 696 µg/day vs. 158 µg/day and 4.6 mg/day vs. 1.1 mg/day, respectively. The test subjects who were part of the highest quintile for both vitamin B_6 and folate had an RR of 0.55 when compared with the low extremes. Multivitamins reduced the risk of CHD (RR = 0.76; 95% CI, 0.65-0.90) as did vitamin B_6 and folate intake. Those women who had up to 1 serving of alcohol daily also had a low RR (RR = 0.69) compared to nondrinkers. The same was true of those who had more than 1 drink daily (RR = 0.27).

Conclusion.—Consumption of folate and vitamin B_6 by women could be an important preventive measure against CHD.

▶ Observations in children with homocysteinuria, and more basic information at a cellular level, were followed by clinical and epidemiologic studies, which led to the development of the homocysteine theory of atherosclerosis.[1] This report from the Nurses Health Study demonstrated a significant inverse relationship between dietary intake of folate and vitamin B_6 and the mortality and morbidity of cardiovascular disease over a 14-year period. Moreover, the association was strengthened by controlling for other cardiovascular risk factors such as smoking, hypertension, intake of alcohol, fiber, vitamin E, and saturated, polyunsaturated, and *trans* fat. As far as I can tell, however, no data on lipid profiles were obtained.

The results are similar to a recent Norwegian study in patients with proved CHD.[2] It appears from this study by Rimm et al. that a daily intake of 400 µg of folate and 3 mg of vitamin B_6 are required to minimize cardiovascular mortality. This supports the view that currently recommended dietary allowances for these nutrients need to be increased.

What is of additional interest in this study is that moderate alcohol intake was accounted for by the greatest reduction in cardiovascular risk among women with the highest folate intake. The interactions between alcohol and homocysteine metabolism are, however, unclear.

In summary, it would certainly appear that increased dietary intake of folate and vitamin B_6, better food processing methods, and perhaps fortification of foods with these nutrients will be beneficial, and from a theoretical standpoint, folate supplementation in individuals with low folate levels makes sense, particularly in the presence of coronary artery disease. Nonetheless, a definitive trial of the benefits and risks, if any, of folate supplementation in patients with low folate levels remains to be determined, and we do not know to what extent and at what level folate supplementation should be introduced.

B.J. Gersh, M.B., Ch.B., D.Phil, F.R.C.P.

References

1. McCully KS: Homocysteine, folate, vitamin B$_6$ and cardiovascular disease (editorial). *JAMA* 279:392-393, 1998.
2. Nygard O, Nordrehaug JE, Ressum HM et al: Plasma homocysteine levels and mortality in patients with coronary heart disease. *N Engl J Med* 337:230-236, 1997.

Risk Factors for 5-Year Mortality in Older Adults: The Cardiovascular Health Study

Fried LP, for the Cardiovascular Health Study Collaborative Research Group (Johns Hopkins Med Institutions, Baltimore, Md)
JAMA 279:585-592, 1998

4–25

Introduction.—Little is known regarding the joint contributions of diseases and disability to mortality. Few population-based studies have information on objectively measured clinical or subclinical diseases to provide insight into how multiple factors contribute to mortality in older adults. In community-dwelling men and women aged 65 years or older, the disease, functional, and personal characteristics that jointly predict mortality were determined.

Methods.—There were 5,201 men and women aged 65 years or older from 4 U. S. communities. Also studied were a supplemental cohort of 685 African-American men and women. Demographic characteristics, self-assessed health status, health habits, physical activity, physical function, and medications used were recorded, as well as a self-report of physician diagnosis of myocardial infarction, angina, congestive heart failure, hypertension, stroke, transient ischemic attack, asthma, emphysema, diabetes, intermittent claudication, renal disease, arthritis, hearing impairment, visual impairment, and cancer. Other measures included cardiovascular and pulmonary diseases and blood pressure

Results.—Within 5 years, there were 646 deaths (12%). Twenty of 78 characteristics were significantly and independently associated with mortality, including increasing age, income less than $50,000 per year, male sex, lack of moderate or vigorous exercise, low weight, high brachial (greater than 169 mm HG) and low tibial (127 mm Hg or less) systolic blood pressure, smoking for more than 50 pack-years, elevated fasting glucose level (greater than 7.2 mmol/L [130 mg/dL]), diuretic use by those without hypertension or congestive heart failure, elevated creatinine level (106 µmol/L or greater [1.2 mg/dL]), low albumin level (37 g/L or less), aortic stenosis and abnormal left ventricular ejection fraction, low forced vital capacity (2.06 mL or less), stenosis of internal carotid artery, major electrocardiographic abnormality, difficulty in any instrumental activity of daily living, congestive heart failure, and low cognitive function by Digit Symbol Substitution test score. Mortality was not associated with high-density or low-density lipoprotein cholesterol. The association between age and mortality diminished after adjustment for other factors, but the reduction in mortality with female sex continued.

Conclusion.—Objective measures of subclinical disease and disease severity were independent and joint predictors of 5-year mortality in older adults. Other predictors were male sex, relative poverty, smoking, physical activity, indicators of frailty, and disability. Objective, quantitative measures of disease were better predictors of mortality than was a clinical history of disease, except for a history of congestive heart failure.

▶ This is an important analysis of the Cardiovascular Health Study, a prospective study designed to determine the risk factors for and consequences of cardiovascular disease in older adults. There are many interesting facets to this analysis, including the fact that the lower mortality in women persisted, even after adjustment for objective measures of disease status and risk factors. This suggests that there must be other, less tangible or unidentified factors contributing to the greater longevity in women, and it does appear that female survival advantage in women persists into old age, even without estrogen. As stated in an accompanying editorial, "women do not catch up to men."

In contrast, however, the association between older age and mortality became weaker after adjustment for risk factors and other measures of disease. This would suggest that with appropriate risk factor modification and attention to co-existing diseases, older people might live considerably longer—although in the elderly, what is perhaps more important is not the predictors of death, but the quality of life before death.

B.J. Gersh, M.B., Ch.B., D.Phil., F.R.C.P.

Reference

1. Barrett-Connor E, Stuenkel CA: Questions of life and death in old age (editorial). *JAMA* 279:622, 1998.

Relationship of Leisure-time Physical Activity and Mortality: The Finnish Twin Cohort
Kujala UM, Kaprio J, Sarna S, et al (Inst of Biomedicine, Helsinki; Univ of Helsinki; Univ of Turku, Finland)
JAMA 279:440-444, 1998   4–26

Introduction.—Premature mortality may be reduced by high physical activity or fitness. High levels of physical activity or fitness may be achieved by genetic section or early childhood experiences and favor the individual with longevity. Further clarification is needed regarding the relative importance of factors over which the individual has little or no control, such as sex, intrauterine and childhood environment, and family history, compared with factors that can be modified, such as diet, smoking, and physical activity. Distinguishing between physical activity and genetic and other familial factors can be clarified by studies of twins, who share some or all of the same genes and nearly always the same childhood environment. Leisure physical activity as a predisposing or preventive factor for premature mortality was investigated in a cohort of twins.

Methods.—A questionnaire on physical activity habits and known predictors of morality was filled out by 7,925 healthy men and 7,977 healthy women aged 25 to 64 years.

Results.—Among the entire cohort, 1,253 died, representing a hazard ratio for death, adjusted for age and sex, of 0.71 in occasional exercisers and 0.57 in conditioning exercisers, compared with those who were sedentary. The odds ratio for death was 0.66 in occasional exercisers and 0.44 in conditioning exercisers, compared with those who were sedentary, among the twin pairs who were healthy at baseline and discordant for death (434). After controlling for other predictors of mortality, the beneficial effect of physical activity remained.

Conclusion.—Even after genetic and other familial factors are taken into account, leisure-time physical activity is associated with reduced mortality.

▶ These results are consistent with others that demonstrate an inverse association between baseline physical activity and premature mortality.[1] The objective of this study was to evaluate the hypothesis that genetic or other factors explain the association between leisure, physical activity, and mortality. A previous study of Danish twins reported that longevity was moderately inheritable.[2] The study reported here was confined to twin pairs who were healthy at baseline and discordant at death and provides further evidence that familial factors do not explain the mortality differences by physical activity.

This is an interesting study, but the only conclusion that can be drawn is the same clear message as from other studies that increased physical fitness is associated with reduced mortality. The beneficial effect remained after controlling for other predictors of mortality, such as hypertension and smoking.

B.J. Gersh, M.B., Ch.B., D.Phil., F.R.C.P.

References

1. Paffenbarger RS Jr, Hyde RT, Wing AL, et al: The association of changes in physical-activity level and other lifestyle characteristics with mortality among men. *N Engl J Med* 328:538-545, 1993.
2. Herskind AM, McGue M, Holm NV, et al: The inheritability of human longevity: A population-based study of 2872 Danish twin pairs born 1870 to 1900. *Human Genetics* 97:319-323, 1996.

Differences in Prevalence of and Risk Factors for Subclinical Vascular Disease Among Black and White Participants in the Cardiovascular Health Study

Kuller L, Fisher L, McClelland R, et al (Univ of Pittsburgh, Pa; Cardiovascular Health Study Coordinating Ctr, Seattle; Johns Hopkins Univ, Baltimore, Md; et al)

Arterioscler Thromb Vasc Biol 18:283-293, 1998   4–27

Introduction.—Whether the relationship between risk factors and cardiovascular disease is similar among different races, sexes, and ethnic groups is still unknown. White populations have been the primary focus of previous studies. Among a larger sample of black and white participants in the Cardiovascular Health Study, the risk factors for a composite measure of subclinical disease were determined to see whether there are any differences in key risk factors between blacks and whites.

Methods.—The prevalence of subclinical disease was measured in previous reports of 5,201 participants who were recruited from 4 communities in the United States. In year 4 of the study (1992-1993), a larger cohort of 424 black women and 2,489 black men was added. The prevalence of subclinical disease among blacks and whites and the association with cardiovascular risk factors were compared in this study.

Results.—For all participants, the prevalence of subclinical disease was 41.3% for white women, 39.7% for black women, and 41.9% for white men, and 43.7% for black men, all aged 65 years or older. With age, the prevalence increased. Among blacks and whites, the risk factor associations for subclinical disease were similar. Among black and white women, the age, systolic blood pressure, low-density lipoprotein cholesterol, smoking, and family history of myocardial infarction were independently associated with subclinical disease. For white men, subclinical disease was related to systolic blood pressure, use of antihypertensive medication, smoking, body mass index, and diastolic blood pressure. Subclinical disease was associated with blood triglyceride level, use of antihypertensive medications, and family history of myocardial infarction in black men.

Conclusion.—Body mass index was not significantly associated with subclinical disease compared to no disease for black and white women and for black men. Among premenopausal and younger perimenopausal and postmenopausal women, weight gain and obesity may be more important risk factors. It must still be determined whether the composite index is a better predictor of clinical disease compared to any of the specific components of subclinical disease, such as carotid artery wall thickness, ankle/brachial blood pressure, or traditional risk factors such as cholesterol and blood pressure.

▶ One of the important contributions of the Cardiovascular Health Study is the development of a composite measure of subclinical vascular disease, based on the extent of intimal-medial thickness of the carotid artery; the ankle/brachial blood pressure ratio; major ECG abnormalities; echocardiographic abnormalities of wall motion and ejection fraction; and a positive response on the Rose questionnaire for either claudication or possible angina pectoris.

In this large prospective, observational study confined to patients aged 65 years and older, the prevalence of subclinical disease for all participants was high, with little difference according to gender or race. The prevalence did increase with age and the risk factors associated with subclinical disease were also similar among blacks and whites. What was of interest was that body mass index was not significantly associated with subclinical disease compared to no disease for black men and both black and white women, and it is possible that weight gain and obesity are more important risk factors for cardiovascular disease among premenopausal and younger perimenopausal and postmenopausal women than among older women.[1] Furthermore, it was pointed out that body mass index or waist measurements may be an inadequate measure of body fatness among older individuals, particularly in the presence of osteoporosis.

What is clearly evident, however, is that the major risk factors for *subclinical* disease are similar to those for *overt* disease and include hypertension, cigarette smoking, and, in black males, high blood triglyceride levels. What was of interest and has been noted in other studies is the absence of a strong association of low-density lipoprotein (LDL) cholesterol to either subclinical or clinical cardiovascular disease, which may relate to decreasing LDL cholesterol in individuals with other comorbid conditions, e.g., malignancies, or to selective survival to old age in that individuals with high LDL-cholesterol levels have already died before reaching old age.[2, 3]

B.J. Gersh, M.B., Ch.B., D.Phil., F.R.C.P.

References

1. Stevens J, et al: The effect of age on the association between body mass index and mortality. *N Engl J Med* 338:1-7, 1998.
2. Newschaffer CJ, Bush TL, Hale WE: Aging and total cholesterol levels: Cohort, period and survivorship effects. *Am J Epidemiol* 1:23-24, 1992.
3. Manson JE, Willett WC, Stampfer MJ, et al: Body weight and mortality among women. *N Engl J Med* 333:677-685, 1995.

Reduction of Plasma Homocyst(e)ine Levels by Breakfast Cereal Fortified With Folic Acid in Patients With Coronary Heart Disease
Malinow MR, Duell PB, Hess DL, et al (Oregon Health Sciences Univ, Portland; Providence St Vincent Med Ctr, Portland, Ore; Fox Chase Cancer Ctr, Philadelphia)
N Engl J Med 338:1009-1015, 1998   4–28

Objective.—The research finding that folic acid supplementation can prevent congenital neural tube defects has led to folic acid supplementation of cereal-grain products in the U.S. food supply. At the fortification level recommended by the Food and Drug Administration (FDA), folic acid intake would increase by 80 to 100 µµg/day in women of childbearing age, and by 70 to 120 µg/day in adults older than 50 years. Plasma homocyst(e)ine, or plasma total homocysteine, is commonly elevated in patients with arterial occlusive disease and can be reduced by folic acid supplementation. Whether folic acid fortification can reduce plasma homocyst(e)ine levels in patients with coronary artery disease was determined.

Methods.—The randomized, controlled trial included 75 adult patients with coronary artery disease. They were randomly assigned to receive breakfast cereals fortified with 3 levels of folic acid—127, 499, and 665 µg—along with the recommended daily allowances of vitamins B_6 and B_{12}. The patients ate cereal containing 1 of the 3 folic acid levels or placebo for the first 5 weeks; after a 5-week washout period, they were switched to the alternate cereal. The effects of the different levels of folic acid fortification on plasma folic acid and homocyst(e)ine levels were assessed.

Results.—As the level of folic acid fortification increased, so did plasma folic acid and plasma homocyst(e)ine. The 127-µg folic acid level, chosen to approximate the results of the FDA's recommended fortification level, produced a 31% increase in plasma folic acid, but only a 4% decrease in plasma homocyst(e)ine. The 499-µg level of folic acid increased plasma folic acid by 65% and reduced plasma homocyst(e)ine by 11%. The 665-µg level increased plasma folic acid by 106% while reducing plasma homocyst(e)ine by 14%.

Conclusions.—Fortification of cereal grains with folic acid could lead to increased plasma folic acid levels and reduced plasma homocyst(e)ine levels. To achieve this effect, higher levels of folic acid supplementation than those currently recommended by the FDA may be required. Additional studies are needed to determine whether folic acid fortification can prevent vascular disease.

▶ It is well established that an elevated plasma homocyst(e)ine level is a risk factor for arterial occlusive disease, and this issue has been addressed frequently in previous issues of the YEAR BOOK.[1] This small randomized trial of patients with coronary artery disease takes the subject a step further by demonstrating that folic acid fortification could actually reduce plasma homocyst(e)ine levels. From this study, it appears that a consumption of at least 400 µg of supplemental folic acid is required per day to lower the blood homocyst(e)ine concentration in most of the population. This can be provided for conveniently, easily, and safely by a standard multivitamin tablet or a serving of a fully fortified breakfast cereal. This ensures a daily intake of 400 µg per day, which will prevent birth defects in addition to other potential benefits regarding coronary artery disease.

B.J. Gersh, M.B., Ch.B., D.Phil., F.R.C.P.

Reference

1. Mayer EL, Jacobson DW, Robinson K: Homocysteine and coronary atherosclerosis. *J Am Coll Cardiol* 27:517-527, 1996.

Increasing Burden of Cardiovascular Disease: Current Knowledge and Future Directions for Research on Risk Factors

Hennekens CH (Harvard Med School, Boston)
Circulation 97:1095-1102, 1998

4–29

Background.—Heart disease is the leading cause of death for men aged 45 and older and for women aged 65 and older. One in 3 deaths results from heart disease, and there is evidence that cardiovascular disease mortality may be rising. Evidence on the burden of cardiovascular disease is reviewed, along with the direction of current and future research regarding risk factors.

Burden of Cardiovascular Disease.—Mortality from coronary heart disease (CHD) is higher in blacks than in whites, with age-adjusted rates of 264.1/100,000 for black men, 190.3/100,000 for white men, 162.4/100,000 for black women, and 98.1/100,000 for white women. Though mortality from CHD is decreasing, the decline is not as great among blacks as among whites. For U.S. adolescents, the rates of smoking and obesity are increasing, as the rate of physical activity declines. These trends will have long-lasting consequences for overall and cardiovascular morbidity and mortality. Cardiovascular disease is increasing in importance as a cause of morbidity and mortality worldwide. This increase is related largely to the aging of the population in the developing world and to dramatic increases in cigarette smoking. All of these trends emphasize the need to intensify policy and research efforts in cardiovascular disease treatment and prevention.

Risk Factors.—Though genetic factors make their contribution, environmental factors clearly play a role in cardiovascular disease risk. There is proof that cardiovascular disease risk can be reduced through modification of certain risk factors, including cigarette smoking, high cholesterol, and hypertension (Table 2). Other risk factors are also proven, though the possibility of modification is unclear. About half of patients with an episode of CHD have no known risk factors. Thus, interventions for treatment and primary prevention, including antioxidant vitamins, low-dose aspirin, and hormone replacement therapy for women have been studied. Studies of the multifactorial causes of CHD have identified potential new disease markers, including the primarily atherogenic marker

TABLE 2.—Causal and Preventive Risk Factors for Cardiovascular Disease

Causal	Preventive
Cigarette smoking	Low-dose aspirin?
Elevated cholesterol	Estrogen replacement therapy in women?
Hypertension	Antioxidant vitamins?
Obesity	
Physical inactivity	
Diabetes	

(Courtesy of Hennekens CH: Increasing burden of cardiovascular disease: Current knowledge and future directions for research on risk factors. *Circulation* 97:1095-1102, 1998.)

TABLE 3.—Potential New Risk Factors for Cardiovascular Disease

Atherosclerotic and/or Thrombotic	Genetic
Homocysteine	Arterial
Plasma fibrinogen	MTHFR gene
Factor VII	ACE gene
Endogenous tissue-type plasminogen activator	Angiotensinogen
Plasminogen activator inhibitor	Venous
D-Dimer	Factor V mutation
Lipoprotein(a)	

(Courtesy of Hennekens CH: Increasing burden of cardiovascular disease: Current knowledge and future directions for research on risk factors. *Circulation* 97:1095-1102, 1998.)

homocysteine, the primarily thrombotic marker fibrinogen, and primarily inflammatory markers such as C-reactive protein (Table 3). Though measurements of environmental and genetic factors will probably become common in the future, such a focus is unlikely to replace the current focus on established risk factors. Public education is an essential part of the attack on the epidemic of cardiovascular disease. One in 3 women will die of heart disease, compared with 1 in 25 who will die of breast cancer; yet 46% of women perceive breast cancer as their major health risk, compared with 4% who perceive heart disease as the major risk.

Discussion.—Available information on the burden of cardiovascular disease is reviewed, along with the present state and future direction of research. Clinical and policy efforts addressing the known risk factors for cardiovascular disease must be intensified. Steady funding will be needed to continue to advance our ability to prevent and treat cardiovascular disease.

▶ This article, a transcript of Dr. Hennekens' presentation of the Lewis A. Conner Memorial Lecture at the 1996 Annual Scientific Sessions of the American Heart Association, is a "must" read. He emphasizes not only that the war against cardiovascular disease is far from being won, but that the burden of cardiovascular disease is increasing, both in the United States and around the world, including developing countries. In terms of years of life lost, cardiovascular disease will jump in ranking from fourth to first between 1990 and 2020; and as a cause of premature death and disability, its ranking will change from fifth to first. These projected increases in the importance of cardiovascular disease worldwide are related principally to 2 trends in developing countries: the eradication of malnutrition and infectious disease, which will allow the population to age, and marked increases in cigarette smoking. Dr. Hennekens provides a fascinating discussion of the factors underlying the "totality of evidence" and of the contributions made by epidemiology, clinical trials, clinical investigation, and basic science.

His discussion on the emergence of nontraditional risk factors for coronary artery disease is highly topical and provocative. In regard to the well-established risk factors, we are urged to redouble our clinical and public policy efforts to implement and expand public education about the growing epidemic of cardiovascular disease.

B.J. Gersh, M.B., Ch.B., D.Phil., F.R.C.P.

Triglyceride Concentration and Ischemic Heart Disease: An Eight-Year Follow-up in the Copenhagen Male Study

Jeppesen J, Hein HO, Suadicani P, et al (Copenhagen Univ Hosp; Glostrup Univ Hosp, Denmark)
Circulation 97:1029-1036, 1998   4–30

Background.—There is continuing debate about the significance of triglycerides (TG) as a risk factor for ischemic heart disease (IHD). Most epidemiologic studies have found a positive relationship between TG level and IHD risk; however, after adjustment for high-density lipoprotein cholesterol (HDL-C), the predictive value of TG is eliminated or diminished. Data from a large prospective study were evaluated to assess the relationship between fasting TG level and IHD risk.

Methods.—The analysis included data on 2,906 white men, aged 53 to 74 years, from the Copenhagen Male Study. All patients were free of overt cardiovascular disease at baseline, when measurements of fasting lipids and other IHD risk factors were obtained. Eight-year follow-up data were analyzed to examine the effect of TG level or risk of IHD, compared with the effect of HDL-C level.

Results.—An initial IHD event occurred during follow-up in 229 men. The rate of such events was 4.6% for men in the lowest third of triglyceride level, 7.7% for those in the middle third, and 11.5% for those in the highest third. After adjustment for other risk factors—including age, body mass index, alcohol, smoking, physical activity, hypertension, non–insulin-dependent diabetes mellitus, social class, low-density lipoprotein cholesterol, and HDL-C, patients with higher TG levels were at higher risk for IHD. Relative risks were 1.5 (95% confidence interval, 1.0-2.3) for men in the middle third of TG levels and 2.2 (95% confidence interval, 1.4-3.4) for men in the highest third. After stratification by HDL-C level, IHD risk clearly increased within each level of HDL-C. This was so even among men with a high HDL-C level, which is believed to be a protective factor against IHD.

Conclusions.—An elevated fasting TG level is an important risk factor for IHD, suggests this study of middle-aged and elderly white men. The impact of TG is independent from that of other risk factors, including HDL-C. Measurement of fasting serum TG should be included in risk factor profiles, with increased attention to levels of 1.6-2.5 mmol/L.

▶ Most studies have demonstrated an association between triglyceride levels and coronary artery disease, but this finding has not stood up to multivariate analyses, which control for HDL levels.[1] The role of serum triglyceride concentrations as a screening test has therefore remained controversial. The methodo ogic limitations of multivariate models, including both HDL-C and triglyceride levels, were avoided by this Danish study, in which triglyceride levels were categorized according to terciles from the lowest to the highest levels. Using this analysis after stratification by HDL levels, a clear gradient of risk with increasing triglycerides was noted, even among men with favorably high HDL levels. Elevated triglycerides also appeared to be a marker for the presence of several other risk factors.[2] I tend to agree, on the basis of this study, that triglyceride levels should be measured and treated if elevated, and this approach is consistent with the concept of global risk assessment, in which tryglicerides and other risk factors are considered part of a comprehensive evaluation of the role of coronary artery disease.

B.J. Gersh, M.B., Ch.B., D.Phil., F.R.C.P.

References

1. Austin MA: Plasma triglyceride and coronary heart disease. *Arterioscler Thromb Vasc Biol* 11:2-14, 1991.
2. Gotto AM: Triglyceride: The forgotten risk factor. *Circulation* 97:1027-1028, 1998.

Persistence of Use of Lipid-Lowering Medications: A Cross-National Study
Avorn J, Monette J, Lacour A, et al (Harvard Med School, Boston; Université de Montréal)
JAMA 279:1458-1462, 1998   4–31

Introduction.—The clinical usefulness of lipid-lowering regimens has been documented in reducing rates of cardiac morbidity and mortality. Little is known about how these drugs are taken outside managed care settings, among the poor, among minorities, and in those older than 65 years. Reasons for stopping use of a drug including a patient's noncompliance or a physician's decision to discontinue therapy if adverse effects outweigh benefits. Predictors of persistence with therapy for lipid-lowering drug regimens were estimated in typical populations of patients in Canada and the United States.

Methods.—There were 5,611 Medicaid patients in the United States and 1,676 patients older than 65 years in Canada who were studied for 1 year. The proportion of days during the study year for which patients had filled prescriptions for lipid-lowering drugs was followed as well as predictors of good vs. poor persistence with therapy. The drugs taken included clofibrate, colestipol, cholestyramine, gemfibrozil, niacin, probucol, and 3-hydroxy-3-methylglutaryl coenzyme.

Results.—For about 40% of the study year, patients did not fill prescriptions for lipid-lowering drugs in both populations. There were significantly higher persistence rates with 3-hydroxy-3-methylglutaryl coenzyme A reductase inhibitors than with cholestyramine (64.3%) compared with 36.6% of days with drug available. Significantly higher rates of persistence were seen with patients with hypertension, diabetes, or coronary artery disease. Lower rates of drug use were seen among the poorest patients compared with the less indigent, despite virtually complete drug coverage. Only 52% of surviving patients were still filling prescriptions for this drug class when rates of use were measured in the U.S. population for the 5 years after the study.

Conclusion.—For more than one third of the study year, on average, patients who were prescribed lipid-lowering drug regimens did not fill prescriptions. In choice of agent prescribed, comorbidity, socioeconomic status, and rates of persistence varied substantially despite universal coverage of prescription drug costs. Lipid-lowering therapy was stopped altogether by about half the surviving original cohort in the United States after 5 years.

▶ This is a rather discouraging paper, but perhaps the results should not come as a surprise given previous data demonstrating poor persistence with antihypertensive medications despite unequivocal evidence of efficacy from randomized trials.[1] The dramatic effects of lipid-lowering therapy in reducing clinical events in a wide spectrum of patients has been one of the most dramatic and satisfying developments during the last few years. These data suggest we have a long way to go if we are to translate these benefits so clearly demonstrated in the clinical trials to the community as a whole.

B.J. Gersh, M.B., Ch.B., D.Phil., F.R.C.P.

Reference

1. Monane M, Bohn RL, Gurwitz JH, et al: Compliance with antihypertensive therapy among elderly medicaid enrollees. *Am J Public Health* 96:1805-1808, 1996.

Obesity and Risk of Adverse Outcomes Associated With Coronary Artery Bypass Surgery

Birkmeyer NJO, for the Northern New England Cardiovascular Disease Study Group (Dartmouth Med School, Hanover, NH; Optima Health Care, Manchester, NH; Eastern Maine Med Ctr, Bangor; et al)
Circulation 97:1689-1694, 1998   4–32

Introduction.—For perioperative morbidity and mortality with cardiac surgery and other major surgical procedures, obesity is thought to be a risk factor. These perceptions are contributed by factors associated with obesity, such as hypertension, hypercholesterolemia, and diabetes, all of which contribute to the severity of coronary disease. The independent contribution of obesity to risks of in-hospital death, intraoperative/postoperative cerebrovascular accident, postoperative bleeding, and sternal wound infection associated with coronary artery bypass grafting was assessed.

Methods.—There were 11,101 patients having coronary artery bypass grafting, for which data was collected on age, sex, height, weight, medical

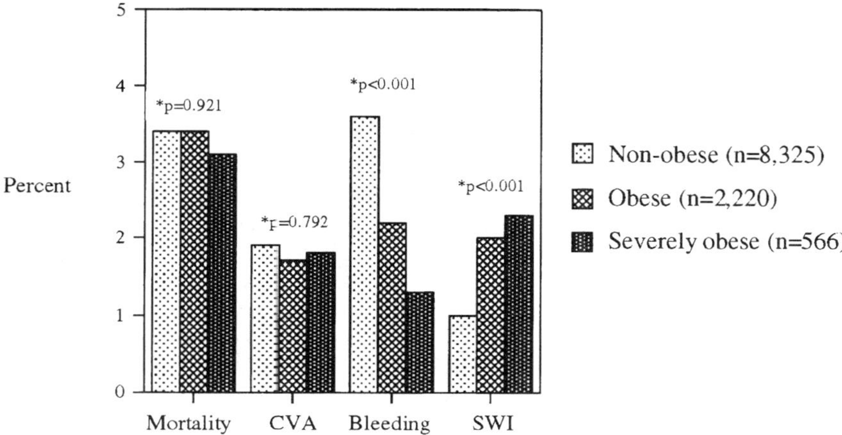

FIGURE 2.—Incidence of in-hospital adverse outcomes (death, cerebrovascular accident [*CVA*]), bleeding, and sternal wound infection (*SWI*) of coronary artery bypass infection. *χ^2 test for association. (Courtesy of Birkmeyer NJO, for the Northern New England Cardiovascular Disease Study: Obesity and risk of adverse outcomes associated with coronary artery bypass surgery. *Circulation* 97:1689-1694, 1998.)

history, current clinical status, and treatment factors. Body mass index was used as the measure of obesity. Nonobese was categorized as first to 74th percentiles, obese was categorized as 75th to 94th percentiles, and severely obese was categorized as 95th to 100th percentiles. Factors that were defined prospectively included adverse outcomes occurring in-hospital, death, intraoperative/postoperative cerebrovascular accident, postoperative bleeding, and sternal wound infection. Logistic regression was used to assess associations between obesity and postoperative outcomes to adjust for potentially confounding variables.

Results.—Increased mortality rate or postoperative cerebral vascular accident were not associated with obesity, but risks of sternal wound infection were substantially increased in the obese and severely obese (Fig 2). In the obese and severely obese, rates of postoperative bleeding were significantly lower.

Conclusion.—The perception among clinicians that obesity predisposes to various postoperative complications with coronary artery bypass grafting is not supported, with the exception of sternal wound infection. To understand the apparent protective effect of obesity on risks of postoperative bleeding, further work is needed.

▶ This interesting study from the very large Northern New England Cardiovascular Disease Study Group is the largest to examine the impact of obesity on operative mortality after bypass surgery. As is the case with other studies,[1] obesity is not an independent risk factor for operative mortality. Nonetheless, obesity is a powerful risk factor for sternal wound infection, which in itself is associated with increased perioperative mortality rate and a lengthy postoperative stay. This needs to be borne in mind, particularly in the presence of other risk factors for wound infection, including diabetes mellitus and bilateral internal mammary artery implants. A surprising feature of this study is the lower risk of postoperative bleeding in obese patients, but the reasons for this protective effect are unclear.

B.J. Gersh, M.B., Ch.B., D.Phil., F.R.C.P.

Reference

1. Moulton MJ, Crewell LL, Mackey ME, et al: Obesity is not a risk factor for significant adverse outcomes after cardiac surgery. *Circulation* 94(Suppl II):II-87-II-92, 1996.

Association of Fibrinogen, C-reactive Protein, Albumin, or Leukocyte Count With Coronary Heart Disease: Meta-analyses of Prospective Studies

Danesh J, Collins R, Appleby P, et al (Univ of Oxford, England)
JAMA 279:1477-1482, 1998   4–33

Introduction.—Associations between coronary heart disease and blood levels of fibrinogen, C-reactive protein, and albumin and leukocyte count have been reported. The short term can be influenced by insults that trigger acute-phase reactions. A meta-analysis of the available evidence from published prospective epidemiologic studies was conducted to determine the nature of the associations between coronary heart disease and fibrinogen, C-reactive protein, and albumin and leukocyte count.

Methods.—MEDLINE searches were conducted to find long-term prospective studies published before 1998 that reported on correlations between coronary heart disease and blood levels of fibrinogen, C-reactive protein, or albumin or leukocyte count. Other sources of information were from scanning of relevant reference lists, hand searching of cardiology, epidemiology, and other relevant journals, and discussions with authors of relevant reports.

Results.—There were 4,018 patients with coronary heart disease in 18 studies in which fibrinogen was studied. Patients in the top third were compared with those in the bottom third of the baseline measurements. A combined risk ratio of 1.8 associated with a difference in long-term usual mean fibrinogen levels of 2.9 μmol/L (0.1 g/dL) between the top and bottom thirds (10.3 vs. 7.4 μmol/L [0.35 vs. 0.25 g/dL]). There were 1,053 patients with coronary heart disease in 7 studies in which C-reactive protein was studied. The result was a combined risk ratio of 1.7 that was associated with a difference of 4 g/L (38 vs. 42 g/L for an inverse association). There were 5,337 patients with coronary heart disease in the 7 largest studies in which the leukocyte count was measured. The result was a combined risk ratio of 1.4 associated with a difference of 2.8×10^9/L (8.4 vs. 5.6×10^9/L). The overall results found that each of them was highly significant.

Conclusion.—There are moderate but highly statistically significant associations with coronary heart disease. Further study of the relevance of these factors to the causation of coronary heart disease is warranted, even though the mechanisms that might account for these associations are not clear.

▶ This detailed meta-analysis of long-term prospective studies of coronary heart disease is interesting in that the published results are remarkably consistent, indicating a moderate but highly significant association with coronary heart disease. These data should also be a strong incentive for further study. The mechanisms that account for the associations of these risk factors with each other and with coronary heart disease are not yet clear, and it is possible that fibrinogen, C-reactive protein, and albumin or leukocyte counts may be an indicator of another underlying process that is more relevant to the disease. If, in the future, specific treatments that affect these risk factors have become available, one might see randomized trials; but for the present, we need to accept that these highly significant relations to a condition that is a major underlying cause of death is of interest, even if the mechanisms are not well understood.

B.J. Gersh, M.B., Ch.B., D.Phil., F.R.C.P.

Acute Respiratory-Tract Infections and Risk of First-Time Acute Myocardial Infarction

Meier CR, Jick SS, Derby LE, et al (Boston Univ)
Lancet 351:1467-1471, 1998   4–34

Introduction.—More deaths occur from cardiovascular diseases, especially acute myocardial infarction (AMI), in winter than in summer, an association that may be explained by the greater number of acute respiratory-tract infections during cold weather. A large, population-based study explored the link between acute respiratory-tract infections and AMI.

Methods.—Data were obtained from the UK General Practice Research Database. Cases were patients with a first-time diagnosis of AMI during a 3-year period (1994-1996), no history of clinical risk factors, and were age 75 years or younger. Four controls were matched to each case on the basis of age, sex, and practice attended. In both groups, the date of the last respiratory-tract infection before the index date was identified. In a case-crossover analysis, cases acted as their own controls.

Results and Conclusion.—The final dataset consisted of 1,922 cases. In 1994 and 1995, more cases of AMI occurred in the winter, with the highest number (175) in January and the lowest (110) in June. Significantly more cases than controls had an acute respiratory-tract infection in the 10 days before the index date (2.8% vs. 0.9%). After adjustment for smoking and body-mass index, the odds ratio for first-time AMI in association with an infection was 3.6 when the infection occurred 1 to 5 days before the index

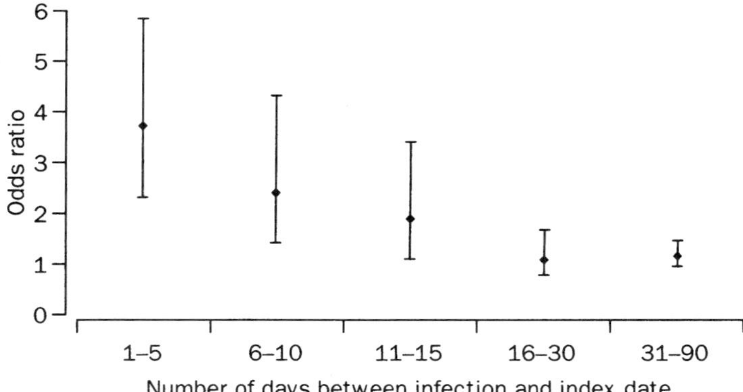

FIGURE 1.—Risk of AMI in relation to timing of previous acute respiratory tract infection. *Vertical bars*, 95% confidence interval. (Courtesy of Meier CR, Jick SS, Derby LE, et al: Acute respiratory-tract infections and risk of first-time acute myocardial infarction. *Lancet* 351:1467-1471, 1998. Copyright by The Lancet, Ltd.)

date (Fig 1). The relative risk for AMI was 2.7 in the case-crossover analysis when the infection occurred in the 10 days before the index date. Although cause and effect cannot be assumed, findings suggest that there is a seasonal variation in AMI.

▶ This epidemiologic case control and case-crossover study documents an association between recent upper respiratory-tract infections and myocardial infarction. The findings of this large study of almost 10,000 patients suggest that in acute respiratory-tract infection there is a risk factor for acute myocardial infarction in that the risk of AMI was 3 times higher among patients who had had an acute respiratory tract infection in the previous 10 days compared with those who had not. This increase in risk, however, fell away in patients who had respiratory tract infections 11 to 30 days before the indexed infarction. It is of interest that there was no increased risk of acute myocardial infarction in relation to acute urinary tract infections.

One should bear in mind, however, that an association does not imply incrimination or a direct cause and effect relation. Nonetheless, these data support other studies suggesting that there is a seasonal variation to myocardial infarction that is common in the winter[1] as well as other studies that suggest that death rates from cardiovascular disease increase during epidemics of influenza.[2]

The inflammatory theory of atherosclerosis and the role of inflammation in acute coronary syndromes has created intense interest, and we already have 2 small randomized trials of macrolide antibiotics that have reported possible benefits in regard to the secondary prevention of coronary disease.[3] There are many possible pathophysiologic mechanisms whereby an acute infection might trigger myocardial infarction, and these include changes in circulating clotting factors, increased concentrations of inflammatory cytokines that alter endothelial function, or the presence of leukocytosis and other factors that may cause plaque rupture—but at present the relations are speculative.

B.J. Gersh, M.B., Ch.B., D.Phil., F.R.C.P.

References

1. Woodhouse PR, Khaw K-T, Plummer M, et al: Seasonal variations of plasmofibrinogen and factor VII activity in the elderly: Winter infections and death from cardiovascular disease. *Lancet* 343:435-439, 1994.
2. Tillett HE, Smith JWG, Gooch CD: Excess deaths attributable to influenza in England and Wales: Age of death and certified cause. *Int J Epidemiol* 12:344-352, 1983.
3. Gurfinkel E, Bozovitch G, Daroca A, et al: Randomized trial of roxithromycin in non-Q-wave coronary syndromes: ROXIS pilot study. *Lancet* 350:404-407, 1997.

Randomized Trial of Estrogen Plus Progestin for Secondary Prevention of Coronary Heart Disease in Postmenopausal Women
Hulley S, for the Heart and Estrogen/Progestin Replacement Study (HERS) Research Group (Univ of California, San Francisco; Johns Hopkins Univ, Baltimore, Md; Wake Forest Univ, Winston-Salem, NC; et al)
JAMA 280:605-613, 1998   4–35

Background.—Observational studies report that coronary heart disease (CHD) rates are lower in postmenopausal women who take estrogen than in those who do not. However, this potential has not been confirmed in clinical trials. The effect of estrogen plus progestin therapy on the risk of CHD events in postmenopausal women with established coronary disease was investigated in a randomized, blinded, placebo-controlled, secondary prevention trial.

Methods.—A total of 2,763 women with CHD seen in outpatient and community settings at 20 U.S. clinical centers were included. All were younger than 80 years, with a mean age of 66.7 years. All were postmenopausal and had an intact uterus. The women were given either daily doses of 0.625 mg of conjugated equine estrogens plus 2.5 mg of medroxyprogesterone acetate or placebo. The mean follow-up was 4.1 years. Eighty-two percent of the women assigned to hormone treatment were still using the therapy at the end of 1 year, and 75% at the end of 3 years.

Findings.—The occurrence of nonfatal myocardial infarction or death from CHD was comparable in the 2 groups, despite a net 11% lower low-density lipoprotein cholesterol level and a 10% higher high-density lipoprotein cholesterol level in the hormone group. There was a significant time trend, with more CHD events occurring in the hormone group than in the placebo group within the first year and fewer in years 4 and 5. A greater proportion of the women in the hormone group had venous thromboembolic events and gallbladder disease. Several other end points, for which the statistical power was limited, were also comparable between groups, including fractures, cancer, and total mortality.

Conclusion.—This hormone treatment did not decrease the overall rate of CHD events in postmenopausal women with established coronary disease. However, it did increase the rate of thromboembolic events and gallbladder disease. Based on the finding of no overall cardiovascular benefit and a pattern of early increase in the risk of CHD events, this treatment is not recommended for the secondary prevention of CHD. However, continuing this treatment in women already receiving it may be appropriate.

▶ This negative result came as a surprise, given the overwhelming evidence from observational studies of estrogen replacement therapy and CHD in women with and without overt CHD.[1] This randomized trial reinforces the need to be cautious about observational studies and their confounding effects, e.g., "prevention bias."[2] In other words, perhaps the benefit of estrogen in the observational studies is the result of "compliance," which, in turn, is associated with other healthy behaviors or factors that may not be taken into account in the analysis of observational studies because they are not measured, are poorly measured, or are unmeasurable.

The authors raise the possibility that hormone replacement therapy may have detrimental prothrombotic effects that offset the beneficial effects on lipids and endothelial function. Fortunately, other trials are ongoing, and the results of this study may not apply to estrogen replacement therapy alone, to different regimens of hormone replacement therapy, or to different progestins in women with CHD, nor to the use of hormone replacement therapy as primary prevention.[2] Given the trend or the benefit after a longer duration of therapy, the author of the accompanying editorial agrees with the authors of the study that there is no reason for women currently receiving hormone replacement therapy (particularly in the presence of congestive heart disease) to abruptly stop taking the drugs, based upon the results of this study.

The second question is whether hormone replacement therapy, using this combination of drugs, should be started for the purposes of secondary prevention of CHD. This trial would suggest not. It would appear that the hormone replacement therapy issue remains a subject for randomized trials, and we are fortunate that several large, randomized trials in different patient populations are ongoing.

B.J. Gersh, M.B., Ch.B., D.Phil., F.R.C.P.

References

1. Grady D, Ruben SM, Petitti DB, et al: Hormone therapy to prevent disease and prolong life in post menopausal women. *Ann Intern Med* 117:1016-1037, 1992.
2. Petitti DB: Hormone replacement therapy and heart disease prevention, experimentation/transobservation (editorial). *JAMA* 280:650-652, 1998.

Effect of Pravastatin on Cardiovascular Events in Women After Myocardial Infarction: The Cholesterol and Recurrent Events (CARE) Trial
Lewis SJ, Sacks FM, Mitchell JS, et al (Portland Cardiovascular Inst, Ore; Harvard Med School, Boston; Baylor Univ, Dallas; et al)
J Am Coll Cardiol 32:140-146, 1998   4–36

Introduction.—Because most participants in clinical trials of the effect of lipid-lowering treatment on cardiovascular disease have been men, there is little direct evidence of the benefits of this treatment in women. The Cholesterol and Recurrent Events (CARE) trial, which included 576 postmenopausal women, showed that pravastatin reduces the risk of cardiovascular events in women after myocardial infarction (MI).

Methods.—Women in the CARE trial had a total cholesterol level of less than 240 mg/dL and a low-density lipoprotein level of 115 to 174 mg/dL. All entered the trial between 3 and 20 months after MI and were randomized to pravastatin (40 mg/day) or matching placebo. Patients were followed for a median of 5 years for combined coronary events, coronary death or nonfatal MI, and stroke.

Results.—Compared with men in the CARE trial, women were older at randomization (61 vs. 58) and had a significantly higher prevalence of certain risk factors (including hypertension and diabetes). Pravastatin had a similar effect on plasma lipids in women and men, with an average decrease of approximately 20% over 5 years. Women had a risk reduction of 43% for coronary death or nonfatal MI, 46% for combined coronary events, and 56% for stroke. The overall risk reduction was 46% for women and 20% for men (Fig 2).

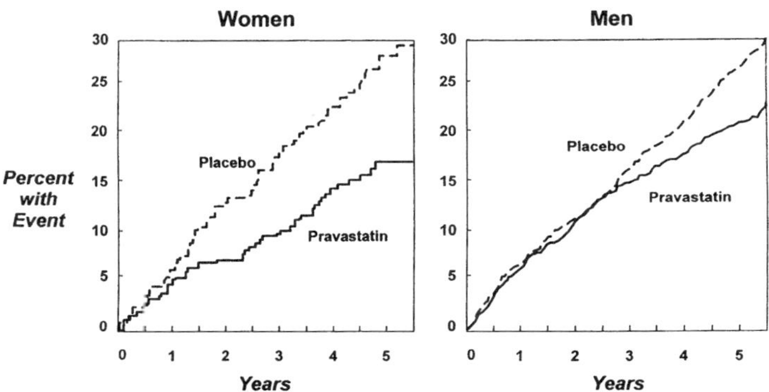

FIGURE 2.—Coronary events in women and men treated with pravastatin or placebo (overall risk reduction: 46% for women, 20% for men, P = 0.001 for both). (Reprinted with permission from the Amerian College of Cardiology from Lewis SJ, Sacks FM, Mitchell JS, et al: Effect of pravastatin on cardiovascular events in women after myocardial infarction: The Cholesterol and Recurrent Events (CARE) trial. *J Am Coll Cardiol* 32:140-146, 1998.)

Conclusion.—Pravastatin therapy resulted in a strong, early reduction in recurrent coronary events in women with MI and with average cholesterol levels before treatment.

▶ Coronary artery disease is the leading cause of death in women but, in general, women have been under-represented in clinical trials, including those of lipid-lowering therapy.[1] Although the trials of lipid-lowering therapy showed a trend toward reduction in events in women, because of the relatively small numbers of women enrolled, this did not result in statistical significance. Guidelines for cholesterol-lowering in women are by and large extrapolated from data in men.

The Scandinavian Simvastatin Survival Study demonstrated a significant reduction in coronary events in hypercholesterolemic women with prior myocardial infarction or angina.[2] This important substudy from the CARE trial extends these observations and demonstrates unequivocally the benefits of pravastatin in women survivors of a myocardial infarction who have average cholesterol levels. Whether the apparently greater benefit in women is real or a result of post-hoc subset analyses is unknown.

B.J. Gersh, M.B., Ch.B., D.Phil., F.R.C.P.

References

1. Gurwitz JH, Col MF, Avorn J: The exclusion of the elderly and women from clinical trials in acute myocardial infarction. *JAMA* 268:1417-1422, 1992.
2. Miettinen TA, Pyorala K, Olsson AG, et al: Cholesterol-lowering therapy in women and elderly patients with myocardial infarction or angina pectoris. *Circulation* 96:4211-4218, 1997.

Trends in the Incidence of Myocardial Infarction and in Mortality Due to Coronary Heart Disease, 1987 to 1994
Rosamond WD, Chambless LE, Folsom AR, et al (Univ of North Carolina, Chapel Hill; Univ of Minnesota, Minneapolis; Natl Heart, Lung, and Blood Inst, Bethesda, Md; et al)
N Engl J Med 339:861-867, 1998   4–37

Introduction.—Although mortality from coronary heart disease (CHD) is known to have declined steadily in the United States in recent years, there is less information about the incidence of CHD during this period. Accurate measures of the incidence of CHD are needed to distinguish the effects of primary prevention from those of treatment. Researchers studied population-based trends in mortality from CHD and in the incidence of myocardial infarction from 1987 to 1994.

Methods.—Data were obtained from the Atherosclerosis Risk in Communities study, which examined the incidence of CHD in 4 areas of varying size in the United States. Included in a surveillance of hospital admissions for myocardial infarction and of in-hospital and out-of-hospital deaths caused by CHD were 35- to 74-year-old residents of the 4

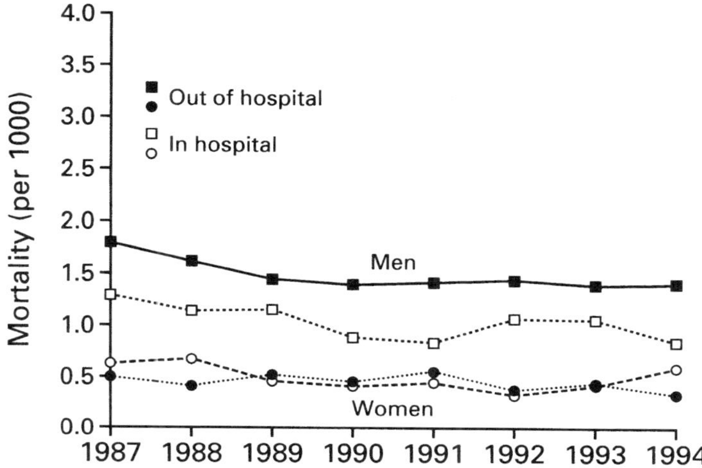

FIGURE 2.—Age-adjusted mortality from coronary heart disease among men and women aged 35 to 74, from 1987 to 1994, according to whether death occurred in or out of the hospital. (Reprinted by permission of *The New England Journal of Medicine* from Rosamond WD, Chambless LE, Folsom AR, et al: Trends in the incidence of myocardial infarction and in mortality due to coronary heart disease, 1987 to 1994. *N Engl J Med* 339:861-867. Copyright 1998, Massachusetts Medical Society. All rights reserved.)

communities. For the period between 1987 and 1994, it was estimated that there were 11,869 hospital admissions for myocardial infarction (on the basis of 8,572 admissions sampled) and 3,407 fatal coronary events (3,023 sampled).

Results.—White men showed the largest average annual decrease in CHD mortality (−4.9%), followed by white women (−4.5%), black women (−4.1%), and black men (−2.5%). In-hospital mortality from CHD fell by 5.1% and out-of-hospital mortality by 3.6% per year (Fig 2). The incidence of hospitalization for a first myocardial infarction remained stable overall and increased among black women (7.4% per year) and black men (2.9% per year). Survival after myocardial infarction improved and recurrence rates decreased.

Conclusion.—The incidence of hospitalization for myocardial infarction was stable or increased slightly from 1987 to 1994. Mortality from CHD, however, decreased significantly each year. Both medical care and secondary prevention have contributed to the decline in CHD mortality.

▶ This article about 4 communities in the United States highlights an apparent paradox: the declining mortality of coronary heart disease is not accompanied by an expected reduction in incidence. There is little doubt that the decline in mortality was the result of a reduction in case fatality rates, which is an encouraging testament to advances in therapy, including aspirin, reperfusion strategies, β blockers, angiotensin converting enzyme inhibitors, and lipid-lowering drugs. At first glance, the lack of any reduction in incidence could imply that primary prevention strategies have failed, although much of the decline in mortality over the past 30 years is related to primary prevention efforts. An accompanying editorial points out that the incidence rates in this study may have actually declined but may not be reflected in the data for a variety of reasons that apply to all surveillance studies of trends in the incidence of myocardial infarction. For example, a greater public awareness of the symptoms of myocardial infarction may result in more frequent diagnoses and hospitalization rates, in addition to other factors.[1]

Of concern are the differences between blacks and whites both in mortality rates and in the increasing incidence of first myocardial infarctions in black women. Studies of trends and the severity of disease and changes in risk factors may shed further light on the mechanisms underlying these encouraging statistics.

B.J. Gersh, M.B., B.Ch., D.Phil., F.R.C.P.

Reference

1. Levy D, Thom TJ: Death rates from coronary disease: Progress and a puzzling paradox (editorial). *N Engl J Med* 339:915-916, 1998.

Percutaneous Transluminal Coronary Angioplasty and Devices

Long-term Follow-up After Deferral of Percutaneous Transluminal Coronary Angioplasty of Intermediate Stenosis on the Basis of Coronary Pressure Measurement

Bech GJW, De Bruyne B, Bonnier HJRM, et al (Catharina Hosp, Eindhoven, The Netherlands; Cardiovascular Ctr, Aalst, Belgium)
J Am Coll Cardiol 31:841-847, 1998   4–38

Purpose.—Patients who have persistent typical or atypical chest pain with angiographically intermediate stenosis but without inducible ischemia pose a clinical challenge. Although these patients are at increased risk of a coronary event, the extent of that risk is unknown. Some reliable technique of evaluating the functional significance of intermediate lesions would be useful in making decisions about the need for dilation. The use of coronary pressure measurement and myocardial fractional flow reserve (FFR_{myo}) in deciding the need for percutaneous transluminal coronary angioplasty (PTCA) in patients with intermediate stenosis was examined retrospectively.

Methods.—During a 4-year period, guide wire–based coronary pressure measurements of FFR_{myo} were obtained in more than 600 patients. Of these, 100 patients were referred for PTCA of an intermediate stenosis in the middle or proximal part of a native coronary artery but had the procedure deferred because of a pressure-derived FFR_{myo} of 0.75 or greater. This level was regarded as showing that myocardial perfusion was adequate, and that the lesion could not be causing the patient's chest pain. Subsequent management decisions were left to the referring physician. Follow-up clinical data were available in all patients; mean follow-up was 18 months.

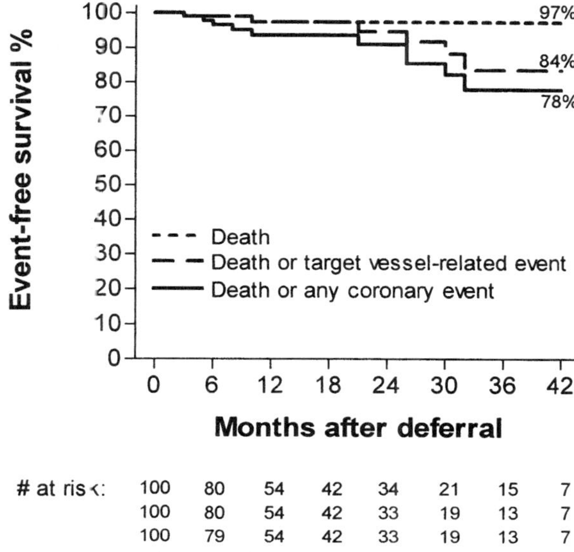

FIGURE 3.—Estimated survival and event-free survival curves (Kaplan-Meier) of all patients in whom the planned percutaneous transluminal coronary angioplasty of an intermediate coronary stenosis was deferred on the basis of a pressure-derived myocardial fractional flow reverse of 0.75 or greater. *Numbers below the x-axis* represent patients at risk at 0, 6, 12, 18, 24, 30, 36, and 42 months after deferral of angioplasty for survival; survival or target vessel-related event; and survival or any coronary event, respectively. (Courtesy of Bech GJW, De Bruyne B, Bonnier HJRM, et al: Long-term follow-up after deferral of percutaneous transluminal coronary angioplasty of intermediate stenosis on the basis of coronary pressure measurement. *J Am Coll Cardiol* 31:841-847, 1998. Reprinted with permission from the American College of Cardiology.)

Results.—Mean percent diameter stenosis in this group of patients was 47%. Two patients died of noncardiac causes during follow-up. Only 4 patients had an event related to the target vessel; 1 had a myocardial infarction caused by disease progression in the target vessel at 26 months. At 42 months, estimated survival was 97%, survival without target vessel-related events was 84%, and survival without any coronary event was 78% (Fig 3).

Conclusions.—Percutaneous transluminal coronary angioplasty can be safely deferred in patients with intermediate stenosis who have an FFR$_{myo}$ of 0.75 or greater. Although no control group was studied, the clinical event rate with deferral is much lower than expected if PTCA had been performed as originally planned. A large, randomized trial is being performed to confirm the safety of PTCA deferral in this group of patients.

▶ This is an extremely provocative study and consistent with a prior study of an insurance claims database of patients younger than 65 years, which suggests that 60% or more of coronary interventions are performed without objective evidence of ischemia.[1] The only indications for PTCA in patients with single-vessel disease are to relieve symptoms or ischemia. There is no evidence that dilation of a lesion in the *absence* of clear-cut symptoms or objective evidence of ischemia is of value, because "future culprit" lesions cannot be defined purely on the basis of their angiographic appearance.[2]

This is a retrospective study confined to patients with stenoses of intermediate severity and single-vessel disease in 60%, double-vessel disease in 34%, and triple-vessel disease in only 6% of patients. Nonetheless, in this selected patient population, after deferral of PTCA on the basis of a measurement of adequate coronary/myocardial flow reserve, the subsequent event rate was low—much lower than expected had PTCA been performed in all patients. What would be fascinating, but more difficult to put to the test, would be the outcomes of a conservative approach in patients who had an abnormal coronary flow reserve consistent with ischemia, given that so many of them had negative exercise tests and single-vessel disease and stenosis of apparently moderate severity.

B.J. Gersh, M.B., Ch.B., D.Phil., F.R.C.P.

Reference

1. Topol EJ, Ellis SG, Delos M, et al: Analysis of coronary angioplasty practice in the United States with an insurance-claims data base. *Circulation* 87:1489-1497, 1993.
2. Mann JM, Davies MJ: Vulnerable plaque. Relation of characteristics to degree of stenosis in human coronary arteries. *Circulation* 94:928-931, 1996.

Comparison of Antiplatelet Effects of Aspirin, Ticlopidine, or Their Combination After Stent Implantation
Rupprecht HJ, Darius H, Borkowski U, et al (Johannes Gutenberg Univ, Mainz, Germany)
Circulation 97:1046-1052, 1998   4–39

Background.—With combined antiplatelet therapy using ticlopidine and aspirin to prevent subacute stent thrombosis, stenting has become a widely used interventional cardiology technique. Given the side effects of ticlopidine and aspirin—particularly neutropenia and gastrointestinal bleeding, respectively—it may be questioned whether these 2 drugs, alone or in combination, are sufficient to counteract platelet activation and aggregation after stenting. The effects of aspirin and/or ticlopidine on platelet activation and aggregation parameters were compared after stent implantation.

Methods.—A total of 61 patients who underwent successful implantation of a single Palmaz-Schatz stent in a native coronary artery were studied. They were randomly assigned to 1 of 3 groups: group A received aspirin, 300 mg/day plus, ticlopidine, 2 × 250 mg/day; group B received ticlopidine only; and group C received aspirin only. Measures of platelet activation—flow cytometric measurement of CD62p (p-selectin) expression and binding of fibrinogen to the platelet surface glycoprotein IIb/IIIa receptor—were assessed on days 1, 7, and 14. Platelet aggregation in response to adenosine 5'-diphosphate (ADP) and collagen was also evaluated.

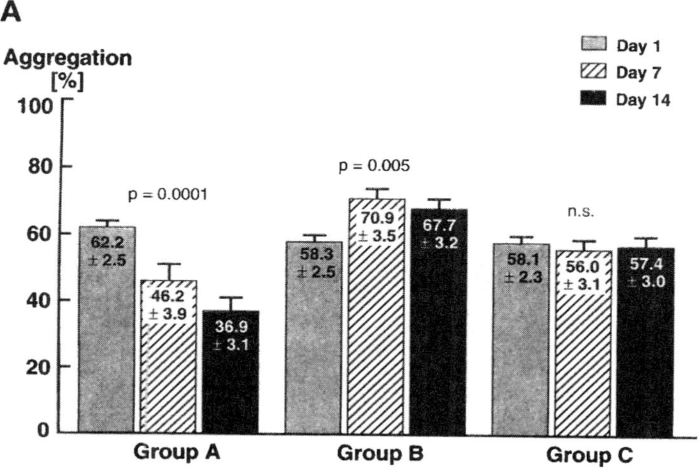

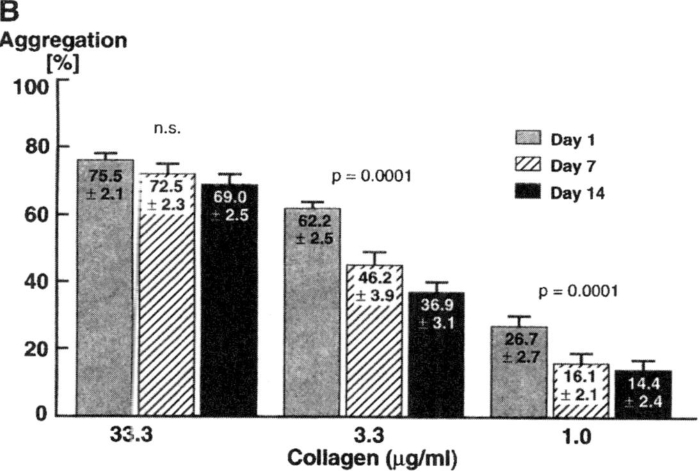

FIGURE 1.—A, time-dependent alterations in collagen-induced platelet aggregation (collagen 3.3 µg/mL) measured as percentage of light transmittance in group A (ticlopidine + aspirin), group B (ticlopidine), and group C (aspirin). *Numbers within bars* represent mean ±1 SEM. Probability values relate to differences between different time points in each treatment group. Comparison of treatment groups by analysis of variance (ANOVA) revealed a value of *P* < 0.0001. **B,** dose-dependent platelet stimulatory effects of collagen (33.3, 3.3, or 1.0 µg/mL) in patients of group A receiving ticlopidine and aspirin. *Numbers within bars* represent mean ±1 SEM. Probability values relate to differences between different time points in each treatment group. (Courtesy of Rupprecht HJ, Darius H, Borkowski U, et al: Comparison of antiplatelet effects of aspirin, ticlopidine, or their combination after stent implantation. *Circulation* 97:1046-1052. Copyright 1998, American Heart Association. Reproduced with permission.)

Results.—From day 1 to day 14, collagen-induced platelet aggregation decreased from 62% to 37% in group A and from 68% to 58% in group B, with no significant change in group C (Fig 1). Platelet aggregation induced by ADP also decreased significantly in groups A (from 75% to 55%) and B (from 72% to 53%), but not in group C. Expression of

CD62p decreased from 68% to 41% in group A and from 65% to 39% in group B; fibrinogen binding decreased from 61% to 36% in group A and from 58% to 39% in group B. Neither measure of platelet activation was significantly changed in group C.

Conclusions.—In patients after stent implantation, ticlopidine and aspirin have synergistic and accelerated platelet inhibitory effects when given in combination. This combination is clearly superior to monotherapy with either drug in its effects on platelet aggregation and platelet activation. Aspirin plus ticlopidine is the antiplatelet therapy of choice for patients undergoing stent implantation.

▶ Since the introduction of coronary stents by Sigwart, the problem of subacute stent thrombosis led to advances in stent deployment techniques and in antithrombotic therapy.[1] What came about as somewhat of a surprise, was the failure of oral anticoagulants (warfarin) to reduce stent thrombosis in comparison with platelet inhibitors. Two large multicenter trials demonstrated the superiority of aspirin and ticlopidine over aspirin alone, and outcomes in both trials were significantly worse with oral anticoagulants.[2, 3]

This trial of 61 patients provides a theoretical underpinning for the results of the larger trials. The combination of aspirin and ticlopidine is clearly superior in terms of platelet aggregation parameters and markers of platelet activation, in comparison with monotherapy with either aspirin or ticlopidine. Other basic investigations have shown that fibrinogen receptor activity and platelet surface expression of p-selectin is enhanced (an unfavorable response) by oral anticoagulants in contrast with ticlopidine.

Given the known associations between ticlopidine and neutropenia, the next question is whether clopidogrel, the likely successor to ticlopidine, has similar platelet antiaggregatory effects.[4]

B.J. Gersh, M.B., Ch.B., D.Phil., F.R.C.P.

References

1. Sigwart U, Puel A, Mirkovitch V, et al: Intravascular stents to prevent occlusion and restenosis after transluminal angioplasty. *N Engl J Med*, 316:701-706, 1987.
2. Leon MB, Baim DS, Gordon P, et al: Clinical and angiographic results from the stent anticoagulation regimen study (STARS). *Circulation* 94:685S, 1996.
3. Bertrand M, LeGrand V, Boland J, et al: Full anticoagulation versus ticlopidine plus aspirin after stent implantation: A randomized multicenter European study: The FANTASTIC Trial. *Circulation* 94:685S, 1996.
4. CAPRIE Steering Committee. A randomized blinded trial of clopidogrel versus aspirin in patients at risk of ischemic events [CAPRIE]. *Lancet* 348:1329-1339, 1996.

Predictors of Restenosis After Coronary Stent Implantation
Bauters C, Hubert E, Prat A, et al (Univ of Lille, France; INSERM CJF, Lille, France)
J Am Coll Cardiol 31:1291-1298, 1998   4–40

Introduction.—For patients with coronary artery disease, balloon angioplasty has become an established treatment, but so has the problem of restenosis. Coronary stenting is a newer alternative form of coronary revascularization, which has demonstrated relatively low rates of angiographic and clinical restenosis. A high proportion of patients having repeat percutaneous transluminal coronary angioplasty has had coronary stenting performed because of recent improvements in the technique of stent implantation. The technique has been used in diabetic patients, in rescue situations, in vessels smaller than 3 mm, for the treatment of chronic coronary occlusions, and in infarct-related lesions. The 6-month angiographic outcome of lesions in patients having successful coronary stenting was analyzed.

Methods.—There were 463 patients who had successful coronary stenting in 500 lesions. They all received antiplatelet therapy. There were 19% of patients with diabetes mellitus, 71% who were smokers, 38% with hypertension, 59% with hypercholesterolemia, 49% with family history of coronary artery disease, and 36% with unstable angina. Restenosis was correlated with clinical, qualitative, and quantitative angiographic variables.

Results.—In 26% of the 405 lesions at the angiographic follow-up, restenosis was present and defined as the presence of more than 50% diameter stenosis in the dilated segment. During the follow-up period, the mean late lumen loss was 0.79 ± 0.64 mm. A higher late lumen loss was associated with implantation of multiple stents and a high acute gain. A lower late lumen loss was associated with the use of high-inflation pressure and Palmaz-Schatz stents. Independent predictors of restenosis were implantation of multiple stents, stenosis length, smaller reference diameter, and stent type other than Palmaz-Schatz when restenosis was defined as a qualitative variable (Table 9).

TABLE 9.—Multiple Logistic Regression Analysis for the Dependent Variable of Restenosis*

Independent Variable	Coeff	SE	p Value	OR (95% CI)
No. of stents	0.83	0.26	0.001	2.29 (1.37-3.82)
Palmaz-Schatz stent	-0.68	0.25	0.007	0.50 (0.31-0.83)
Stenosis length (mm)	0.05	0.02	0.008	1.06 (1.01-1.10)
Ref diam (mm)	-0.58	0.26	0.02	0.56 (0.34-0.93)

*Diameter stenosis greater than 50% at follow-up. *CI,* Confidence interval; *OR,* odds ratio; *Ref diam,* reference diameter. (Courtesy of Bauters C, Hubert E, Prat A, et al: Predictors of restenosis after coronary stent implantation. *J Am Coll Cardiol* 31:1291-1298, 1998. Reprinted with permission from the American College of Cardiology.)

Conclusion.—An unacceptable restenosis rate is associated with coronary stenting in an unselected patient group. The risk of restenosis was not related to most of the variables tested, although some of the risk factors were identified. In terms of restenosis, coronary stenting may have superiority over balloon angioplasty, which may apply to subgroups of patients who were not included in these studies.

▶ Although previous studies have examined factors predictive of stent restenosis, the strength of this study lies in its large size and its relevance to current practice. All the patients in this study underwent high-pressure inflation of balloon-expandable stents and were subsequently treated with a combination of aspirin and ticlopidine, whereas in many of the previous studies oral anticoagulant agents were given for at least 2 months after the procedure. The rate of subacute thrombosis was high and the importance of high-pressure inflation for adequate stent deployment has not been widely appreciated.

The overall rate of restenosis was 26%, and the major predictors were periprocedure variables, namely multiple stents, smaller vessels, the particular stent used, and the degree of stenosis. What I found to be of particular interest, however, was the lack of any effect on restenosis variables primarily associated with restenosis after balloon angioplasty, such as diabetes, unstable angina, pretreatment total occlusions, and intervention in an infarct-related artery. Perhaps in these subgroups of patients there is a particular benefit from coronary stenting, and randomized trials should soon provide us with more definitive answers. The potential role of coronary stenting in diabetics is of great clinical interest given the results of the Bypass Angioplasty Revascularization Investigation (BARI Trial) of patients with multivessel disease, in which bypass surgery was shown to be superior to PTCA in diabetics.[1]

It remains to be seen what proportion of diabetics with multivessel disease will have vessels large enough for coronary stenting since this study and others show a small vessel diameter is a powerful predictor of restenosis in patients with coronary stents.

B.J. Gersh, M.B., Ch.B., D.Phil., F.R.C.P.

Reference

1. The Bypass Angioplasty Revascularization Investigation (BARI) investigators: Comparison of coronary bypass surgery with angioplsty in patients with multivessel disease. *N Engl J Med* 335:275-277, 1996.

Coronary Artery Bypass Surgery

Renal Dysfunction After Myocardial Revascularization: Risk Factors, Adverse Outcomes, and Hospital Resource Utilization

Mangano CM, for the Multicenter Study of Perioperative Ischemia Research Group (Stanford Univ, Calif; Ischemia Research and Education Found, San Francisco; Emory Univ, Atlanta, Ga; et al)
Ann Intern Med 128:194-203, 1998   4–41

Purpose.—The effects of cardiac surgery on renal function remain unclear. Renal function abnormalities can result from nonpulsatile blood flow, increased catecholamine and inflammatory mediator levels, renal embolic insults, and release of free hemoglobin from traumatized erythrocytes. Renal dysfunction was studied in a large population of patients undergoing cardiopulmonary bypass and myocardial revascularization.

Methods.—A total of 2,222 patients undergoing myocardial revascularization at 24 research hospitals were studied. Their rates of postoperative renal failure (defined as the need for dialysis) and of renal dysfunction (defined as a postoperative serum creatinine level of 177 µmol/L or greater and an increase in serum creatinine of 62 µmol/L or greater from the preoperative to postoperative period) were assessed.

Results.—By these definitions, postoperative renal dysfunction occurred in 7.7% of patients and renal failure in 1.4%. Mortality was 0.9% for patients with neither adverse renal outcome, compared with 19% for those with renal dysfunction and 63% for those with renal failure. The risk of renal failure increased steadily with age: doubled for patients in their 70s and tripled for patients in their 80s, compared with younger patients. Factors associated with renal dysfunction were type 1 diabetes mellitus, preoperative glucose level, congestive heart failure, previous coronary artery bypass grafting, and preoperative creatinine level of 124 to 177 µmol/L. More than 80% of patients with renal dysfunction had intraoperative or postoperative hemodynamic instability or hemorrhage.

Conclusions.—An 8% rate of renal dysfunction or failure was documented in patients undergoing myocardial revascularization. Renal risk is related to patient-specific factors, probably reflecting diffuse atherosclerosis. The findings have implications for preoperative communication of risk, treatment with potential nephrotoxic drugs, and surgical technique.

▶ This is the largest study published on this important subject. As stated by the authors, on the basis of 600,000 coronary bypass procedures performed annually throughout the world, and assuming a 7.7% incidence of renal dysfunction (defined by a postoperative serum creatinine-level of 2.0 mg/dL (≥ 177 µmol/L) and a 0.70 mg/dL (≥ 62 µmol/L) rise in serum creatinine from the preoperative to postoperative period), it is estimated that approximately 46,000 patients will develop postoperative renal dysfunction and 8,000 will require dialysis. The impact of this upon the utilization of health care resources, both early and late, is substantial and quite sobering.

The predictors of postoperative renal dysfunction are primarily patient specific and reflect many characteristics indicative of diffuse atherosclerosis. This does not help us much clinically, other than to provide a more realistic estimate of the risks of bypass surgery when communicating with the patient. However, the potential to reduce preoperative renal dysfunction exists by maximizing cardiac output and perfusion pressure, avoiding nephrotoxic drugs, and allowing time for contrast-induced renal dysfunction to stabilize. Intraoperatively, the surgeon has to balance the benefits of a more comprehensive procedure against the risks of prolonging cross-clamp time. Attention to serum glucose levels and both volume and inotropic status is clearly part of the routine management.

The increasing number of elderly patients undergoing bypass surgery results in a burgeoning population that is particularly vulnerable to the deleterious effects of cardiac surgery and cardiac pulmonary bypass upon renal function. As we push the envelope of cardiac surgery fuller, by including an expanding population of high-risk patients, perhaps the difference between success and failure may increasingly depend upon attention to detail.

This study identifies targets for therapy; whether we can modify outcomes by addressing these in high-risk, elderly, and diabetic patients undergoing bypass surgery remains to be seen. The alternative of withholding surgical treatment is not the answer. The risks of bypass surgery in such patients are greater, but the potential benefits are substantial.

B.J. Gersh, M.B., Ch.B., D.Phil., F.R.C.P.

Prediction of Death and Myocardial Infarction by Screening With Exercise-Thallium Testing After Coronary-Artery-Bypass Grafting

Lauer MS, Lytle B, Pashkow F, et al (Cleveland Clinic Found, Ohio)
Lancet 351:615-622, 1998   4–42

Background.—Coronary artery bypass grafting is becoming more common in the treatment of patients with coronary heart disease. The value of myocardial-perfusion imaging in determining risk in patients without symptoms after coronary artery bypass grafting is controversial. Clinical guidelines of the American Heart Association/American College of Cardiology do not recommend routine screening of such patients but do allow for screening of selected patients without symptoms.

Methods.—The independent and incremental value of exercise thallium-201 single-photon emission CT in predicting death and nonfatal myocardial infarction was determined in 873 patients. The mean patient age was 64 years; 9% were women. All patients had undergone coronary artery bypass grafting, and none had recurrent angina or other major intercurrent coronary events. Follow-up was 3 years.

Results.—Analysis showed that 508 patients had myocardial-perfusion defects. A total of 57 patients died and 72 patients experienced major events. Patients with thallium-perfusion defects had a higher rate of death

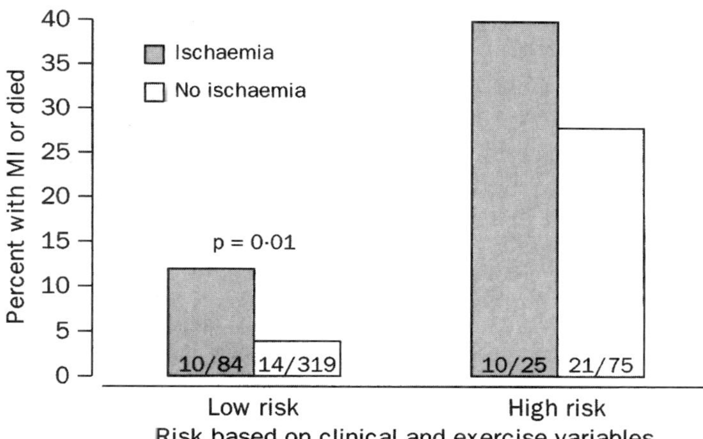

FIGURE 5.—Three-year major event (death or nonfatal myocardial infarction [*MI*]) rates according to prethallium risk stratification and the presence of reversible thallium defects. Prethallium risk stratification was based on a logistic regression model predicting events as a function of clinical and exercise variables only. Within both low risk and high risk categories, patients with reversible thallium-perfusion defects had higher 3-year event rates. The *numbers within the columns* are the number of patients with events (*numerators*) and the total number of patients within each category (*denominators*). (Courtesy of Lauer MS, Lytle B, Pashkow F, et al: Prediction of death and myocardial infarction by screening with exercise-thallium testing after coronary artery bypass grafting. *Lancet* 351:615-622, copyright 1998, The Lancet Ltd.)

and of major events. Fixed defects only were not associated with risk of death or major events. Reversible defects were associated with death and major events and with higher event rates in low-risk and high-risk patients (Fig 5). Impaired exercise capacity was the exercise variable with the strongest predictive power; poor exercise capacity was predictive of death (18% vs. 4%, $P < 0.0001$) and death or nonfatal myocardial infarction (19% vs. 5%, $P < 0.0001$). Thallium-perfusion defects were predictive of death and major events after adjusting for baseline clinical variables, surgical variables, time since coronary artery bypass grafting, and standard cardiovascular risk factors. Impaired exercise was strongly predictive of death and major events after adjusting for confounding variables. The sensitivity of thallium-perfusion defects for predicting major events was 82%; specificity was 43%, positive predictive value was 15%, and negative predictive value was 95%. The sensitivity of reversible thallium-perfusion defects for predicting major events was 36%; specificity was 80%, positive predictive value was 18%, and negative predictive value was 91%.

Discussion.—In these patients, thallium-perfusion defects and impaired exercise capacity were strong, independent predictors of death or nonfatal myocardial infarction. Based on these findings, it is recommended that the current guidelines against routine screening with exercise myocardial-perfusion tests in patients without symptoms after coronary artery bypass grafting be reconsidered. The cost of identifying patients with a higher risk of events seems reasonable. Although the cost per high risk patient identified increased from \$553 to \$1,285 with thallium scintigraphy, it also identified patients for whom coronary angiography would not be indicated. This brings the cost to about \$1,000 per patient who might be considered a candidate for aggressive revascularization.

▶ This excellent study provides, to my mind, more questions than answers. Clearly, reversible thallium perfusion defects in asymptomatic patients post bypass surgery are an independent risk factor for late death and myocardial infarction. Nonetheless, the positive predictive value of 15% (for fixed or reversible defects) or 18% (reversible defects alone) limits the clinical utility of such an approach. Although the negative predictive value is high, it should be appreciated that these are asymptomatic patients to begin with.

In regard to the cost effectiveness of adding thallium to the clinical and exercise variables, one also needs to take into account the cost of angiography, which will be performed in a majority of patients with positive thallium study results in whom no events occurred during follow-up. In this study, the analysis was confined to the costs of the stream tests and not the "downstream" implications.

How often should one perform exercise testing in asymptomatic patients post bypass surgery? We do not know the answer, but I agree with the authors that this should be performed some time during the first 3 to 6 years (the earlier the better), and it is reasonable to add scintigraphic imaging at this time. There are no data, however, to support the routine use of thallium imaging or any other form of stress imaging on an annual or biannual basis in asymptomatic patients.

B.J. Gersh, M.B., Ch.B., D.Phil., F.R.C.P.

Patients Treated by Cardiologists Have a Lower In-Hospital Mortality for Acute Myocardial Infarction
Casale PN, Jones JL, Wolf FE, et al (Lancaster Heart Found, Pa; Pennsylvania Health Care Cost Containment Council, Harrisburg; Messiah College, Grantham, Pa)
J Am Coll Cardiol 32:885-889, 1998   4–43

Introduction.—Acute myocardial infarction (AMI) is a common illness treated by both primary care physicians and specialists. A recent study of Medicare patients suggests that outcome of AMI is better when a cardiologist admits a patient, an effect attributed to the cardiologist's greater use of life-saving therapies. A retrospective study analyzed in-hospital mortality for AMI patients admitted by cardiologists vs. that for patients admitted by primary care physicians.

Methods.—Data were analyzed from 30,175 direct hospital admissions for the treatment of AMI in Pennslyvania in 1993. A risk-adjusted model of in-hospital mortality was developed by testing 20 clinical and demographic variables, including age, medical history, and test results. In addition, physician-, hospital-, and primary payer-related characteristics were entered into the model.

Results.—Multiple logistic regression analysis identified independent predictors of lower in-hospital mortality to be treatment by a cardiologist (odds ratio = 0.83) and by physicians treating a high volume of AMI patients (odds ratio = 0.89). Compared to treatment by primary care physicians, treatment by cardiologists was associated with a significantly shorter stay for both medically treated patients and those undergoing revascularization.

Conclusion.—Although limiting access to specialists is recommended as a means of reducing the cost of health care, both in-hospital mortality and hospital length of stay were reduced in those AMI patients treated by a cardiologist.

▶ Good news, but it should not come as a surprise to cardiologists. The management of acute myocardial infarction is complex but rewarding. The decisions to be made are many and involve the emergency room as well as primary care physicians. Nonetheless, the importance of the cardiologist (as self-serving as this may sound) is understandable when treatment strategies involve multiple decisions, including those about acute reperfusion therapy, β blockers, angiotensin converting enzyme inhibitors, and heparin as opposed to the newer antithrombotic or antiplatelet agents. Other issues include the role of stress testing and the preferred modality, and the role of an invasive as opposed to a conservative strategy in post-infarct survivors.

As we work through these major issues in the current climate of health care reform, approaches to the management of acute myocardial infarction have important implications, which extend beyond the immediate horizons of our own practices. Let these be evidence-based; the consequences are too far-reaching for us to resort to the comforting bulwark of "clinical experience."

B.J. Gersh, M.B., Ch.B., D.Phil., F.R.C.P.

Pharmacologic Therapy

Effect of HMGcoA Reductase Inhibitors on Stroke: A Meta-analysis of Randomized, Controlled Trials
Bucher HC, Griffith LE, Guyatt GH (Kantonsspital Basel, Switzerland; Mc-Master Univ, Hamilton, Ont, Canada)
Ann Intern Med 128:89-95, 1998   4–44

Background.—Scientists have not adequately determined the correlation of hypercholesterolemia and stroke. This study examines the relationship between stroke and the administration of antilipidemic interventions.

Methods.—Researchers searched MEDLINE and EMBASE through October 1996 to find controlled, randomized studies of cholesterol-lowering interventions. Selection of studies was based on random assignment of treatment, use of control, and reporting of cases of stroke, death from coronary disease, and overall mortality. Researchers took differences in antilipidemic treatments into account and reviewed each trial for criteria, methods, and outcomes. Twenty-eight total trials were used. The intervention group numbered 49,477, and the control group numbered 56,636. Researchers combined data for fatal and non-fatal strokes.

Results.—Researchers tabulated risk ratios at 0.95 (95% CI, 0.86 to 1.05; test of heterogeneity, $P = 0.2$) for total risk, 0.76 (CI, 0.062 to 0.92; test of heterogeneity, $P = 0.2$) for HMGcoA reductase inhibitors, and 1.0 for interventions other than HMGcoA including fibrates, resins, and dietary interventions. Summary estimate differences between HMGcoA reductase inhibitors and other interventions were statistically significant and clinically important. Rates of overall mortality and death from coronary heart disease were also reduced in HMGcoA trials.

Conclusion.—According to this meta-analysis, HMGcoA reductase inhibitors reduce the incidence of stroke by lowering cholesterol much more effectively than do older drugs.

▶ Although cholesterol-lowering drugs have been shown to reduce emphatically the incidence of non-fatal and fatal myocardial infarction in both primary and secondary prevention, a previous meta-analysis study found no reduction in stroke-related morbidity and mortality.[1] This review, however, did not include the more recent trials using the HMGcoA reductase inhibitors. This review suggests that HMGcoA reductase inhibitors do reduce incidence of non-fatal and fatal strokes, but other less potent lipid-lowering agents are not effective in regard to this specific end point. Whether a marked lowering of serum cholesterol by the "statins" could increase the risk for hemorrhagic stroke cannot be answered by the data. Nonetheless, indirect evidence would suggest that in populations with a significant risk for cardiovascular disease, the risk of hemorrhage is outweighed by the benefits of cholesterol-lowering on overall cardiovascular events. Whether this applies to patients at lower risk of cardiovascular disease, remains to be seen.

There are numerous limitations to this analysis. These are addressed extensively by the authors in the discussion. One has to conclude that in regard to the new generation of lipid-lowering drugs, all the news so far is good.

B.J. Gersh, M.B., Ch.B., D.Phil., F.R.C.P.

Reference

1. Atkins D, Psaty BM, Koepsell TD, et al: Cholesterol reduction and the risk of stroke in men. A meta-analysis of randomized control trials. *Ann Inter Med*, 119:136-145, 1993.

Thrombosis Prevention Trial: Randomised Trial of Low-Intensity Oral Anticoagulation With Warfarin and Low-Dose Aspirin in the Primary Prevention of Ischaemic Heart Disease in Men at Increased Risk

Meade TW, for the Medical Research Council's General Practice Research Framework (Wolfson Inst of Preventive Medicine, London)
Lancet 351:233-241, 1998   4–45

Purpose.—The relation of factors VII and VIIc activity to the incidence of ischemic heart disease (IHD), particularly fatal IHD, prompted a thrombosis prevention trial, which assessed the effects of low-intensity warfarin anticoagulation on the incidence of IHD. Soon after the start of this trial, aspirin's value in the secondary prevention of IHD became apparent. However, aspirin's primary preventive value remains unknown. The original thrombosis prevention trial was expanded into a factorial comparison of low-intensity warfarin anticoagulation and low-dose aspirin, alone and in combination, for primary prevention of IHD.

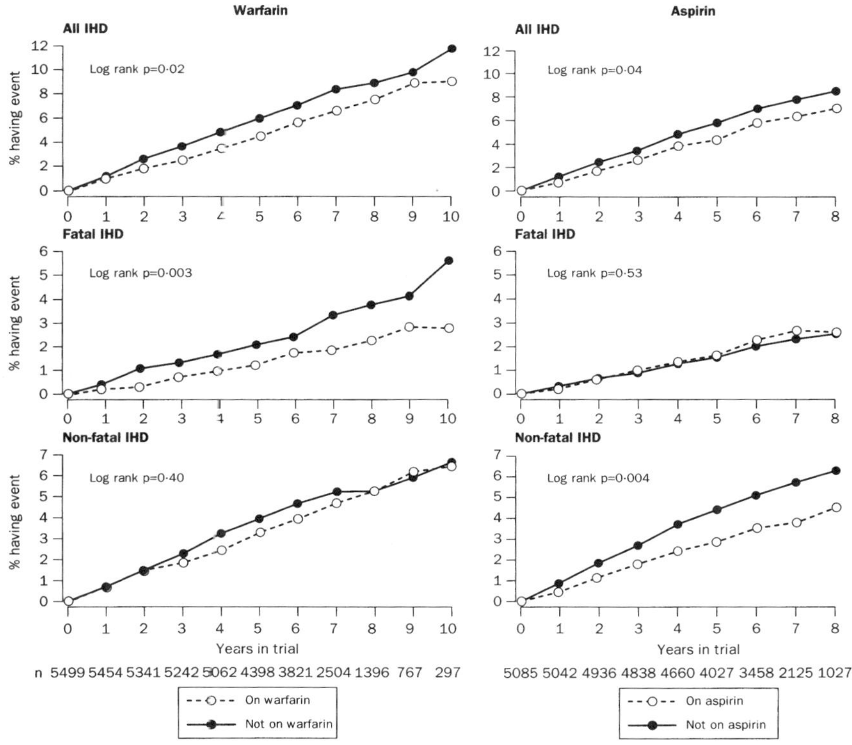

FIGURE 2.—Cumulative proportion (%) of men with IHD, main effects. *Abbreviation: n,* number in trial for specified duration of follow-up. (Courtesy of Meade TW, for the Medical Research Council's General Practice Research Framework: Thrombosis prevention trial: Randomised trial of low-intensity oral anticoagulation with warfarin and low-dose aspirin in the primary prevention of ischaemic heart disease in men at increased risk. *Lancet* 351:233-241, copyright by The Lancet Ltd., 1998.)

Methods.—The initial trial included 5,499 men aged 45 to 69 years from 108 U.K. general practices. One thousand four hundred twenty-seven subjects were randomized to warfarin or placebo. Of these, 1,013 were subsequently moved to the factorial trial, in which they continued taking their assigned warfarin or placebo and were further randomized to aspirin or placebo. Including another 4,072 subjects entering the factorial trial directly, there were 5,085 subjects. The warfarin plus aspirin group included 1,277 patients, the placebo plus aspirin group 1,268 patients, the warfarin plus placebo group 1,268 patients, and the placebo plus placebo group 1,272 patients. The 4 groups were compared for the overall incidence of IHD, including coronary deaths and fatal and nonfatal myocardial infarctions.

Results.—Patients taking warfarin had a mean International Normalized Ratio (INR) of 1.47, on a mean warfarin dose of 4.1 mg/day. Of 410 incidents of IHD, 268 were nonfatal and 142 fatal. Warfarin reduced all IHD by 21%, mainly through a 39% reduction in fatal events. Warfarin reduced the death rate from all causes by 17%. Aspirin reduced all IHD by 20%, almost all through a 32% reduction in nonfatal events (Fig 2). Warfarin reduced IHD by 2.6 per 1,000 person-years and aspirin by 2.3/1,000 person-years. Patients taking warfarin plus aspirin had a 34% reduction in IHD compared with patients taking placebo plus placebo. However, they had an increased rate of hemorrhagic stroke and fatal stroke. There were 15 cases of ruptured aortic or dissecting aneurysm in patients taking warfarin, compared with 3 cases in patients not taking warfarin.

Conclusions.—Aspirin and warfarin each reduce the incidence of IHD—aspirin by reducing nonfatal IHD and warfarin mainly by reducing fatal events. The combination of aspirin and warfarin is more effective than either agent on its own. Future antithrombotic regimens should consider the possibility that differing components of the hemostatic system govern the thrombotic contribution to fatal and nonfatal events.

▶ This complex trial provides further evidence that aspirin is effective in the primary prevention of myocardial infarction in men. Similar results were obtained in the Physician's Health Study,[1] although the much smaller British Male Doctors' Study,[2] which also used a higher dose of aspirin, did not demonstrate a benefit.

Another finding from the Thrombosis Prevention Trial demonstrated a protective benefit from low-intensity oral anticoagulants. Nonetheless, the increased risk of bleeding and the need for regular monitoring of the International Normalized Ratio (INR) makes this approach impractical, except possibly for patients at high risk for myocardial infarction who are intolerant to aspirin. Even in that event, it is difficult to see a role of warfarin as a primary preventive agent, particularly with the availability of other drugs such as clopidogrel.

Should aspirin be advised for everybody in the prevention of myocardial infarction? The answer is no, because there is a significant incidence of gastrointestinal bleeding and in some cases intracranial hemorrhage. The risk of disabling stroke, while low, is not trivial in relationship to the number of myocardial infarctions prevented.[3] Furthermore, the benefits to date have only been demonstrated in males and we await the results of the United States Women's Health Study, which has recruited over 40,000 healthy middle-aged women. Finally, among low-risk patients, the absolute risk of myocardial infarction is low (less than 0.5% per year).[4] For patients at high risk, the role of aspirin is undisputed, but it should be used in conjunction with other preventive measures—for example, smoking cessation, weight reduction, exercise, dietary modification, control of blood pressure, and in the year of the "statins," a low threshold for the pharmacologic treatment of hyperlipidemia.

B.J. Gersh, M.B., Ch.B., D.Phil, F.R.C.P.

References

1. Steering Committee of the Physicians Study Research Group. Final report on the aspirin component of the ongoing physicians study. *N Engl J Med* 321:129-135, 1989.
2. Peto R, Gray R, Collins R, et al.: Randomized trial of prophylactic baby aspirin in British male doctors. *BMJ* 296:313-316, 1998.
3. Hennekens CH, Peto R, Hutchison GB, et al: An overview of the British and American studies. *N Engl J Med* 318:923-924, 1988.
4. Verheugt FWA: Aspirin, the poor man's statin? *Lancet* 351:227-228, 1998.

Socioeconomic Issues

Mortality Differences Between Black and White Men in the USA: Contribution of Income and Other Risk Factors Among Men Screened for the MRFIT

Davey Smith G, for the MRFIT Research Group (Univ of Bristol, England)
Lancet 351:934-939, 1998   4–46

Background.—Although many studies have been done on the causes of differences in adult mortality in black and white U.S. residents, these studies have been limited by small size. This study investigated the effect on mortality of socioeconomic differences in black and white men.

Methods.—Between 1973 and 1975, researchers screened 361,662 men in 22 sites during the Multiple Risk Factor Intervention Trial (MRFIT). This trial gathered information on previous treatment for diabetes, previous heart attacks, cigarette smoking, blood pressure, age, and serum cholesterol levels. Information on median family income was also gathered by zip code on 20,224 black men and 300,685 white men. This study followed up on MRFIT test subjects and categorized causes of death. The death rates and causes of death for black and white men were compared with and without adjustment for many risk factors, including differences in income.

Results.—By December 1990, 10.6% of white men and 14.5% of black men had died (black-white relative risk, 1.37). After adjustment for age, this relative risk became 1.47 (95% confidence interval, 1.42-1.53). This decreased to 1.40 after adjustment for previous hospital treatment for heart attack, cigarette smoking, diabetes, serum cholesterol, and diastolic blood pressure. Relative risk was much lower after adjustment for age and income (1.19; confidence interval, 1.14-1.24). The relative risk did not change with further adjustment for risk factors. However, when income and age were adjusted for, the sites showed little difference in relative risk for black men and white men ($P = 0.12$). The difference in relative risk was exaggerated in men age 35 to 44 years at baseline. When considering death related to cardiac problems, age-adjustment yielded a relative risk of 1.24. Further adjustment for income decreased this number to 1.00, and adjustment for other risk factors yielded 0.97.

Conclusion.—The elevated risk of mortality for black men was decreased substantially by adjusting for income.

▶ Differences in death rates between black and white men in the United States are substantial and increasing.[1] Similar trends are apparent for black and white women. This inequality is a major public health concern which has been recognized for most of this century.[2] This large study of over 300,000 men screened for a randomized trial in the 1970s emphasizes the substantially higher mortality rates in black men compared with white men, and coronary heart disease was the most frequent cause of death. Adjustment for income substantially, but not completely, accounted for the increased risk among black men. These data support other studies emphasizing the huge impact of socioeconomic status on mortality, particularly that caused by cardiovascular disease. Other factors, such as diet, alcohol consumption, exercise, occupational exposure, and access to health care were not, however, measured in this study.

The interplay between socioenvironmental factors and coronary heart disease is complex and multifactorial. Nonetheless, it is reasonable to assume that an overall improvement in socioeconomic status in economically disadvantaged groups will result in a lessening of these troubling differences in mortality rates.

B.J. Gersh, M.B., Ch.B., D.Phil., F.R.C.P.

References

1. Kochenek KD, Maurer JD, Rosenberg HM: Why did black life expectancy decline from 1984-1989 in the USA? *Am J Public Health* 84:938-944, 1994.
2. Trask JW: The significance of the mortality rate of the colored population of the United States. *Am J Public Health* 6:254-260, 1916.

Causes of Declining Life Expectancy in Russia

Notzon FC, Komarov YM, Ermakov SP, et al (Natl Ctr for Health Statistics, Hyattsville, Md; MedSocEconomInform and Ministry of Health of Russia, Moscow; Univ of Illinois at Urbana-Champaign; et al)
JAMA 279:793-800, 1998   4–47

Background.—The correlation between the major causes of death in Russia and the decline of life expectancy in the 1990s has not been measured. This study analyzes the effect of many major causes of death on the Russian decline in life expectancy.

Method.—Researchers gathered 1990 to 1994 mortality and natality data from Russian and American vital statistics systems. They analyzed mortality rates and life expectancy for the whole Russian population and determined the contribution of mortality factors to life expectancy. The U.S. data served as a basis for comparison. Life expectancy for each year was generated using standard life-table methods. The contribution of specific mortality factors was assessed using a partitioning method.

Results.—After age-adjustment, Russian mortality rates rose nearly 33% from 1990 to 1994. Life expectancy declined from 63.8 to 57.7 years for men and from 74.4 to 71.2 years for women. Comparatively, U.S. life expectancy rose from 71.8 to 72.4 years for men and 78.8 to 79.0 years for women. Increased mortality rates for those aged 25 to 64 years was responsible for more than 75% of the Russian decline in life expectancy. Sixty-five percent resulted from cardiovascular disease (32.8% from decline in men, 21.8% from decline in women) and injuries (41.6% from decline in women, 33.4% from decline in men). A 5.8% decline resulted from infectious disease; 2.4% resulted from chronic liver disease and cirrhosis; 19.6% was related to other alcohol-related diseases; and 0.7% resulted from cancer.

Conclusion.—In 4 years, Russian life expectancy declined a total of 5 years. Factors that have contributed to this decline include depression, a deteriorating health care system, poor nutrition, alcohol and tobacco consumption, and economic instability.

▶ This is a very disturbing paper. The phenomenal rise in mortality rates in Russia between 1990 and 1994 is way beyond the peacetime experience of other industrialized countries, and the implications are staggering. Overall, cardiovascular disease (heart and stroke) accounted for 65% of the decline in life expectancy—most of this in the 25- to 64-year-old age group. These statistics tell a dismal tale and emphasize the interaction of environmental factors (economic and social instability; depression; deterioration of the health care system) with other more traditional risk factors, e.g., tobacco, alcohol abuse, and poor nutrition.[1] For all causes combined, the Russian mortality rate during this period was almost double that of the United States and, as the authors point out, this cannot be blamed upon the quality of the data.

The final message from the authors is worth repeating: Life expectancy can decline and, in certain circumstances, this may be surprisingly rapid and large. It will take years to restore the life expectancy of the Russian population to its level of 1990 and, even at that time, the age adjusted mortality rates were depressingly high in comparison with the United States.

B.J. Gersh, M.B., Ch.B., D.Phil., F.R.C.P.

Reference

1. Pratt LA, Ford DE, Crum RM, et al: Depression, psychotropic medication and risk of myocardial infarction. *Circulation* 94:3123-3129, 1996.

Pathophysiology

Angina Pectoris Caused by Coronary Microvascular Spasm
Mohri M, Koyanagi M, Egashira K, et al (Kyushu Univ, Higashi-ku, Japan)
Lancet 351:1165-1169, 1998   4–48

Introduction.—Exercise-induced myocardial ischemia in patients with syndrome X may result from inadequate microvascular dilation in response to increased demand for myocardial oxygen. Many patients with the syndrome, however, have angina at rest. Researchers tested the hypothesis that myocardial ischemia at rest results from primary hyperconstriction (spasm) of coronary microvessels.

Methods.—Study participants were 117 consecutive patients with chest pain at rest and/or during exertion, and with no flow-limiting (greater than 50%) organic stenosis in the large epicardial coronary arteries. Because acetylcholine induces coronary artery spasm in patients with variant angina, graded acetylcholine doses of 10 µg, 30 µg, and 100 µg were infused over 30 seconds into the left coronary artery of the patients. One minute after each dose, systemic arterial pressure, heart rate, and 12-lead ECG were recorded and coronary arteriography undertaken. The metabolism of myocardial lactate during acetylcholine administration was examined in 36 patients by measuring lactate in paired blood samples from the coronary artery and coronary sinus vein.

Results.—Sixty-three patients (54%) had large-artery spasm, 29 (25%) had microvascular spasm, and the remaining 25 (21%) without atypical chest pain did not have angina, ischemic ECG changes, or coronary artery spasm. These 3 groups of patients did not differ significantly in age or type of chest pain, but more men than women had large-artery spasm. Those patients with microvascular spasm had angina-like chest pain or ischemic ECG changes, which appeared after acetylcholine administration in 27 patients and spontaneously in 2 (Fig 2), but without spasm of the large epicardial coronary arteries. Overall, 27 patients in the microvascular spasm group had angina, 24 had ischemic ECG changes, and 20 had both.

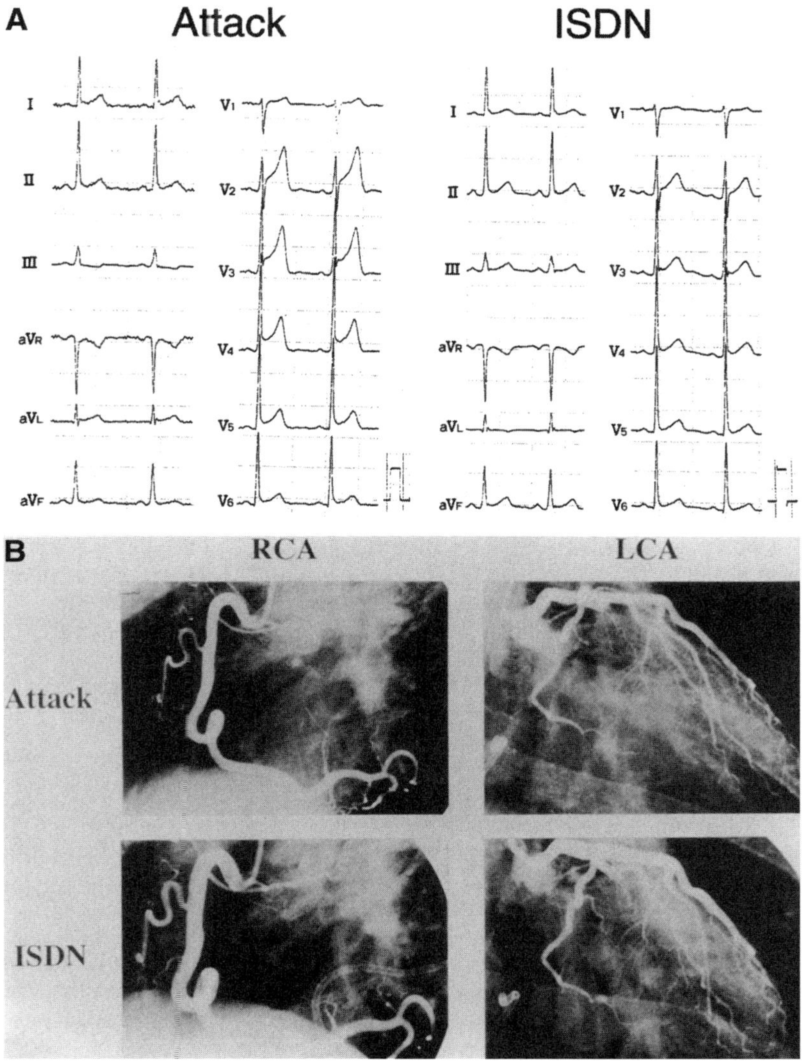

FIGURE 2.—Twelve-lead ECG (**A**) and coronary arteriograms (**B**) of 39-year-old man with a history of angina on exertion ard at rest. (Courtesy of Mohri M, Koyanagi M, Egashira K, et al: Angina pectoris caused by coronary microvascular spasm. *Lancet* 351:1165-1169, 1998. Copyright 1998, The Lancet Ltd.)

In 9 of 11 patients with microvascular spasm, paired blood samples showed that lactate was produced during an angina attack.

Conclusion.—In a subgroup of patients with microvascular angina, chest pain may be caused by coronary microvascular spasm and resultant myocardial ischemia. The spasm may be related to reduced availability of nitric oxide or to vascular hypersensitivity.

▶ Syndrome X is a common and troubling disorder, and although the prognosis for survival is excellent, the morbidity is high.[1] The syndrome has been extensively investigated and perhaps the only consensus after years of effort is that it is heterogenous, encompassing multiple pathophysiological mechanisms.[2] At one end of the spectrum, the syndrome has been attributed to a central abnormality of pain perception, and at the other end, to microvascular dysfunction with true ischemia. Other explanations include endothelial dysfunction, estrogen deficiency, and esophageal abnormalities. Obviously the therapeutic approaches may also be radically different, depending upon the underlying cause. The authors of this article make a strong case for microvascular dysfunction as a cause of ischemia and lactate production, but it should be emphasized that the methodology does not allow the authors actually to demonstrate microvascular spasm (as opposed to dysfunction), or to rule out an additional component of diffuse epicardial coronary vasoconstriction secondary to endothelial dysfunction, albeit not necessarily spasm. As any clinician knows, not only is it difficult to treat patients with "angina pectoris" and normal coronary arteries, but it is also frustrating that we are unable to provide the patients with a sensible explanation for their symptoms. For the present, we need to appreciate the multiple causes of this syndrome, and hope that we can identify the subgroup to which patients belong, and treat them accordingly.

B.J. Gersh, M.B., Ch.B., D.Phil., F.R.C.P.

References

1. Cannon RO, Camici PG, Epstein SE: Pathophysiological dilemma of syndrome X. *Circulation* 85:883-892, 1992.
2. Kaski JC: Chest pain and normal coronary anteriograms: Role of "microvascular spasm." *Lancet* 351:1144-1145, 1998.

Increased Plasminogen Activator Inhibitor Type 1 in Coronary Artery Artherectomy Specimens From Type 2 Diabetic Compared With Nondiabetic Patients: A Potential Factor Predisposing to Thrombosis and Its Persistence
Sobel BE, Woodcock-Mitchell J, Schneider DJ, et al (Univ of Vermont, Burlington; Massachusetts Gen Hosp, Boston)
Circulation 97:2213-2221, 1998   4–49

Introduction.—Compared with nondiabetic individuals, patients with type 2 diabetes have a fourfold or greater prevalence of coronary artery disease and reduced survival after angioplasty. Researchers hypothesized that a factor contributing to the poorer outcome among patients with type

2 diabetes is a disproportionate elevation of plasminogen activator inhibitor type 1 (PAI-1) in vascular wall components and atheroma.

Methods.—Two groups of patients, both with clinical indications for directional coronary atherectomy, were studied. Twenty-five had type 2 diabetes and 18 had no clinical evidence of diabetes. Treatment was the same and directional coronary atherectomy was successful in all cases. Atherectomy samples were analyzed for urokinase plasminogen activator (u-PA) and PAI-1 and assayed for cellularity.

Results.—The 2 groups were similar in demographic variables and severity of coronary artery disease. Tissue from diabetic patients showed significantly more PAI-1 and appeared to exhibit less u-PA than tissue from patients without diabetes. These differences were consistent in patients with primary and restenotic lesions and regardless of the treatment of diabetes.

Conclusion.—Atherectomy samples from patients with diabetes showed consistently more PAI-1 and consistently less u-PA than samples from patients without diabetes, a finding consistent with increased gene expression of PAI-1 in vessels. This increase may contribute to accelerated or persistent thrombosis and could be modified by reducing insulin resistance and stringently controlling hyperglycemia.

▶ It is well established that even in well-controlled patients with type 2 diabetes, the risk of cardiovascular disease is increased. Moreover, the presence of type 1 or type 2 diabetes has a negative impact on the results of both percutaneous transluminal coronary angioplasty (pTCA) and coronary bypass surgery, but this appears to be proportionately greater among patients undergoing PTCA.[1]

The prothrombotic effects of PAI-1, which is associated with reduced fibrinolysis and accelerated atherosclerosis, have been previously demonstrated, as has the effect of insulin in raising PAI-1 levels.[2] This elegant study on atherectomy specimens provides an additional mechanistic explanation for the effects of diabetes and insulin resistance on the development of vascular disease and the results of PTCA. The disproportionate elevation of PAI-1 compared with u-PA reflects a thrombogenic milieu and subsequent vascular disease exacerbated by plaque-associated mitogens in the vessel wall.

B.J. Gersh, M.B., Ch.B., D.Phil., F.R.C.P.

References

1. Writing group for the Bypass Angioplasty Revascularization Investigation (BARI) investigators: Five-year clinical and functional outcomes comparing bypass surgery and angioplasty in patients with multivessel coronary disease: A multicenter randomized trial. *JAMA* 177:715-721, 1997.
2. McGill JB, Schneider DJ, Arfkin CL, et al: Factors responsible for impaired fibrinolysis in obese subjects and in NIDDM patients. *Diabetes* 43:104-109, 1994.

Angiogenesis Is Enhanced in Ischemic Canine Myocardium by Transmyocardial Laser Revascularization

Yamamoto N, Kohmoto T, Gu A, et al (Columbia Univ, New York)
J Am Coll Cardiol 31:1426-1433, 1998   4–50

Purpose.—There is growing interest in transmyocardial laser revascularization (TMLR) because of its ability to relieve angina and improve myocardial infarction in patients with diffuse, otherwise untreatable coronary artery disease. The concept behind this therapy is to use the laser to create channels through the myocardial wall that penetrate into the ventricular chamber, thus reducing reliance of myocardial perfusion on the epicardial arteries. However, experimental evidence suggests that this is not the true mechanism of clinical benefit. Using a dog model of chronic

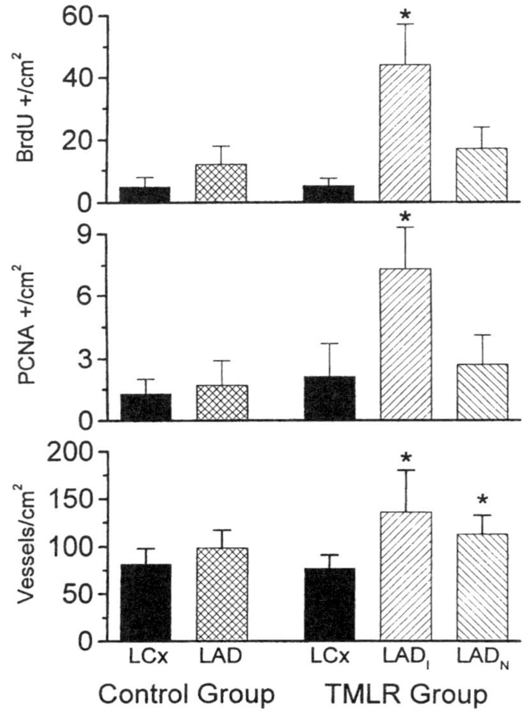

FIGURE 6.—Quantitative analysis of bromodeoxyridine, proliferating cell nuclear antigen, and vessel density in control and TMLR-treated hearts. *LCx*, Data from nonischemic, normally perfused left circumflex territory; *LAD*, data from ischemic anterior wall of control hearts; LAD_I, data from anterior wall myocardium immediately surrounding channel remnants (i.e., confined between edge of remnant and an ellipse with minor and major axes of 0.6 and 1.0 cm, respectively); LAD_N, data from anterior wall myocardium neighboring the channel remnants (i.e., confined between the first ellipse and a second concentric ellipse with axes of 1.0 and 1.4 cm). Each *bar graph* represents mean value ± SD of observations made from 21 observations (3 from each heart studied). *$P < 0.05$ by analysis of variance with the Student-Newmann-Keuls post hoc test. (Courtesy of Yamamoto N, Kohmoto T, Gu A, et al: Angiogenesis is enhanced in ischemic canine myocardium by transmyocardial laser revascularization. *J Am Coll Cardiol* 31:1426-1433, 1998. Reproduced by permission from the American College of Cardiology.)

myocardial ischemia, this study evaluated the possibility that TMLR stimulates angiogenesis.

Methods.—Ameroid constrictors were placed on the proximal left anterior descending arteries of dogs to create a clinically relevant ischemic condition. Some of the animals were then treated with TMLR of the anterior wall, creating transmural channels from the epicardial surface into the ventricular chamber over the left anterior descending artery territory. Channel density was approximately 1 channel per square centimeter. The remaining dogs were left untreated as ischemic controls. Acutely and after 2 months, myocardial blood flow was assessed at rest with colored microspheres and during chemical stress with adenosine. Bromodeoxyridine incorporation and proliferating cell nuclear antigen studies were performed to assess vascular proliferation.

Results.—The acute assessments showed no change in blood flow after TMLR. By 2 months, both groups showed an increase in resting blood flow to the anterior wall to approximately 80% of normal. At the same time, dogs in the TMLR group had a 40% increase in blood flow under adenosine stress in the ischemic territory. Laser treatment was associated with approximately a 4-fold increase in vascular proliferation. On examination, the myocardium surrounding the TMLR channel remnants showed a 40% increase in the density of blood vessels with at least 1 smooth muscle cell layer compared with control ischemic tissue (Fig 6).

Conclusions.—In this study of dogs with induced chronic myocardial ischemia, TMLR appears to lead to significant increases in angiogenesis. Laser-treated animals showed increased numbers of smooth muscle cell–lined vessels, increased vascular proliferation markers, and increased blood flow capacity under stress. Thus, TMLR may lead to a novel pattern of vascular growth rather than creating channels directly from the ventricular chamber.

▶ Several series have documented that TLMR may provide significant relief of angina in addition to an apparent improvement in myocardial perfusion.[1] What is extremely puzzling are the potential mechanisms of benefit because it has been shown that the laser channels, which were designed to provide myocardial perfusion directly from the ventricular chamber, do not conduct blood. Furthermore, these channels do not remain patent but are occluded by thrombus and infiltrated by granulation tissue within a few weeks.[2, 3]

This and other studies suggest that angiogenesis may be a major factor underlying the clinical benefits after TLMR. What is particularly relevant are the observations that active vascular growth occurs in the normal myocardium surrounding TLMR channel remnants. The results of the present study provide the strongest evidence to date that angiogenesis is enhanced by TLMR, to the extent that this may augment collateral blood flow to ischemic myocardium.

I suspect that the original hypothesis that TLMR would work by creating channels mimicking the reptilian heart have been discounted. Future research will focus upon the role of myocardial injury, the subsequent inflammatory response, and the role of growth factors in the stimulation of angiogenesis. It is likely that alternative methods of inducing angiogenesis will become identified, and pilot studies involving transcatheter approaches are already well underway.

B.J. Gersh, M.B., Ch.B., D.Phil., F.R.C.P.

References

1. Horvath KA, Mannting F, Cummings N, et al: Transmyocardial laser revascularization: Operative techniques and clinical results at two years. *J Thorac Cardiovasc Surg* 111:1047-1053, 1996.
2. Kohmoto T, Fisher PE, Gu A, et al: Physiology, histology and two-week morphology of acute transmyocardial laser channels made with a CO_2 laser. *Ann Thorac Surg* 63:1275-1283, 1997.
3. Burkhoff D, Fisher PE, Apfelbaum M, et al: Histological appearance of transmyocaridal laser channels after 4 weeks. *Ann Thorac Surg* 61:1532-1535, 1996.

Miscellaneous

Prognostic Significance of Exercise-Induced Left Bundle-Branch Block
Grady TA, Chiu AC, Snader CE, et al (Cleveland Clinic Found, Ohio)
JAMA 279:153-155, 1998   4–51

Objective.—Whereas 0.5% of individuals experience exercise-induced left bundle-branch block (LBBB) during exercise stress tests, the significance of LBBB during exercise has not been well studied. A matched control cohort study examined whether exercise-induced LBBB is an independent predictor of major cardiovascular morbidity and mortality.

Methods.—Between September 1990 and February 1994, 70 of 17,277 patients undergoing an exercise stress test at the Cleveland Clinic experienced LBBB. These patients were matched with patients of the same age, sex, test date, prior history of coronary artery disease, hypertension, diabetes, smoking, and β-blocker use who did not experience exercise-induced LBBB. Outcome measures included all-cause mortality, percutaneous or surgical revascularization, nonfatal myocardial infarction, and need for a permanent pacemaker, an implantable pacemaker, or an implantable cardiac defibrillator with documented symptomatic or sustained ventricular tachycardia or ventricular fibrillation by either telemetry or Holter monitor.

Results.—Patients were observed for an average of 3.7 years. There were 28 events in 17 patients with exercise-induced LBBB and 9 events in 8 control patients (risk ratio, 2.78). Of the patients with a history of coronary artery disease, 5 patients with exercise-induced LBBB and 2 control patients had coronary artery bypass surgery. Ten patients with exercise-induced LBBB and 5 control patients had percutaneous intervention. Five patients with exercise-induced LBBB and 2 control patients died. Event-free survival rates at 4 years were 19% for patients with exercise-induced LBBB and 10% for control patients.

Conclusion.—Although exercise-induced LBBB is rare, it is an independent predictor of serious cardiac events and increased mortality.

► New-onset LBBB on the resting electrocardiogram may be due to isolated conduction disease (Lenègre's disease), but in many patients this is a marker of severe coronary artery disease or structural heart disease, (e.g., dilated cardiomyopathy or hypertensive heart disease). In the Framingham study, over an 18-year period of observation, LBBB developed in 1.1%, among whom 50% died within 10 years and only 11% remained free of clinically apparent cardiovascular events.[1] On the other hand, right bundle-branch block is not associated with an adverse prognosis.

In this matched control study, the incidence of *exercise-induced* LBBB was only 0.41% (70 cases) out of 1,727 patients undergoing symptom-limited treadmill exercise testing, an incidence similar to that reported previously.[2] After a mean follow-up of only 3.7 years, 28 cardiovascular events occurred in 17 patients (24%), and the majority of events were death or revascularization. The adjusted risk ratio for cardiovascular events vs. controls was 2.78 with 95% confidence intervals ranging from 1.16 to 6.65; $P = 0.02$.

Despite the existence of bias in this study, in that patients with this abnormality may have undergone more stringent follow-up and a greater likelihood of coronary angiography, the data do suggest that exercise-induced LBBB warrants an additional cardiac evaluation, which may include coronary angiography. That exercise-induced LBBB may occur in patients with normal coronary arteriograms is well established, but I suspect that this occurs in a minority, given the relatively high incidence of events in this study. The same principles apply to patients with new-onset LBBB on the resting echocardiogram, in whom structural heart disease other than isolated conduction disease needs to be excluded.

B.J. Gersh, M.B., Ch.B., D.Phil., F.R.C.P.

References

1. Schneider J, Thomas H, Kreger B, et al: Newly acquired left bundle branch block: The Framingham study. *Ann Intern Med* 90:303-310, 1979.
2. Williams M, Esterbrooks D, Nair C, et al: Clinical significance of exercise-induced bundle branch block. *Am J Cardiol* 61:346-348, 1988.

Constitutive Expression of phVEGF$_{165}$ After Intramuscular Gene Transfer Promotes Collateral Vessel Development in Patients With Critical Limb Ischemia
Baumgartner I, Pieczek A, Manor O, et al (Tufts Univ, Boston)
Circulation 97:1114-1123, 1998   4–52

Introduction.—A large proportion of patients with critical limb ischemia are not candidates for operative or percutaneous revascularization. Amputation is often recommended in such cases, despite its associated

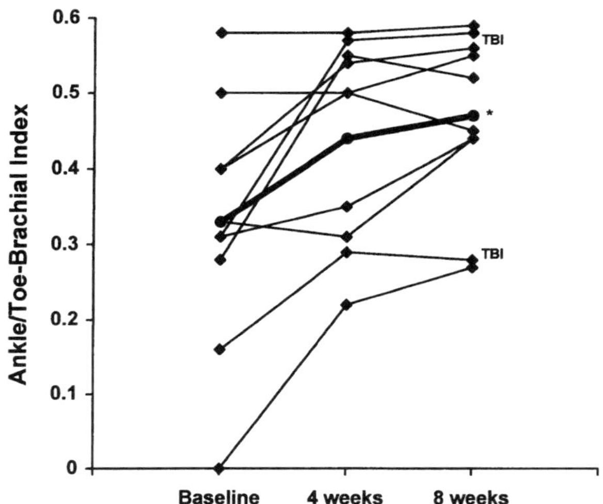

FIGURE 2.—Gain in ABI and/or TBI in 10 limbs, 4 and 8 weeks after intramuscular phVEGF$_{165}$ gene transfer. *Mean values, P=.02. *Abbreviations: ABI,* ankle-brachial index; *TBI,* toe-brachial index; *phVEGF$_{165}$,* the 165-amino-acid isoform of human vascular endothelial growth factor. (Courtesy of Baumgartner I, Pieczek A, Manor O, et al: Constitutive expression of phVEGF$_{165}$ after intramuscular gene transfer promotes collateral vessel development in patients with critical limb ischemia. *Circulation* 97:1114-1123, 1998.)

morbidity and mortality. An alternative treatment strategy, therapeutic angiogenesis, has the potential to stimulate the development of collateral arteries. A phase 1 clinical trial was conducted to document the safety and feasibility of intramuscular gene transfer, using naked plasmid DNA encoding an endothelial cell mitogen, and to evaluate outcome in patients with critical limb ischemia.

Methods.—Study participants were 9 patients with 10 involved limbs. Seven limbs had nonhealing ischemic ulcers and all were affected by rest pain. In gene transfer, a total dose of 4,000 µg of naked plasmid DNA, encoding the 165-amino-acid isoform of human vascular endothelial growth factor, was injected directly into the muscles of the ischemic limb. A transient increase in serum levels of vascular endothelial growth factor, as monitored by enzyme-linked immunosorbent assay, confirmed gene expression. Patients were studied weekly for the first 8 weeks, then monthly.

Results.—A significant increase in ankle-brachial index, from a mean of 0.33 to a mean of 0.48, was recorded after gene transfer (Fig 2). Contrast angiography documented newly visible collateral blood vessels in 7 limbs, and MR angiography showed qualitative evidence of improved distal flow in 8. In 4 of the 7 limbs with ischemic ulcers, therapy produced healing or marked improvement of the ulcers. Three of these patients had been advised to have below-knee amputation. Limb salvage was possible in a 33-year-old woman who had undergone 7 unsuccessful surgical reconstructions at another hospital. Eight weeks after gene transfer, she underwent a split-thickness skin graft that healed successfully. Tissue specimens from an amputee showed foci of proliferating endothelial cells 10 weeks after gene therapy.

Discussion.—Preliminary data from a small patient group support the strategy of intramuscular gene therapy and the concept of therapeutic angiogenesis for critical limb ischemia. Spontaneous resolution of rest pain and/or healing of an ischemic ulcer in such patients has not been reported previously.

▶ This is a very exciting article which should be read in conjunction with the sentinel article by Schumacher, et al., in which the authors describe the results of the angiogenic protein acidic fibroblast growth factor injected into the myocardium after coronary bypass surgery.[1] Both studies have demonstrated the growth of collaterals, but what are particularly notable in this article from Isner's group are the clinical outcomes. It would appear that the growth of collaterals resulted in substantial clinical benefit, as measured by improvements in ankle-brachial index, healing of ischemic ulcers in some patients, limb salvage in 3 patients scheduled for amputation, and angiographic evidence of improved distal flow. An accompanying editorial[2] addresses many of the unresolved issues, from both a theoretical and a clinical standpoint, including the possibility that the intramuscular transfer of angiogenic growth factor could stimulate pathological angiogenesis at remote sites, e.g. ocular angiogenesis or tumor angiogenesis. This raises the possibility of induction of corneal neovascularization or tumor growth or metastases. Fortunately, the evidence to date on the systemic administration of fibroblast growth factor or vascular endothelial growth factor is reassuring, but these are still early days.

One cannot escape the impression that we are on the threshold of a real therapeutic breakthrough. Perhaps, in the future, the introduction of angiogerm growth factors into the human heart could be administered through minimally invasive or videoscopic techniques.

B.J. Gersh, M.B., Ch.B., D.Phil., F.R.C.P.

References

1. Schumacher B, Pescher P, VonSpecht BU, et al: Induction of neoangiogenesis in ischemic myocardium by human growth factor: First clinical results in the new treatment of coronary heart disease. *Circulation* 97:645-650, 1998.
2. Folkman J: Therapeutic angiogenesis in ischemic limbs (editorial). *Circulation* 97:1108-1110, 1998.

Induction of Neoangiogenesis in Ischemic Myocardium by Human Growth Factors: First Clinical Results of a New Treatment of Coronary Heart Disease

Schumacher B, Pecher P, von Specht BU, et al (Klinikum Fulda, Germany; Universitätsklinik Freiburg, Germany)
Circulation 97:645-650, 1998

4–53

Introduction.—The limitations of bypass materials currently used for the treatment of coronary heart disease have led researchers to search for alternatives. Attention has been directed toward natural angiogenesis and growth factors that can induce angiogenesis. Reported here are results of animal studies and of first clinical applications of a new treatment for coronary heart disease, using the human growth factor FGF-1 (basic fibroblast growth factor) to induce neoangiogenesis in the ischemic myocardium.

Methods.—Genetic engineering was used to produce human FGF-1 from apathogenic strains of *Escherichia coli.* The growth factor was then isolated and highly purified. The apathogenic action and neoangiogenic potency of this factor were demonstrated in several series of animal experiments. In clinical applications, 20 patients with 3-vessel coronary disease had FGF-1 (0.01 mg/kg body weight) injected close to the vessels, after completion of internal mammary artery /left anterior descending coronary artery anastomosis. Patients also had additional peripheral stenoses of the left anterior descending coronary artery or 1 of its diagonal branches. The internal mammary artery bypasses were selectively imaged 12 weeks later using intra-arterial digital subtraction angiography.

Results.—The animal studies provided unequivocal proof of induced neoangiogenesis. Histological examination of the rat heart myocardium revealed a three-fold increase in capillary density per square millimeter around the site of the FGF-1 injection. As in the animal experiments, neoangiogenesis and the development of a normal vascular appearance were demonstrated angiographically when FGF-I was first used on the human heart. Formation of capillaries was found around the site of injection, in all cases and a capillary network arising from the proximal part of the artery had bypassed the stenoses and rejoined the distal parts of the vessel. Results of electronic data processing-assisted digital gray value analysis for quantification of the neoangiogenesis yielded a mean gray value of 124 for the vessels.

Conclusion.—Neoangiogenesis induced by FGF-I offers new possibilities for the treatment of ischemic myocardial disease. When combined with operative myocardial revascularization, FGF-I may enhance outcome for patients with additional peripheral stenoses that cannot be treated surgically.

► This landmark article complements other clinical studies of the administration of vascular endothelial growth factor to patients with severe lower extremity peripheral vascular disease.[1] This article is noteworthy for its description of the development of recombinant human fibroblast growth factor-1, but also for the authors' randomized controlled clinical trial in 20 patients. The exciting aspect of this approach is that it induces local angiogenesis but appears to avoid high levels of circulating angiogenic activity that could possibly stimulate plaque angiogenesis, which in turn could have detrimental effects by stimulating angiogenesis and growth in pre-existing coronary plaques.[2] What is also fascinating is that neovascularization persisted for at least ´2 weeks after only a single set of intramyocardial injections of the angiogenic protein. There are several theoretical explanations for this, as postulated by Folkman in an accompanying editorial. The results of this study are impressive, but the end points are primarily anatomic, and we will have to wait longer to see whether the growth of new blood vessels can be transplanted into an improvement in symptoms, functional class, and ultimately survival. Perhaps we really are on the threshold of an exciting new era in which developments in the molecular biology of the endothelial cell and smooth muscle will be transplanted into a dramatic new form of therapy.

B.J. Gersh, M.B., Ch.B., D.Phil., F.R.C.P.

References

1. Isner JM, Pieczek A, Schainfeld R, et al: Clinical evidence of angiogenesis after arterial gene transfer of phVEGF165 in patients with ischaemic limbs. *Lancet* 348:373-374, 1996.
2. Folkman J: Angiogenic therapy of the human heart (editorial). *Circulation* 97:628-629, 1998.

Prognostic Value of Vasodilator Myocardial Perfusion Imaging in Patients With Left Bundle-Branch Block

Wagdy HM, Hodge D, Christian TF, et al (Mayo Clinic, Rochester, Minn)
Circulation 97:1563-1570, 1998   4–54

Introduction.—Patients with left bundle-branch block appear to be at increased risk for cardiac abnormalities. One study reported that 10-year cardiovascular mortality after the onset of left bundle-branch block was 50%. Treadmill exercise tests and exercise perfusion scintigraphy with thallium-201 and technetium-99m sestamibi have not been useful in the diagnosis of coronary artery disease in such patients. This study examined the prognostic value of tomographic myocardial perfusion imaging in patients with left bundle-branch block.

Methods.—Patients were seen at the Mayo Clinic between December 1986 and December 1993. All had complete left bundle-branch block at the time of stress perfusion imaging with dipyridamole (153 patients) or adenosine (92 patients). Patients were prospectively classified into high- and low-risk groups. Those patients considered at high risk had a large severe fixed defect (28 patients), a large reversible defect (36 patients), or cardiac enlargement and either increased pulmonary uptake (thallium) or

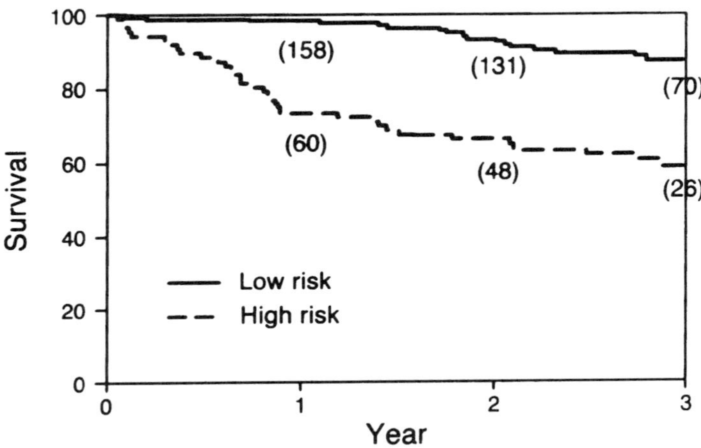

FIGURE 1.—Overall survival for the low- *(solid line)* and high- *(dotted line)* risk groups. There was a highly significant difference (P less than .0001) between the 2 groups. The curves are truncated at 3 years because there were fewer than 10 patients studied for 4 years in the low-risk group. (Courtesy of Wagdy HM, Hodge D, Christian TF, et al: Prognostic value of vasodilator myocardial perfusion imaging in patients with left bundle-branch block. *Circulation* 97:1563-1570, 1998.)

a decreased resting ejection fraction (sestamibi) (20 patients). The 161 patients without these findings (66%) were considered at low risk.

Results.—The study group included 125 men and 120 women with a mean age of 69. More men were in the high-risk group, and there were significantly higher incidences of insulin-requiring diabetes, smoking, and previous myocardial infarction in this group. Three-year overall survival (Fig 1) was significantly lower in the high-risk group (57%) than in the low-risk group (87%). The 2 groups also differed significantly in survival free of cardiac death/nonfatal myocardial infarction/cardiac transplantation (55% in the high-risk vs. 93% in the low-risk group). After adjustment for age, sex, diabetes, and previous myocardial infarction, high-risk findings at imaging had a significant incremental prognostic value. Survival for patients with left bundle-branch and a low-risk scan did not differ significantly from that for an age-matched U.S. population.

Conclusion.—Vasodilator perfusion imaging was successful in predicting outcome in patients with left bundle-branch block. Outcome in those with high-risk imaging features and other cardiac risk factors differs significantly from outcome in patients without these findings.

▶ It is well established that the prognosis of asymptomatic left bundle-branch block is poor, and that the condition is a marker in many patients of serious underlying structural heart disease.[1] Nonetheless, there is a subset of patients in whom left bundle-branch block is probably a manifestation of isolated conduction system disease, and in these patients the prognosis is favorable, providing they have no other cardiac risk factors.[2]

In patients with a new diagnosis of left bundle-branch block, it is imperative to exclude underlying high-risk cardiac disease (e.g. cardiomyopathy, ischemic heart disease, and hypertension). This large study from the Mayo Clinic demonstrates the clinical utility of pharmacologic perfusion imaging with thallium-201 or sestamibi, and other investigators have suggested that pharmacologic stress may be preferable to exercise stress in patients with left bundle-branch block, at least for the detection of coronary artery disease. A particularly useful finding in this study is the excellent prognosis, even in patients with an abnormal study, providing they did not demonstrate any of the "high risk" scintigraphic features. These data would certainly support the use of perfusion imaging as a first step in patients with new onset left bundle-branch block, and angiography could then be confined to those patients with evidence of coronary artery disease.

B.J. Gersh, M.B., Ch.B., D.Phil., F.R.C.P.

References

1. Schnieder JF, Thomas HE Jr, Sorlie P, et al: Comparative features of newly acquired left and right bundle branch block in the general population: The Framingham Study. *Am J Cardiol* 47:931-940, 1981.
2. Smith RF, Jackson DH, Hawthorne JW, et al: Acquired bundle branch block in a healthy population. *Am Heart J* 80:746-751, 1970.

Effects of Exposure to Altitude on Men With Coronary Artery Disease and Impaired Left Ventricular Function

Erdmann J, Sun KT, Masar P, et al (Clinic for Rehabilitation Gais, Switzerland)
Am J Cardiol 81:266-270, 1998
4–55

Introduction.—Every year, 35 million Americans travel to altitudes of more than 2,400 m. Of these, about half a million have symptomatic coronary artery disease and about 2.9 million have systemic hypertension. Little is known about the effects of exposure to altitude. Men with coronary disease and impaired left ventricular function were studied at an altitude of 2,500 m.

Methods.—There were 23 patients with coronary artery disease who had a mean age of 51 ± 9 years and a mean ejection fraction of 39% ± 6%. They were compared with 23 normal controls. A maximal symptom-limited bicycle stress test was conducted at 1,000 m and 2 days later at 2,500 m for both groups. The first stage was set at 60 W with increments of 30 W every 2 minutes. A continuous recording was taken with a 12-lead electrocardiogram. After each stage, measurements were taken of blood pressure, heart rate, oxygen saturation, lactate concentration, and perceived intensity of exertion. Exercises were performed until participants could not continue because of fatigue or dyspnea.

Results.—Exercise capacity decreased significantly for both groups. The coronary artery disease group at 1,000 m measured 162 ± 28 W and at 2,500 m measured 155 ± 28 W. The control group at 1,000 m measured 205 ± 28 W and at 2,500 m measured 198 ± 25 W. No difference was found in maximal heart rate and blood pressure between 1,000 and

2,500 m. At rest and during exercise, oxygen saturation remained unchanged. The test was terminated more often at 2,500 meters because of dyspnea, but the level of perceived exertion was similar to that at 1,000 meters. No complications or signs of ischemia were seen.

Conclusion.—Good tolerance to exposure to altitude was found among patients with coronary artery disease with impaired left ventricular function. The risk for an adverse event is not increased among patients with coronary heart disease, and the effects in patients are comparable to those in a group of normal subjects.

▶ Apparently 35 million Americans travel to altitudes greater than 2,400 m every year.[1] This height corresponds to the altitude at many Rocky Mountain resorts. This study is both useful and reassuring in that it demonstrates that patients with coronary artery disease and left ventricular dysfunction, without overt ischemia or heart failure, can tolerate the stress of exposure to higher altitudes without adverse effects. Many patients who have been successfully revascularized or survived a myocardial infarction fall into this category. One should emphasize that patients with angina or overt ischemia and patients with congestive heart failure were appropriately excluded from this study, and in my own clinical practice I believe that exposure to high altitude is contraindicated in such patients. An additional caveat applies to individuals going skiing. The additional stresses of skiing at higher altitudes in conjunction with exposure to cold might not be well tolerated. This study, however, was carried out under different conditions. Moreover, the base may be at 8,000 feet, but the summits of many of our mountains are more than 12,000 to 14,000 feet—a very different set of circumstances.[2] As is the case in many clinical situations, the science and the data need to be adapted to the individual. At least this study provides us with some data.

B.J. Gersh, M.B., Ch.B., D.Phil., F.R.C.P.

References

1. Moore LG: Altitude-aggravated illness: Examples in pregnancy and prenatal life. *Ann Emerg Med* 16:965-973, 1987.
2. West JB: The effects of high altitude after coronary bypass surgery. *JAMA* 260:2218, 1988.

Response Times and Outcomes for Cardiac Arrests in Las Vegas Casinos
Karch SB, Graff J, Young S, et al (Univ of Nevada, Las Vegas)
Am J Emerg Med 16:249-253, 1998 4–56

Introduction.—The mean time from 911 activation to arrival at the scene of out-of-hospital cardiac arrest varies greatly from city to city and between urban and rural areas. Cardiac arrests that occurred at Las Vegas casino-hotels between January 1993 and June 1996 were reviewed to measure emergency medical services response times and the relation between those times and the probability of survival.

Methods.—During the study period, 206 of 736 cases collected had complete data sets. Response times were calculated with all 736 patients, whereas regression analysis was limited to the 206 patients for whom all nodal events were recorded.

Results.—Sixty patients (29.3%) were resuscitated and survived to hospital discharge. The mean elapsed time from 911 activation to delivery of the first defibrillatory shock was 9.88 minutes for survivors vs. 12.46 minutes for nonsurvivors. The 2 groups did not differ significantly in time from 911 activation to arrival of paramedics. Model fitting showed a 911-to-shock time of 4 minutes yielded a survival probability of 36%. Odds decreased by 5% each minute, to 19% after 23 minutes. There was a strong trend to increased survival rate with ventricular fibrillation as the initial rhythm.

Conclusion.—Delay in reaching the patient is an important reason for nonsurvival after out-of-hospital cardiac arrest and CPR, but there is a limit to how fast emergency medical services systems can respond. A possible solution might be to have police cruisers carry an automatic external defibrillator.

▶ If you have to have a cardiac arrest, perhaps a Las Vegas casino is a better location than most. On an average, the response time from dialing 911 to arrival at the hotel was 4.8 to 5.6 minutes, but the elapsed time from dialing 911 to the first shock was 9.88 minutes in survivors vs. 12.46 minutes in nonsurvivors. These times are consistently better than other published reports for large emergency medical service systems (particularly the vertical response time, which is the time from arrival on scene to arrival at the patient's side). In comparison with studies from New York and Chicago in which overall survival was 2%, the survival rates in this Las Vegas study were 29.3%.[1] Whether significantly shorter response times are achievable is debatable, and despite the encouraging trend in this study, one has to realize that for 71.7% of patients having a cardiac arrest in a Las Vegas casino, the odds are not in their favor.

B.J. Gersh, M.B., Ch.B., D.Phil., F.R.C.P.

Reference

1. Becker L, Ostander M, Barrett J, et al: Outcome of CPR in the large metropolitan area: Where are the survivors? *Ann Emerg Med* 20:355-361, 1991.

Systematic Direct Angioplasty and Stent-Supported Direct Angioplasty Therapy for Cardiogenic Shock Complicating Acute Myocardial Infarction: In-Hospital and Long-term Survival
Antoniucci D, Valenti R, Santoro GM, et al (Careggi Hosp, Florence, Italy)
J Am Coll Cardiol 31:294-300, 1998   4–57

Introduction.—Several articles have reported improved outcome when percutaneous transluminal coronary angiography (PTCA) is used to treat

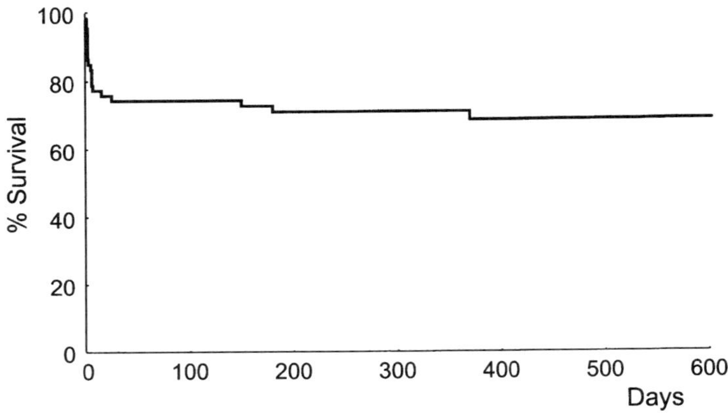

FIGURE 1.—Actuarial survival of 66 patients with AMI complicated by cardiogenic shock who were treated by direct PTCA. *Abbreviations: AMI,* acute myocardial infarction; *PTCA,* percutaneous transluminal coronary angioplasty. (Reprinted with permission from the American College of Cardiology from Antoniucci D, Valenti R, Santoro G, et al: Systematic direct angioplasty and stent-supported direct angioplasty therapy for cardiogenic shock complicating acute myocardial infarction: In-hospital and long-term survival. *J Am Coll Cardiol* 31:294-300, 1998.)

patients with acute myocardial infarction complicated by cardiogenic shock. A prospective study examined the impact of a systematic direct PTCA strategy on mortality in such patients.

Methods.—Direct PTCA was performed in 364 consecutive patients during the study; 66 had cardiogenic shock. All patients were pretreated with aspirin, and heparin (10,000 U) was administered immediately after sheath insertion. Direct PTCA and coronary stenting were accomplished with standard techniques. An optimal immediate angiographic result was defined as a residual stenosis (30%) associated with Thrombolysis in Myocardial Infarction grade 3 flow. Patients returned to an outpatient clinic for follow-up at 1, 3, and 6 months.

Results.—Direct PTCA had a success rate of 94% in patients with cardiogenic shock; 85% of patients achieved an optimal angiographic result. Corresponding figures for patients without shock were 98% and 96%. In-hospital mortality for those with shock was 26% (vs. 0.7% without shock). In univariate analysis, patient age, chronic coronary occlusion, and completeness of revascularization were significantly related to in-hospital mortality. The survival rate of patients with shock was 71% at 6 months (Fig 1).

Conclusion.—Most patients with acute myocardial infarction and cardiogenic shock can achieve a Thrombolysis in Myocardial Infarction grade 3 flow after systematic direct PTCA. Primary stenting has both initial and long-term benefits.

▶ Earlier articles have reported encouraging results for primary angioplasty in patients with cardiogenic shock, but have not excluded the possibility of selection bias. A recent large prospective international registry showed that the selection of patients for angiography identified a group with a lower mortality, whether or not the patients underwent revascularization.[1] This observational study of consecutive patients (all of whom were offered PTCA) is less subject to bias, although we have no information about those patients who were not referred to this tertiary care hospital. We do know that 4 patients with cardiogenic shock died before they could reach the catheterization laboratory. The proportion of patients undergoing primary PTCA who were classified as having cardiogenic shock is higher than in previous studies, raising the question of the definitions of "shock."

Nonetheless, the in-hospital mortality of 26% is the lowest yet reported and may reflect the frequent use of stenting for a poor or suboptimal angiographic result after conventional PTCA. Thrombolysis in Myocardial Infarction grade 3 flow was achieved in a remarkable 85% of cases. Late outcomes in this study, as in others, were surprisingly good, and here again primary stenting appeared to reduce late events.

The final answer must await the ongoing SHOCK trial, which should determine the benefit of early revascularization, including new support devices in different categories of patients with cardiogenic shock. In the interim, this study of 66 patients treated within 6 hours is encouraging and suggests that improvements in technology have been translated into superior results from mechanical perfusion in the setting of acute myocardial infarction.

B.J. Gersh, M.B., Ch.B., D.Phil., F.R.C.P.

Reference

1. Hochman JS, Boland J, Sleeper LA, et al: Current spectrum of cardiogenic shock and effect of early revascularization on mortality: Results of an international registry. *Circulation* 91:873-881, 1995.

5 Noncoronary Heart Disease in Adults

Prediction of Indications for Valve Replacement Among Asymptomatic or Minimally Symptomatic Patients With Chronic Aortic Regurgitation and Normal Left Ventricular Performance
Borer JS, Hochreiter C, Herrold EMcM, et al (New York Hosp-Cornell Med Ctr)
Circulation 97:525-534, 1998

5–1

Introduction.—Appropriate criteria for valve replacement in the asymptomatic or minimally symptomatic patient with aortic regurgitation are controversial. Both subnormal left ventricular performance at rest and symptoms of early pulmonary vascular congestion—which often occurs with normal resting left ventricular systolic performance—are the currently accepted criteria for operation. The stress of exercise can unmask subnormal performance not found at rest, although the optimal application of this finding in clinical prognostication remains unclear. A determination was made of the absolute and relative strengths of association between descriptors and clinical outcome in patients who were initially asymptomatic or minimally symptomatic and who had normal left ventricular ejection fraction at entry and at rest.

Methods.—In 104 patients, annual assessments were made of clinical variables and measurements of left ventricular size, performance, and end-systolic wall stress by using radionuclide cineangiography at rest and at maximal exercise and by echocardiography at rest. During exercise, end-systolic wall stress was derived.

Results.—Four of 104 patients died suddenly; in 22, symptoms developed operable and in 13, subnormal left ventricular performance with or without symptoms developed. The strongest predictor of progression to any end point or sudden cardiac death alone was change in left ventricular ejection fraction rest to exercise, normalized for change in end-systolic wall stress from rest to exercise, according to multivariate Cox analysis. On the basis of change in left ventricular ejection fraction from rest to exercise, normalized for change in end-systolic wall stress from rest to exercise, symptom status modified prediction. At a rate of 13.3%/year, the

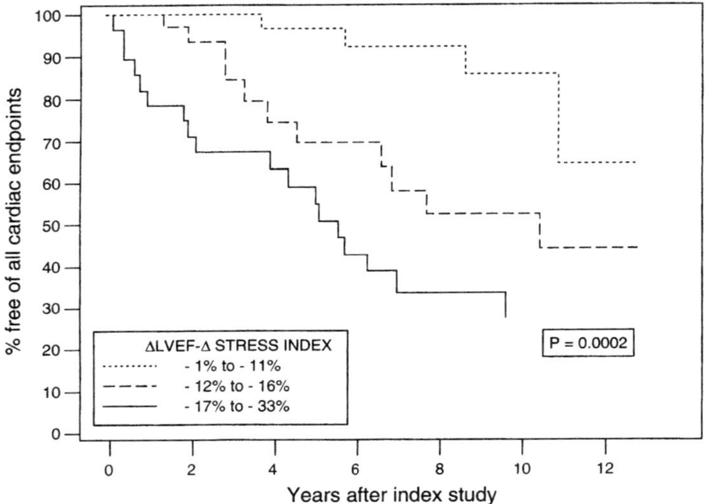

FIGURE 3.—Relation of change in left ventricular ejection fraction–change in end-systolic wall stress (ΔLVEF=ΔSTRESS) index at study entry to occurrence of any cardiac end point (cardiac death, operable symptoms, and/or subnormal left ventricular performance at rest) during follow-up. A population of 88 patients with evaluable data for this analysis has been divided statistically into terciles. The ΔLVEF=ΔSTRESS index boundaries for each tercile are *boxed*. (Courtesy of Borer JS, Hochreiter C, Herrold EMcM, et al: Prediction of indications for valve replacement among asymptomatic or minimally symptomatic patients with chronic aortic regurgitation and normal left ventricular performance. *Circulation* 97:525-534. Reproduced with permission of *Circulation*. Copyright 1998, American Heart Association.)

population tercile at highest risk by this index progressed (Fig 3). The lowest risk tercile progressed at 1.8%/year.

Conclusion.—By using load-adjusted change in left ventricular ejection fraction–change in end-systolic wall stress index—which includes data obtained during exercise—currently accepted symptom and left ventricular performance indications for valve replacement, as well as sudden cardiac death, can be predicted in asymptomatic/minimally symptomatic patients with aortic regurgitation.

▶ In this elegant study, the authors have clearly shown the advantages of evaluating patients with chronic aortic regurgitation by measuring the load-adjusted left ventricular ejection fraction–end-systolic wall stress index, with the measurements made both at rest and during exercise. I suspect that most patients will have a decision made for valve replacement based on easier-to-determine clinical criteria. Hopefully, a number of other centers will verify the results of this study, which makes good physiologic sense. The reader should also be aware of the superb ACC/AHA guidelines published for the management of patients with valvular heart disease.[1] As noted by Cheitlin, to advise surgery in an asymptomatic patient, there must be unequivocal evidence that the future benefits make the real risks of surgery worthwhile.[2]

R.C. Schlant, M.D.

References

1. Bonow RO, Carabello BA, DeLeon AC Jr, et al: ACC/AHA guidelines for the management of patients with valvular heart disease: A report of the American College of Cardiology/American Heart Association Task Force on Practice Guidelines (Committee on Management of Patients With Valvular Heart Disease). *J Am Col Cardiol* 32:1486-1588, 1998.
2. Cheitlin MD: Finding "just the right moment" for operative intervention in the asymptomatic patient with moderate to severe aortic regurgitation. *Circulation* 97:518-520, 1998.

Application of the Proximal Flow Convergence Method to Calculate the Effective Regurgitant Orifice Area in Aortic Regurgitation

Tribouilloy CM, Enriquez-Sarano M, Fett SL, et al (Mayo Clinic and Mayo Found, Rochester, Minn)
J Am Coll Cardiol 32 1032-1039, 1998

5–2

Purpose.—In patients with aortic regurgitation (AR), measurements of the degree of regurgitation play an important role in the decision to perform surgery. Calculation of the aortic effective regurgitant orifice (ERO) is a recently developed noninvasive technique using quantitative Doppler echocardiography. The ERO can also be calculated using the proximal isovelocity surface area (PISA) technique. However, this technique has not been validated in patients with AR. The reliability of the PISA method of calculating the ERO in patients with AR was examined.

Methods.—The prospective study included 71 consecutive patients with AR. The ERO was successfully calculated using the PISA method in 64 of these. At the same time, quantitative Doppler and 2-dimensional echocardiographic measurements were taken for comparison. Angiography was also performed in 12 patients and surgical correlation was available in 18. Ventricular volume measurements were taken in all patients.

Results.—The PISA method of ERO was highly correlated with the reference methods. The PISA method did tend to underestimate ERO: mean values were 24 mm² with PISA vs. 26 mm² with quantitative Doppler and 27 mm² with quantitative echocardiography. However, the underestimation resulted from measurements in 5 patients with a flow convergence angle of greater than 220 degrees. On multivariate analysis, this was the only factor significantly associated with underestimation of ERO. Among patients with a flat flow convergence angle of 220 degrees or less, the PISA method was very highly correlated with the reference methods. The standard error of the estimate was narrow and the trend toward underestimation disappeared: mean values were 22 mm² with PISA vs. 23 mm² with both quantitative Doppler and quantitative echocardiography.

Conclusions.—The PISA method is a feasible way to measure ERO in patients with AR. If the patient has an obtuse flow convergence angle, PISA may underestimate the ERO. However, as long as this angle is relatively flat, PISA measurements are reliable. In most patients, a single

Doppler echocardiographic examination can provide multiple measurements of the ERO area.

▶ A major pitfall of this method is the presence of an obtuse angle of the flow convergence region, due to the geometry of the aortic cusps. In most patients, however, this angle is not present and the proximal flow convergence measure to calculate effective regurgitant orifice should be accurate. It is interesting that the same institution has also recently published descriptions of the assessment of mitral regurgitation utilizing proximal convergence.[1]

R.C. Schlant, M.D.

Reference

1. Chaliki MP, Nishimura RA, Enriquez-Sarano M, et al: A simplified, practical approach to assessment of severity of mitral regurgitation by Doppler color flow imaging with proximal convergence: Validation with concomitant cardiac catheterization. *Mayo Clin Proc* 73:929-935, 1998.

Twenty-Year, Three-Institution Evaluation of the Hancock Modified Orifice Aortic Valve Durability: Comparison of Actual and Actuarial Estimates
Mahoney CB, Miller DC, Khan SS, et al (Univ of Minnesota, Minneapolis)
Circulation 98:II-88-II-94, 1998   5–3

Purpose.—In valve replacement surgery, data on the incidence of structural valve deterioration (SVD) plays an important role in valve selection. The Hancock Modified Orifice valve was introduced in 1976. As it became apparent that the durability of porcine bioprosthetic valves was limited, surgeons began to place them only in patients with an expected survival of less than the durability of the valve. However, it is unclear whether standard actuarial techniques reflect the actual, cumulative incidence of SVD. Actuarial and actual durability estimates for the Hancock Modified Orifice valve were compared.

Methods.—From 1976 to 1985, 3 institutions placed Hancock Modified Orifice valves in 752 patients. Follow-up data were available on 727 patients. The patients were 424 men and 303 women (mean age, 63 years at the time of the first implant). Mean follow-up was 8.5 years, with a total of 6,161 person-years. Patient survival and SVD were calculated by standard actuarial models, the information from which was combined to reach actual estimates of SVD. The 2 types of estimates were compared for various age groups.

Results.—At 5 years, the difference between the 2 methods of calculating incidence of SVD was significant only for the oldest age groups. Thereafter, the difference became more important. The estimated proportion of patients free of SVD at 17 years was 52% by actuarial analysis, compared with 83% by actual analysis. For patients over 65, freedom

Survival

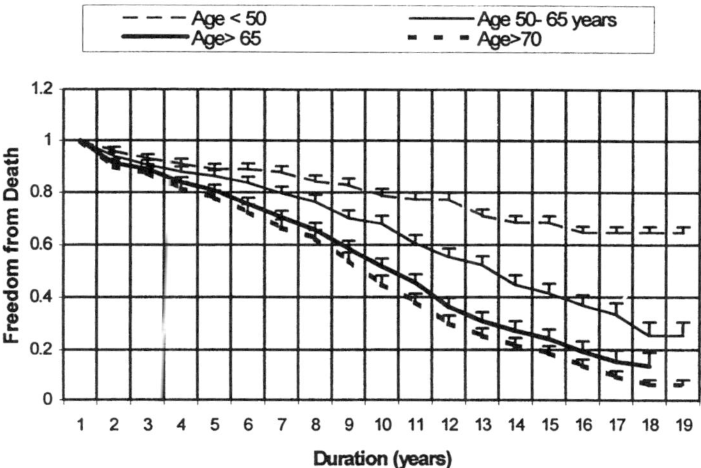

FIGURE 2.—Data presented as % alive at year x. The preimplantation sampling point (T_0) is presented with the consecutive sampling points $(T_0$ *through* $T_{18})$ at years 1 through 18, respectively. Four different age groups of patients are displayed: *bars* at each sampling point represent standard errors at that time. Survival is defined as freedom from death by patient age group. (Courtesy of Mahoney CB, Miller DC, Khan SS, et al: Twenty-year, three-institution evaluation of the Hancock Modified Orifice aortic valve durability: Comparison of actual and actuarial estimates. *Circulation* 98:II-88-II-94, 1998.)

from SVD at 5 years was 98% by actuarial methods vs. 100% by actual methods; by 10 years, it was 93% vs. 96%; and by 17 years, 78% vs. 93%. Actuarial estimates of patient survival were 59% at 10 years and 31% at 15 years. For patients aged 65 and older, survival was 52% at 10 years and 24% at 15 years; for patients aged 70 and older, the figures were 45% and 19%, respectively (Fig 2).

Conclusions.—In patients undergoing porcine bioprosthetic valve implantation, the estimated incidence of SVD varies greatly according to the statistical method used. The actual method suggests a lower risk of SVD in older patients than actuarial analysis does. The data support the current practice of implanting tissue valves in elderly patients. However, the question of generalizability must be considered when data on actual SVD rates are used to guide valve selection decisions in larger populations.

▶ This elegant study demonstrates that the durability of the Hancock Modified Orifice prosthetic valve is reasonably good. The article further illustrates that the particular statistical analysis method used can provide markedly different conclusions.

R.C. Schlant, M.D.

Aortic Root Disease and Valve Disease Associated With Ankylosing Spondylitis

Roldan CA, Chavez J, Wiest PW, et al (Univ of New Mexico, Albuquerque)
J Am Coll Cardiol 32:1397-1404, 1998   5–4

Introduction.—Aortic root disease and valve disease are frequent findings in patients with ankylosing spondylitis (AKS). However, the clinical characterization, relation to clinical features of AKS, evolution, and prognostic implications of aortic root disease and valve disease have not been determined. Their prevalence, characteristics, relation to clinical features, and evolution were examined in 45 patients with AKS.

Methods.—Patients and 30 age- and sex-matched healthy controls underwent initial transesophageal echocardiography and rheumatologic evaluations. At a mean follow-up of 39 months, 25 patients with AKS underwent clinical and echocardiographic re-evaluation.

Results.—Aortic root disease and valve disease were detected in 82% of patients with AKS and 27% of controls, a significant difference. In the patient group, there were findings of aortic root thickening and increased stiffness and dilatation in 61%, 61%, and 25% of patients, respectively. Rates of aortic and mitral valve thickening were 41% and 34%, respectively, and were predominately manifested, in 74% of patients, as nodularities of the aortic cusps and basal thickening of the anterior mitral leaflet (the characteristic subaortic bump). Valve regurgitation was observed in almost half of patients. Moderate lesions were seen in 40%. Aortic root disease and valve disease were not associated with activity, severity, or therapy of AKS, with the exception of duration of AKS. During follow-up, 24% of 25 patients developed new aortic or valve abnormalities, 12% had significant worsening of existing valve regurgitation, and 20% had resolution of abnormalities. In contrast to only 3% of controls, 20% of patients with AKS developed heart failure, underwent valve replacement, had a stroke, or died.

Conclusion.—Aortic root disease and valve disease are frequently seen in patients with AKS, are unrelated to clinical features of AKS, may resolve or progress over time, and are associated with clinically important cardiovascular morbidity.

▶ This remarkable study of 44 patients with AKS found that valve regurgitation, at times requiring valve replacement, was a fairly frequent occurrence. Although most of the patients were asymptomatic, 40% of those with valve regurgitation had moderate lesions; in another 12%, the valve regurgitation progressed significantly. It was not surprising that patients over the age of 45 who had had AKS for more than 15 years had the highest prevalence of cardiovascular disease.

R.C. Schlant, M.D.

Factors Associated With Atrial Fibrillation in Patients With Mitral Stenosis: A Cardiac Catheterization Study
Moreyra AE, Wilson AC, Deac R, et al (UMDNJ-Robert Wood Johnson Med School, New Brunswick, NJ; Tirga-Mures Med School, Romania)
Am Heart J 135:138-145, 1998   5–5

Objective.—Cardiac failure, rheumatic heart disease, valvular heart diseases, and cardiomyopathies contribute to the occurrence of atrial fibrillation (AF). The demographic, hemodynamic, and coronary anatomic variables associated with AF were retrospectively examined in 314 middle-aged patients with mitral stenosis.

Methods.—Between January 1986 and July 1995, 326 of 4,200 patients undergoing cardiac catheterization received a diagnosis of mitral stenosis. Factors associated with AF were determined by univariate and multivariate analysis, and predictors of AF were identified using stepwise logistic multiple regressions.

Results.—The average age of patients with mitral stenosis was 53 (range 28 to 70). Compared with patients in sinus rhythm at the time of catheterization, patients in AF at the time of catheterization were significantly older (51.7 vs. 53.4) and had a significantly lower cardiac index (2.6 vs. 2.3 L/min/m²), a significantly greater systemic resistance, a significantly smaller mitral valve area (1.6 vs. 1.2 cm²), and a significantly smaller index (0.91 vs. 0.61). Compared with patients in normal sinus rhythm, AF patients had significantly more instances of mitral insufficiency (55% vs. 40%) and tricuspid insufficiency (12% vs. 3%) and significantly higher right atrial pressure (9.9 vs. 7.3 mm Hg). Both right atrial mean pressure and decreased mitral valve area were significantly and independently associated with AF, according to multivariate analysis. Age and coronary artery disease were not significantly associated with AF.

Conclusion.—Increased right atrial pressure and decreased mitral valve area were significantly and independently associated with AF in patients with mitral stenosis.

▶ This is a large retrospective analysis of 314 patients with mitral stenosis who were studied by cardiac catheterization. The primary finding that both the severity of mitral stenosis and right atrial pressure were independently associated with atrial fibrillation is not unexpected. It is somewhat surprising, however, that age was not independently associated with atrial fibrillation. Perhaps such a relationship might be shown in a population of more elderly patients.

R.C. Schlant, M.D.

Percutaneous Balloon Versus Surgical Closed and Open Mitral Commissurotomy: Seven-Year Follow-up Results of a Randomized Trial

Farhat MB, Ayari M, Maatouk F, et al (Fattouma Bourguiba Univ, Tunisia)
Circulation 97:245-250, 1998
5–6

Introduction.—Percutaneous balloon mitral commissurotomy has been successfully and safety performed in large series of patients for treatment of rheumatic mitral valve stenosis since its introduction in 1984. Some debate has erupted regarding the advantages and disadvantages of open mitral commissurotomy in comparison with 2 other blind techniques. For the treatment of tight pliable rheumatic mitral valve stenosis, the early invasive and long-term (7 year) clinical and echocardiographic follow-up results of balloon mitral commissurotomy were compared with those of closed mitral commissurotomy and open mitral commissurotomy.

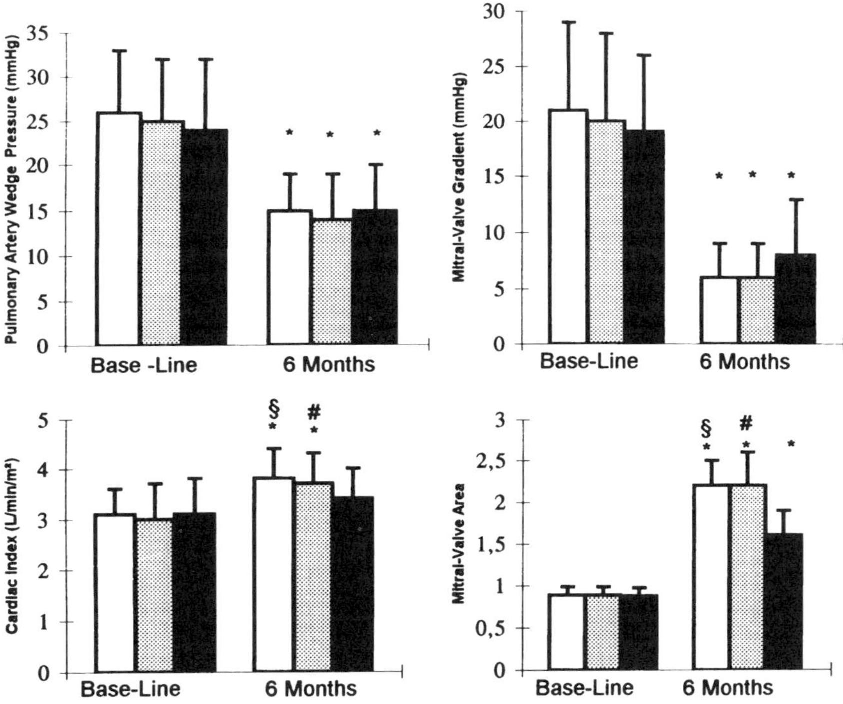

FIGURE 1.—Major hemodynamic variables at baseline and 6 months at rest after balloon mitral commissurotomy (*first white bar*), open mitral commissurotomy (*second white bar*), or surgical closed mitral commissurotomy (*black bar*). *Asterisk* indicates *P* less than 0.001 for comparison of the baseline value with its change at 6 months within each group. *Section mark* indicates *P* less than 0.001 for comparison of balloon mitral commissurotomy vs. closed mitral commissurotomy. *Number symbol* indicates *P* less than 0.001 for comparison of open mitral commissurotomy vs. closed mitral commissurotomy. (Courtesy of Farhat MB, Ayari M, Maatouk F, et al: Percutaneous balloon versus surgical closed and open mitral commissurotomy: Seven-year follow-up results of a randomized trial. *Circulation* 97: 245-250. Reproduced with permission of *Circulation*. Copyright 1998, American Heart Association.)

Methods.—Ninety patients with severe pliable rheumatic mitral valve stenosis participated in a prospective, randomized trial in which the results of percutaneous balloon mitral commissurotomy, surgical closed mitral commissurotomy, and open mitral commissurotomy were compared. There were 30 patients in each group. Clinical and echocardiographic evaluation was conducted initially and throughout the 7-year follow-up period for all patients.

Results.—After balloon mitral commissurotomy, Gorlin mitral valve area increased significantly (from 0.9 ± 0.16 to 2.2 ± 0.4 cm^2). After open mitral commissurotomy, Gorlin mitral valve area increased from 0.9 ± 0.2 to 2.2 ± 0.4 cm^2). After closed mitral commissurotomy, Gorlin mitral valve area increased from 0.9 ± 0.2 to 1.6 ± 0.4 cm^2. After balloon mitral commissurotomy or open mitral commissurotomy, residual rheumatic mitral valve stenosis was 0%. After closed mitral commissurotomy, it was 27%. Among the 3 groups, there was no early or late mortality or thromboembolism. After balloon mitral commissurotomy and open mitral commissurotomy, echocardiographic residual mitral valve area was similar and greater at 7-year follow-up (19.8 ± 0.4 cm^2) than after closed mitral commissurotomy (1.3 ± 0.3 cm^2). After balloon mitral commissurotomy or open mitral commissurotomy, the restenosis rate was 6.6% vs. 37% after closed mitral commissurotomy. In 2 patients in the balloon mitral commissurotomy group, residual atrial septal defect was present, and 1 patient in that group had severe grade 3 mitral regurgitation. After balloon mitral commissurotomy, 87% of patients were in New York Heart Association functional class I; 90% of patients after open mitral commissurotomy were in New York Heart Association functional class I compared with 33% after closed mitral commissurotomy. After balloon mitral commissurotomy, there was 90% freedom from reintervention. After open mitral commissurotomy, there was 93% freedom from intervention, and there was 50% freedom from intervention after closed mitral commissurotomy.

Conclusion.—Excellent and comparable early hemodynamic improvement are produced by balloon mitral commissurotomy and open mitral commissurotomy in contrast to surgical closed mitral commissurotomy (Fig 1). A lower rate of residual stenosis and restenosis and the need for reintervention are associated with balloon mitral commissurotomy and open mitral commissurotomy in contrast to surgical closed mitral commissurotomy. The treatment of choice for patients with tight pliable rheumatic mitral valve stenosis is the balloon mitral commissurotomy because of its good results, lower cost, and elimination of the drawbacks of thoracotomy and cardiopulmonary bypass.

▶ This excellent study compared percutaneous balloon mitral commissurotomy with closed mitral commissurotomy and open mitral commissurotomy for the management of rheumatic mitral valve stenosis. The average age of the patients was 28 years with a range from 11 to 50 years. The majority were women. All had echocardiographic evaluations and evidence of noncalcified, pliable mitral valve leaflets.

The results of this study clearly show that percutaneous balloon mitral commissurotomy produced results comparable with those of surgical open mitral commissurotomy and superior to those of surgical closed mitral commissurotomy. There were no acute complications or deaths associated with percutaneous balloon mitral commissurotomy. The authors noted residual atrial septal defects in only 2 of 30 patients and severe, grade III mitral regurgitation in only 1 patient after percutaneous balloon mitral commissurotomy.

It would now appear in highly selected patients with noncalcified, pliable mitral valve leaflets producing mitral stenosis that percutaneous mitral valve commissurotomy or catheter balloon valvuloplasty would be the procedure of choice when skilled operators are available. In some areas of Europe and North America, the incidence of rheumatic mitral stenosis of this severity is relatively low and the incidence of patients with suitable valve leaflets for balloon mitral commissurotomy is also low. In this situation, open mitral commissurotomy may be the procedure of choice.

R.C. Schlant, M.D.

Retrograde Nontransseptal Balloon Mitral Valvuloplasty: Immediate Results and Intermediate Long-term Outcome in 441 Cases—A Multicenter Experience

Stefanadis CI, Stratos CG, Lambrou SG, et al (Athens Univ, Greece; All India Inst of Med Sciences, New Delhi, India; Onassis Cardiac Surgery Ctr, Athens, Greece; et al)
J Am Coll Cardiol 32:1009-1016, 1998   5–7

Introduction.—Retrograde nontransseptal balloon valvuloplasty (RNBMV) is a purely transarterial technique that was created with the goal of avoiding complications related to transseptal catheterization. To date, only single-center experience with this method has been reported. The immediate and intermediate long-term results of the application of RNBMV were assessed in 4 cooperating centers in Greece and India.

Methods.—Between April 1988 and September 1996, RNBMV was attempted, by independent operators, in 441 patients with mitral stenosis. All patients first underwent a diagnostic workup that included evaluation of clinical status and echocardiographic examination. Determination of functional capacity was based on the criteria of the New York Heart Association (NYHA). Mean pre-procedure echocardiographic score was 7.7 in 320 female and 121 male patients. Mean follow-up of patients with successful immediate outcome of RNBMV was 3.5 years.

Results.—Of 438 patients with completed procedures, a technically successful procedure (increase in mitral valve area of 1.5 cm² or greater and final mitral regurgitation of grade 2+ or below) was achieved in 388 patients (88%). Unfavorable predictors of immediate outcome were pre-procedural mitral regurgitation and prior surgical commissurotomy. There were no occurrences of cardiac perforation, cardiac tamponade, or embolic events. Complications included death, severe mitral regurgitation, and injury of the femoral artery in 0.5%, 3.4%, and 1.1% of patients. Event-free survival rates, which included freedom from cardiac death, mitral valve surgery, repeat valvuloplasty, and symptoms of NYHA class higher than II, for follow-up years 1, 2, 4, and 9, respectively, were 100%, 96.9%, 89.8%, and 75.5%. Significant predictors of intermediate long-term outcome were echocardiographic score, NYHA class, and postprocedural mitral valve area.

Conclusion.—This multicenter experience suggests that RNBMV is a safe and effective approach to the treatment of symptomatic mitral stenosis. As with the transseptal approach, patients with favorable mitral valve anatomy experience the best immediate and intermediate long-term benefit.

▶ This study from 4 hospitals in Greece and India clearly shows that RN-BMV can be successfully performed with minimal morbidity and mortality in carefully selected patients. It appears to be comparable to the transseptal approach. It would be good if a multicenter randomized study could be done comparing the 2 techniques.

R.C. Schlant, M.D.

Disappearance of Mitral and Tricuspid Regurgitation in Haemodialysis Patients After Ultrafiltration

Cirit M, Özkahya M, Soydaş Çinar C, et al (Ege Univ, Izmir, Turkey)
Nephrol Dial Transplant 13:389-392, 1998   5–8

Objective.—Patients with valvular regurgitation who are undergoing dialysis have a poor prognosis. Controlling the resulting volume overload and cardiac dilatation with ultrafiltration may reduce the functional aggravation.

Methods.—Doppler echocardiography detected mitral and tricuspid regurgitation in 21 hemodialysis patients (9 females), aged 17 to 64. Hypertensive drugs were discontinued in the 13 patients receiving antihypertensive therapy. All patients received an intensified ultrafiltration (UF) during dialysis until blood pressure and heart shadow became normal.

Results.—After UF, patients lost an average of 5.4 kg; regurgitation improved in all patients. Mitral regurgitation disappeared in 13 patients, and tricuspid regurgitation disappeared in 14. Significant changes were observed in mean arterial pressure, which declined from 125 to 95 mm Hg, cardiothoracic index (from 0.57 to 0.47), left atrial pressures (from 28 to 22 mm/m^2), left ventricular systolic pressure (from 25 to 21 mm/m^2), left ventricular diastolic pressure (from 31 to 27 mm/m^2), and mitral annular diameters (from 19.4 to 16.6 mm/m^2). Cardiac volume decreased on chest radiograph but never achieved normal size. Left ventricular ejection fraction decreased in most patients during treatment and increased after treatment but remained below 50% in 11 patients.

Conclusion.—Ultrafiltration in dialysis patients can ameliorate the valvular regurgitation and significantly improve cardiac dimensions and blood pressure.

▶ This fine study from Turkey confirms the importance of volume in the pathogenesis of mitral and tricuspid regurgitations in patients undergoing late-term hemodialysis. It is significant that not all of the patients had a complete disappearance of the regurgitation and that three patients with aortic regurgitation had no change with treatment. Since one cannot be assured that a very aggressive approach will be used with each dialysis, I would not be in favor of discontinuing antihypertensive drugs in such patients.

R.C. Schlant, M.D.

The Prevalence of Cardiac Valvular Insufficiency Assessed by Transthoracic Echocardiography in Obese Patients Treated With Appetite-Suppressant Drugs

Khan MA, Herzog CA, St Peter JV, et al (Hennepin County Med Ctr, Minneapolis; Minnesota Heart Clinic, Minneapolis; Univ of Minnesota, Minneapolis)

N Engl J Med 339:713-718, 1998

5–9

Objective.—A number of obese patients taking fen-phen as an appetite suppressant have received a diagnosis of multivalvular disease. Because it was unclear whether valvular insufficiency was a consequence of obesity or was related to the drug combination, the prevalence and severity of valvular dysfunction in obese patients taking appetite suppressants were compared with the prevalence and severity in patients who were not.

Methods.—Echocardiography was used to estimate the prevalence of valvulopathy in age-, sex-, height-, and body mass index-matched obese patients who had taken (n = 257) or had not taken (n = 239) dexfenfluramine alone, phentermine plus fenfluramine, or dexfenfluramine plus phentermine during open-label trials from January 1994 through August 1997. The primary reader of the echocardiograms was blinded to the drug-exposure status of each patient. The presence of mild or moderate mitral valve insufficiency was diagnosed by 2 or more independent cardiologists.

Results.—Of the 233 patients and 233 controls who completed the study, significantly more patients than controls had cardiac valve abnormalities [53 (22.7%) vs. 3 (1.3%)] (odds ratio, 22.6). Age was the only predictor of cardiac valve abnormalities. For dexfenfluramine only, the odds ratio of cardiac valve abnormalities was 12.7; for dexfenfluramine plus phentermine, the odds ratio was 24.5; and for fenfluramine plus phentermine, the odds ratio was 26.3.

Conclusion.—Obese patients who took dexfenfluramine alone, phentermine plus fenfluramine, or dexfenfluramine plus phentermine had a significantly higher prevalence of valvular insufficiency than obese patients who did not take these appetite suppressants.

▶ This article is the first of 3 articles and an editorial[1,2,3] on this subject that were published in the same journal. All 3 articles suggest that there is a slightly higher incidence of aortic and mitral regurgitation in patients treated with appetite-suppressant drugs. The mechanism of the valve dysfunction is not known; it is also not known why some individuals develop valvular abnormalities whereas others do not; and it is not known how long the medications need to be taken to develop valvular regurgitation. Whether any of the valvular abnormalities are reversible is also uncertain.

R.C. Schlant, M.D.

References

1. Jick H, Vasilakis C, Weinranch LA, et al: A population-based study of appetite-suppressant drugs and the risk of cardiac-valve regurgitation. *N Engl J Med* 339:719-724, 1998.
2. Weissman NJ, Tighe JF, Gottdiener JS, et al: An assessment of heart-valve abnormalities in obese patients taking dexfenfluramine, sustained-release dexfenfluramine, or placebo. *N Engl J Med* 339:725-732, 1998.
3. Devereux RB: Appetite suppressants and valvular heart disease (editorial). *N Engl J Med* 339:765-767, 1998.

Modern Management of Prosthetic Valve Anticoagulation
Tiede DJ, Nishimura RA, Gastineau DA, et al (Mayo Clinic Rochester, Minn)
Mayo Clin Proc 73:665-680, 1998   5–10

Objective.—Systemic anticoagulation reduces the incidence of valve thrombosis and systemic embolism in patients with prosthetic heart valves. Although the optimal intensity of anticoagulation is not known, the anticoagulation regimen recommended at the Mayo Clinic, its practical implications, and suggestions for anticoagulation in patients with prosthetic heart valves who are undergoing noncardiac surgical procedures are discussed.

Clinical Implications and Recommendations.—Although higher levels of anticoagulation reduce the risk of thromboembolic events, they increase the risk of bleeding, and guidelines for levels of anticoagulation may need to be adjusted accordingly (Table 1 and Table 2). Although there are few clinical studies on the risk of temporarily discontinuing anticoagulation for noncardiac operations, available data suggest that discontinuing anticoagulation therapy 3 to 5 days before surgery and resuming it 3 to 5 days postoperatively does not increase the risk of thromboembolic events and decreases the risk of serious intraoperative bleeding. Whether aggressive or conventional anticoagulation is recommended depends on the individual patient's risk of thromboembolic events (Table 3). Pregnancy poses a bleeding risk not only to the mother but also to the fetus, because some

TABLE 1.—General Anticoagulation Guidelines for Patients With Prosthetic Valves*

Factor	Target INR†	Aspirin (mg)
Aortic valves		
Newer generation bileaflet mechanical valves	2.5	81
All other mechanical valves	3.0	81
Bioprosthetic valves	2.5 for 3 mo‡	325 indefinitely
Thromboembolic risk factors	2.5 indefinitely	81
Mitral valves		
"First-generation" tilting-disk valves	3.5	81
All other mechanical valves	3.0	81
Bioprosthetic valves	2.5 indefinitely§	81
Low thromboembolic risk and high bleeding risk	2.5 for 3-6 mo	325 indefinitely
Mitral valve repair	2.5 for 3 mo	325 indefinitely
Thromboembolic risk factors	2.5 indefinitely	81

†Ideally, target INR should be lower than ± 0.3.

‡At some medical centers, warfarin is not routinely given after an operation in patients with no concomitant risk factors who have received a bioprosthetic valve in the aortic position.

§At some medical centers, patients who maintain sinus rhythm receive warfarin for only 3 months.

Abbreviation: INR, international normalized ratio.

(Courtesy of Tiede DJ, Nishimura RA, Gastineau DA, et al: Modern management of prosthetic valve anticoagulation. *Mayo Clin Proc* 73:665-680, 1998.)

TABLE 2.—Risk Factors for Thrombosis, Thromboembolism, and Bleeding

Increased risk of thrombosis and thromboembolism
    "First-generation" ball-cage or tilting-disk mitral prostheses (for example,
        Starr-Edwards, Björk-Shiley, Omniscience)[33,85-88]
    Double-position prosthetic valves[87,88]
    Atrial fibrillation[78,79,81,85,87,89-91]
    Severe left ventricular dysfunction[90-92]
    Prior embolic event[16,33,87,90,91,93]
    Hypercoagulable state
Increased risk of bleeding
    Age older than 70 yr[71]
    Prior pronounced bleeding
    Gait instability

(Courtesy of Tiede DJ, Nishimura RA, Gastineau DA, et al: Modern management of prosthetic valve anticoagulation. *Mayo Clin Proc* 73:665-680, 1998.)

TABLE 3.—Anticoagulation With Noncardiac Operation*

Conventional†
    Discontinue warfarin several days preoperatively
    Perform operation when INR is ≤1.5
    Resume warfarin as soon as possible postoperatively
    Administer heparin only if INR is <2.0 for 5 days or more
Aggressive‡
    Discontinue warfarin several days preoperatively
    Administer heparin intravenously when INR is <2.0
    Perform operation when INR is ≤1.5
    Resume warfarin as soon as possible postoperatively
    Resume heparin as soon as possible postoperatively
    Discontinue heparin when INR is ≥2.0

†For patients undergoing mechanical aortic valve replacement who have no other thromboembolic risk factors.

‡For patients undergoing mechanical aortic or mitral valve replacement who have other thromboembolic risk factors.

(Courtesy of Tiede DJ, Nishimura RA, Gastineau DA, et al: Modern management of prosthetic valve anticoagulation. *Mayo Clin Proc* 73:665-680, 1998.)

TABLE 4.—Effects of Common Pharmacologic Agents on Warfarin Anticoagulation*

| | Major Effect | | | | Moderate Effect | | |
Increased	Evidence	Decreased	Evidence	Increased	Evidence	Decreased	Evidence
Amiodarone	A	Barbiturates	A	Propafenone	A	Rifampin	A
Cimetidine	A			Disulfiram	B	Griseofulvin	A
Clofibrate	A			Acetaminophen	B	Phenytoin (late)	B
Itraconazole	A			Phenytoin (early)	B	Cholestyramine	B
Ketoconazole	A			Cephalosporins	C	Carbamazepine	C
Metronidazole	A			Chloramphenicol	C	Ethchlorvynol	C
Miconazole	A			NSAIDs	C	Corticosteroids	D
Sulfinpyrazone	A			Tricyclics	C	Estrogens	D
Sulfonamides	A			Allopurinol	D	Ethanol	D
Aspirin/salicylates	B			Corticosteroids	D	Thiazide diuretics	D
Erythromycin	B			Cyclophosphamide	D	Oral contraceptives	E
Fluconazole	B			Furosemide	D		
Thyroid hormones	B			Isoniazid	D		
Quinidine	C			Omeprazole	D		
Quinine	C			Propoxyphene	D		
Vitamin E	C			Propranolol	D		
Anabolic steroids	D			Quinolones	D		
Penicillins	D			Serotonin reuptake			
Tamoxifen	D			inhibitors	D		
Tetracycline	D			Ascorbic acid	E		
				Influenza vaccine	E		
				Gemfibrozil	E		
				Mineral oil	E		

Abbreviations: A, established: proven in well-controlled trials; B, probable: very likely but not proven; C, suspected: may occur, good data, more study needed; D, possible: could occur, very limited data; E, unlikely: doubtful, no good data; *NSAIDS*, nonsteroidal anti-inflammatory drugs.
(Courtesy of Tiede DJ, Nishimura RA, Gastineau DA, et al: Modern management of prosthetic valve anticoagulation. *Mayo Clin Proc* 73:665-680, 1998.)

TABLE 5.—Common Dietary Sources of Vitamin K

Dietary Source	Vitamin K Content (µg/100 g)
Green tea	712
Turnip greens	650
Avocado	634
Brussels sprouts	317
Chickpeas	220
Broccoli	200
Cauliflower	192
Lettuce	129
Cabbage	125
Kale	125
Beef liver	92
Spinach	89
Watercress	57
Asparagus	57
Green beans	14
Potatoes	3

(Courtesy of Tiede DJ, Nishimura RA, Gastineau DA, et al: Modern management of prosthetic valve anticoagulation. *Mayo Clin Proc* 73:665-680, 1998.)

anticoagulants cross the placental barrier. Drug and diet interactions influence the level of anticoagulation achieved (Table 4 and Table 5).

Conclusion.—A decrease in thromboplastin sensitivity has unnecessarily raised the anticoagulation levels in some patients. These recommendations and guidelines for safe and effective anticoagulation should be adjusted for individual patient risks. Daily aspirin therapy is recommended for its anticoagulation and cardioprotective effects.

▶ This important paper makes recommendations based on the individual characteristics of the prosthetic valve as well as its location. I suspect that most physicians will continue to use the traditional therapeutic range rather than a single-value INR goal. Physicians should review recommendations for patients who undergo elective surgery while taking anticoagulants.[1]

R.C. Schlant, M.D.

Reference

1. Kearon C, Hirsh J: Management of anticoagulation before and after elective surgery. *N Engl J Med* 336:1506-1511, 1977.

Diagnosis and Management of Infective Endocarditis and Its Complications

Bayer AS, Bolger AF, Taubert KA, et al (American Heart Assoc, Dallas)
Circulation 98:2936-2948, 1998
5–11

Introduction.—Infective endocarditis (IE) is associated with high risk of morbidity and mortality. Prompt recognition and treatment are crucial.

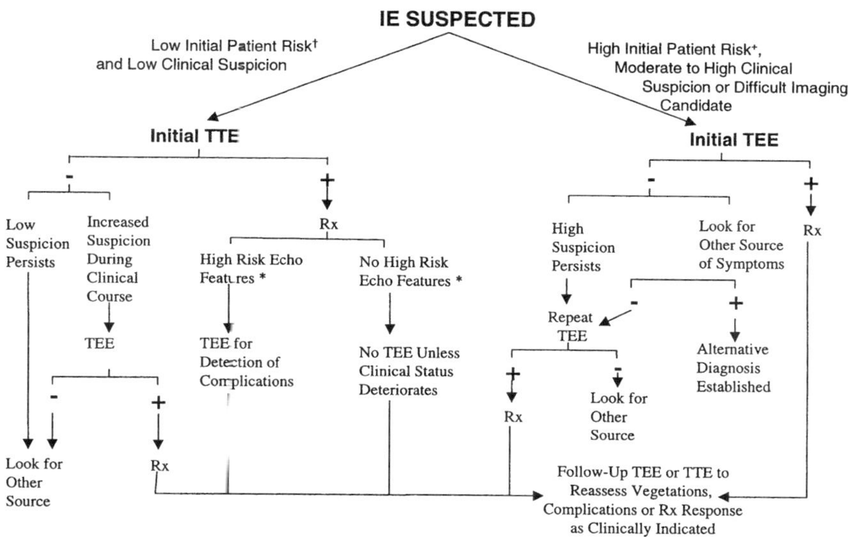

FIGURE.—An approach to the diagnostic use of echocardiography (*echo*). *High-risk echocardiographic features include large and/or mobile vegetations, valvular insufficiency, suggestion of perivalvular extension, and secondary ventricular dysfunction. †Patient with fever and a previously known heart murmur and no other stigmata of infective endocarditis. +High initial patient risks include prosthetic heart valves, many congenital heart diseases, previous endocarditis, new murmur, heart failure, and other stigmata or endocarditis. *Rx*, antibiotic treatment for endocarditis. (Courtesy of Bayer AS, Bolger AF, Taubert KA, et al: Diagnosis and management of infective endocarditis and its complications. *Circulation* 98:2936-2948, 1998.)

Current literature regarding diagnostic challenges and strategies, difficult therapeutic situations, and management choices in patients with IE was reviewed.

Diagnosis.—Diagnosis of IE is specific in patients with classic oslerian manifestations of bacteremia or fungemia, evidence of active valvulitis, peripheral emboli, and immunologic vascular phenomena. For others, classic peripheral stigmata may be few or absent. Variability in the clinical presentation of IE necessitates a diagnostic strategy that is sensitive for disease detection and specific in exclusion. With the Beth Israel criteria, the diagnosis of IE is definitive only with pathological confirmation from surgical or autopsy specimen. Diagnosis is "probable" in the presence of persistent bacteremia and evidence of either new valvular regurgitation or vascular phenomena in the face of underlying valvular heart disease. The Duke criteria use the important diagnostic parameters in the Beth Israel criteria and combine it with echocardiographic findings. There are several refinements pending in the Duke criteria that will use specific serological data to enhance precise determination of culture-negative endocarditis. Echocardiography should not be used as a screening test in patients with fever or blood culture that is unlikely to reflect IE. Some form of echocardiography should be performed in all patients suspected of having IE (Figure).

Management.—The most common cause of prosthetic-valve IE is coagulase-negative staphylococci. Until recently, these organisms have infrequently been associated with native-valve IE. An important subset of patients with coagulase-negative IE have recently been identified: patients with infection caused by *Staphylococcus lugdunensis.* This organism tends to cause a particularly virulent form of IE. Treatment of these and other usual and unusual organisms must be specific to the causative organism. Patients must be monitored closely. Prompt recognition and management of major complications (including heart failure, periannular extension of the infection, splenic abscess, embolism, and mycotic aneurysms) are critical.

Conclusion.—The rising incidence of IE, its significant morbidity and mortality rates, and its substantial prognostic and financial implications make it essential to continue the search for more information on the pathophysiology of the disease and for novel and better treatment and prophylactic strategies.

▶ Major additions in this statement from the American Heart Association include the incorporation of the Duke criteria and the greater use of transesophageal echocardiography. This article should be familiar to all those who may encounter patients with infective endocarditis.

R.C. Schlant, M.D.

Frequency and Phenotypes of Familial Dilated Cardiomyopathy
Grünig E, Tasman JA, Kücherer H, et al (Univ of Heidelberg, Germany; Univ of Lübeck, Germany)
J Am Coll Cardiol 31:186-194, 1998   5–12

Introduction.—Because of the low sensitivity and specificity of diagnostic signs and symptoms of dilated cardiomyopathy, and the low specificity of noninvasive diagnostic procedures, accurate diagnosis of dilated cardiomyopathy is difficult, and the etiology of this disease is still unknown. Up to 25% of index patients were classified as having an inherited disease in recently published prospective studies on patients with dilated cardiomyopathy. A typical phenotype pattern within a single family may often be found after a careful analysis of the family members of patients with dilated cardiomyopathy. Linkage analysis revealed linkage on chromosomes 1p1q1, 3p22-p25 and 9 in families characterized by dilated cardiomyopathy and conduction defects. To determine the frequency of familial disease, segregation analysis in a large cohort of patients with invasively proven dilated cardiomyopathy was performed.

Methods.—To construct pedigrees, detailed family histories were obtained from 445 consecutive patients with angiographically proven dilated cardiomyopathy, and 970 first- and second-degree family members were examined.

Results.—In 48 of the 445 index patients (10.8%), familial dilated cardiomyopathy was confirmed. It was suspected in 108 patients (24.2%). At the time of diagnosis, the 156 patients with suspected or confirmed familial disease were younger and more often revealed electrocardiographic changes, compared with patients with nonfamilial disease. Five phenotypes of familial dilated cardiomyopathy were identified among the families of the 48 index patients with confirmed familial disease. The 5 phenotypes were dilated cardiomyopathy with sensorineural hearing loss; dilated cardiomyopathy with conduction defects; dilated cardiomyopathy with segmental hypokinesia of the left ventricle; juvenile dilated cardiomyopathy with a rapid progressive course in male relatives without muscular dystrophy; and dilated cardiomyopathy with muscular dystrophy.

Conclusion.—An inherited disorder may be found in up to 35% of patients with dilated cardiomyopathy. In some families, distinct clinical phenotypes can be seen, suggesting a common molecular cause of the disease.

▶ The important study by Grünig et al. shows up to 35% of patients with idiopathic cardiomyopathy may have it as an inherited disorder. Actually, the incidence of an inherited genetic predisposition is likely to be much higher. For example, one could argue that there must be an inherited genetic predisposition to explain why idiopathic dilated cardiomyopathy may develop in certain individuals after viral infections and not in others. In the patients studied here, many appeared to have other neuromuscular disorders.

In the somewhat similar paper by Baig et al.[1] from England and Italy, it was found that nearly one third of asymptomatic relatives of patients with idiopathic dilated cardiomyopathy had echocardiographic abnormalities. Over a 3-year period, symptoms developed in a significant number of these patients.

R.C. Schlant, M.D.

Reference

1. Baig MK, Goldman JH, Caforio ALP, et al: Familial dilated cardiomyopathy: Cardiac abnormalities are common in asymptomatic relatives and may represent early disease. *J Am Coll Cardiol* 31:195-201, 1998.

Alcohol Consumption and Idiopathic Dilated Cardiomyopathy: A Case Control Study
McKenna CJ, Codd MB, McCann HA, et al (Mater Misericordiae Hosp, Dublin)
Am Heart J 135:833-837, 1998   5–13

Background.—Alcohol is believed to be a risk factor for idiopathic dilated cardiomyopathy (IDCM). To confirm a causal relationship between excess alcohol intake and IDCM, a case-control study compared the alcohol consumption of patients with IDCM with that of normal, population-based controls.

Methods.—The patients were 100 adults (73 men and 27 women, with a mean age of 54 years) who had IDCM. The controls were 211 adults (86 men and 125 women; mean age, 56 years) who were randomly selected from the population. All participants completed questionnaires that addressed the duration of alcohol intake, average weekly alcohol consumption, and alcohol abuse (via the CAGE questionnaire). Additionally, 200 first-degree relatives of 56 patients with IDCM were examined by echocardiography to identify whether the patients had familial disease. Then risk factors between patients with familial and patients with nonfamilial IDCM were compared.

Findings.—Significantly more of the patients with IDCM (40, or 40%) exceeded the recommended weekly intake of alcohol (21 units for men, 14 units for women) than did the controls (50, or 24%). The average total lifetime consumption of the patients was also significantly greater than that of the controls (31,200 vs. 7,904 units) and significantly more of the patients were alcohol abusers (27, or 27% vs. 33, or 16%). However, when these data were stratified by sex (because the control group contained significantly more women than the patient group), these between-group differences in alcohol consumption and abuse were no longer significant. Of the 56 patients whose relatives were screened, 25 (45% of those examined) had a familial tendency toward IDCM. When these 25 patients were compared with the 31 patients whose disease was nonfamilial, the 2 groups were similar in their risk factors for IDCM (e.g., viral illness, atopy, pregnancy), in alcohol consumption, and in alcohol abuse.

Conclusions.—Alcohol consumption was identified as a possible etiologic agent in 40% of the patients with IDCM. However, 60% of the patients with IDCM were not heavy drinkers, yet they still suffered cardiomyopathy. Thus, alcohol consumption is only one of the risk factors for development of IDCM.

▶ This article confirms an association between excess alcohol intake and dilated cardiomyopathy in many patients with idiopathic dilated cardiomyopathy. The authors are careful to emphasize the limitations of the history of alcohol intake, because many patients tend to report a decrease in this amount.

R.C. Schlant, M.D.

Incidence of Dilated Cardiomyopathy and Detection of HIV in Myocardial Cells of HIV-Positive Patients

Barbaro G, for the Gruppo Italiano per lo Studio Cardiologico dei Pazienti Affetti da AIDS (Univ La Sapienza, Rome; Gen Hosp, Foggia, Italy; Univ of Pavia, Italy)
N Engl J Med 339:1093-1099, 1998

5-14

Background.—The pathogenesis of dilated cardiomyopathy in AIDS is not clear. For a mean of 5 years, these authors studied asymptomatic patients who had HIV infection. Clinical features of dilated cardiomyopathy were correlated with immunologic and virologic parameters.

Methods.—The patients were 952 adults (681 men and 271 women, with a mean age of 28 years) who were HIV-positive. All were New York Heart Association functional class I and Centers for Disease Control and Prevention stage II at enrollment. Every 3 months, patients underwent a clinical examination and a CD4 count, and every 6 months they underwent ECG and echocardiographic studies. An echocardiographic diagnosis of dilated cardiomyopathy was based on the presence of diffuse left ventricular hypokinesia and dilatation (ejection fraction less than 45%, left ventricular end-diastolic volume index more than 80 mL/m²). For patients who developed dilated cardiomyopathy, biopsy specimens were sampled from the right ventricular endomyocardium and submitted for histologic, immunohistologic, and virologic evaluation. Patients were studied for a mean of 5 years.

Findings.—During follow-up, 76 patients (8%) received a diagnosis of dilated cardiomyopathy, at an average of 28 months after enrollment. The mean annual incidence rate was 15.9 cases per 1,000 patients. At diagnosis, 64 patients (84%) were New York Heart Association functional class III and 12 (16%) were class IV. Sixty-three of these 76 patients (83%) had myocarditis. The inflammatory cell infiltrates were primarily CD8 and CD3 lymphocytes, and 54 patients (71%) had intense staining limited to major histocompatibility complex class I antigens. In situ hybridization identified HIV nucleic acid sequences in myocardial cells of 58 of these 76 patients (76%). Thirty-six of these 58 patients (62%) also had myocarditis. Additional viruses found in these 36 patients were coxsackievirus group B, cytomegalovirus, and Epstein-Barr virus. All but 5 of the 76 patients with cardiomyopathy had a CD4 count less than 400 cells/mm³. Furthermore, all 71 of these patients with a low CD4 count had been treated with zidovudine, didanosine, or zalcitabine.

Conclusions.—The extent of immunodeficiency seems to have a major role in the development of dilated cardiomyopathy. Of the 76 patients with dilated cardiomyopathy, 83% had myocarditis, 76% had HIV nucleic acid detected in their myocytes, and 47% had both findings. These results suggest that HIV directly induces myocarditis, although this mechanism does not completely explain the pathogenesis of cardiomyopathy. HIV may also induce an autoimmune process, and the increased expression of major histocompatibility complex class I molecules in the myocardium is consistent with this hypothesis.

▶ This study of 952 asymptomatic HIV-positive patients who were studied for a mean of 5 years found that each year approximately 1.59% of patients developed echocardiographic evidence of dilated cardiomyopathy. Of these patients, approximately 83% had a histologic diagnosis of myocarditis. Some of the many possibilities were infection with HIV itself, coxsackievirus, cytomegalovirus, or Epstein-Barr virus. At present, most HIV-positive patients with dilated cardiomyopathy are best treated with triple therapy for heart failure, since there is no proven therapeutic regimen for viral myocarditis. As patients with AIDS live longer with better therapy, more and more of these patients with a dilated cardiomyopathy will be recognized. Because many of these patients now have a reasonable life expectancy, they should be treated aggressively. It is significant that the incidence of dilated cardiomyopathy was higher in patients with a CD4 count less than 400 cells per millimeter.

R.C. Schlant, M.D.

Resolution of Cardiomyopathy After Ablation of Atrial Flutter
Luchsinger JA, Steinberg JS (Columbia Univ, New York)
J Am Coll Cardiol 32:205-210, 1998   5–15

Background.—Tachycardia-induced cardiomyopathy can lead to congestive heart failure (CHF) and numerous studies have shown that controlling tachycardia improves left ventricular (LV) function. Whether atrial flutter (AFl) is a cause of tachycardia-induced cardiomyopathy is not known. These authors examined the possible contribution of AFl to the development of LV dysfunction and tachycardia-induced cardiomyopathy.

Methods.—The patients were 11 men (mean age, 59 years) with refractory AFl who were undergoing radiofrequency ablation (RFA) of the AFl. Their mean New York Heart Association functional class before RFA was 2.6 ± 0.5. All patients had dilated cardiomyopathy (LV ejection fraction [LVEF] less than 50%) and symptoms of CHF. Furthermore, in each case, the AFl was believed to be caused by structural heart disease. Patients underwent 2-dimensional echocardiography before RFA and again a median of 7 months after RFA to characterize LV function.

Findings.—The RFA was successful in all 11 patients. Before RFA, the mean LVEF was 30.9% ± 11.0%; after RFA, it improved significantly, to 41.3% ± 16% (mean absolute improvement, 17.8%). The mean New York Heart Association functional class also improved significantly after RFA (from 2.6 ± 0.5 to 1.6 ± 0.9). Furthermore, after RFA, all patients experienced a complete resolution of their CHF symptoms, and they were able to discontinue taking medications for CHF. LVEF normalized (more than 50%) in 6 of the 11 patients (55%) after RFA, and all patients reported improvement in functional capacity. Two significant differences were found between patients whose LVEF did and patients whose LVEF did not normalize after RFA: patients whose LVEF did not normalize had a lower preablation LVEF (21.2% ± 2.2% vs. 39.0% ± 8.7%) and a higher New York Heart Association CHF class (3.0 ± 0.0 vs. 2.2 ± 0.4).

Conclusions.—RFA for AFl improved left ventricular function and restored normal sinus rhythm in these patients. Furthermore, dilated cardiomyopathy resolved in about half of the patients after RFA and symptoms of CHF improved in all patients. Thus, AFl appears to have contributed to the development of LV dysfunction and tachycardia-induced cardiomyopathy. AFl may be a more common cause of tachycardia-induced cardiomyopathy than is appreciated, and patients with uncontrolled AFl should seriously consider RFA to prevent or improve cardiomyopathy.

▶ I think that this is an extremely important article. I am afraid that many of us see but do not diagnose left ventricular function caused by rapid heart rate. This can occur with sinus tachycardia, atrial fibrillation, or, as in this report, atrial flutter. It should be noted that of the 11 patients in the present series, only 6 (55%) had complete normalization of LV function, with an LVEF greater than 50% after ablation. I suspect that tachycardia-induced dilated cardiomyopathy is going to turn out to be much more common than is currently recognized.

R.C. Schlant, M.D.

Spontaneous Variability of Left Ventricular Outflow Tract Gradient in Hypertrophic Obstructive Cardiomyopathy

Kizilbash AM, Heinle SK, Grayburn PA (Univ of Texas, Dallas; VA Med Ctr, Dallas)
Circulation 97:461-466, 1998   5–16

Introduction.—Characterized by a broad spectrum of morphologic, functional, and genetic abnormalities, hypertrophic cardiomyopathy is a complex disorder. To evaluate the severity of disease, the presence or absence of left ventricular outflow tract obstruction, and the efficacy of treatment, measurement of the left ventricular outflow tract is often used. In patients with hypertrophic obstructive cardiomyopathy, no data exist on the day-to-day variability of the left ventricular outflow tract gradient. The spontaneous day-to-day variability of rest and provoked left ventricular pressure gradient was examined in stable patients with hypertrophic obstructive cardiomyopathy.

Methods.—In 12 patients with hypertrophic obstructive cardiomyopathy and 5 aortic stenosis controls, the spontaneous variation in the continuous-wave, Doppler-derived pressure gradient was studied on 5 consecutive days.

Results.—The day-to-day variability in resting gradient was small in some patients, whereas in others it varied a great deal. For resting gradient, the 95% confidence interval for attributing a change in left ventricular outflow tract gradient to factors other than random variation is ± 32 mm Hg. For provoked gradient, it is ± 50 mm Hg. For resting gradient, the mean coefficient of variation for gradient across 5 days for the group was 0.52 ± 0.33 and for provoked gradient, it was 0.46 ± 0.16. Changes in heart rate, blood pressure, or left ventricular end-diastolic dimension— each of which had a coefficient of variation of less than 0.11—could not explain the day-to-day variability in pressure gradient. This variability could not be accounted for by technical factors related to the performance or interpretation of the studies because the coefficient of variation for gradient in aortic stenosis was less than 10% and interobserver and intraobserver agreement was excellent.

Conclusion.—In stable patients with hypertrophic obstructive cardiomyopathy, the left ventricular outflow tract pressure gradient varies considerably from day to day. To define the severity of dynamic left ventricular outflow tract obstruction in hypertrophic obstructive cardiomyopathy, a single measurement of pressure gradient is not adequate.

▶ This paper very nicely documents the fairly marked spontaneous variation in the outflow tract pressure gradient that may occur in some patients with hypertrophic obstructive cardiomyopathy. Although this has been recognized by workers in the field for many years, this is the first good documentation of this important phenomenon. Cardiologists need to keep this in mind when evaluating the severity of outflow tract obstruction or the response to therapy.

R.C. Schlant, M.D.

Clinical Features and Prognostic Implications of Familial Hypertrophic Cardiomyopathy Related to the Cardiac Myosin-Binding Protein C Gene

Charron P, Dubourg O, Desnos M, et al (Hôpital Pitié-Salpêtrière, Paris; Hôpital Ambroise Paré, Boulogne, France; Hôpital Boucicaut, Paris; et al)
Circulation 97:2230-2236, 1998   5–17

Introduction.—Familial hypertrophic cardiomyopathy (FHC) is a genetically heterogeneous disease that can result from mutations in several different genes, including the recently discovered cardiac myosin binding protein C (MYBPC3) gene. Preliminary results suggest that these families may have a better prognosis than those with mutations of the β-myosin heavy-chain (β-MHC) gene. However, there are few data on phenotype-genotype associations in cases of FHC related to the MYBPC3 gene. This study examined the clinical findings and prognosis of patients with FHC caused by MYBPC3 mutations.

Methods.—The analysis included 76 patients from 9 families with FHC. The families had 7 different mutations of the MYBPC3 gene. After genotyping, the patients underwent detailed clinical and cardiovascular investigation, including ECG and echocardiography. Phenotypic evaluation included comparison of patients with different mutations of the MYBPC3 gene and comparison of patients with MYBPC3 mutations vs. patients with various mutations of the β-MHC gene.

Results.—Families with different mutations of the MYBPC3 gene showed no significant phenotypic differences from each other. However, prognosis was significantly better for patients with MYBPC3 mutations than for patients with β-MHC mutations. Cumulative survival at age 50 was 95% in the MYBPC3 group vs. 62% in the β-MHC group; by age 60, survival was 76% and 23%, respectively. No patient in the MYBPC3 families died before 40 years of age. Mean age at symptom onset was 41 years in the MYBPC3 group vs. 35 years in the β-MHC group. Before 30 years of age, patients with MYBPC3 mutations had a particularly mild phenotype. Gene penetrance was lower: 41% in the MYBPC3 group vs. 62% in the β-MHC group. Maximal wall thickness was lower: 12 vs. 16 mm. Abnormal T waves were less frequent: 9% vs. 45%.

Conclusions.—The prognosis of FHC appears to be better for families with mutations of the MYBPC3 gene than for families with mutations of the β-MHC gene. Disease onset is delayed in the former group, early death is less likely, and prolonged survival is more likely. Although based on a small number of families, these findings may have important implications for clinical management and genetic counseling of FHC families.

► It is now clear that there are many different genetic abnormalities in patients with FHC. These differences, and perhaps the co-existence of mitochondrial changes in some patients, may help explain the different clinical features and prognoses in different patients with this syndrome. There have been several important studies of the genetic abnormalities in patients with FHC.[1-4] In addition, mitochondrial abnormalities may co-exist.[5]

R.C. Schlant, M.D.

References

1. Anan R, Shono H, Kisanuki A, et al: Patients with familial hypertrophic cardio-myopathy caused by a Phe110IIe missense mutation in the cardiac troponin T gene have variable cardiac morphologies and a favorable prognosis. *Circulation* 98:391-397, 1998.
2. Nimura H, Bachinski LL, Sangwatanaroj S, et al: Mutations in the gene for cardiac myosin-binding protein C and late-onset familial hypertrophic cardiomyopathy. *N Engl J Med* 338:1248-1257, 1998.
3. Bonne G, Carrier L, Richard P, et al: Familial hypertrophic cardiomyopathy: From mutations to functional defects. *Circ Res* 83:580-593, 1998.
4. Maron BJ, Moller JH, Seidman CE, et al: Impact of laboratory molecular diagnosis on contemporary diagnostic criteria for genetically transmitted cardiovascular diseases: Hypertrophic cardiomyopathy, long-QT syndrome, and Marfan syndrome. *Circulation* 98:1460-1471, 1998.
5. Arbustini E, Fasani R, Morbini P, et al: Coexistence of mitochondrial DNA and β myosin heavy chain mutations in hypertrophic cardiomyopathy with late congestive heart failure. *Heart* 80:548-558, 1998.

Screening for Hypertrophic Cardiomyopathy in Young Athletes

Corrado D, Basso C, Schiavon M, et al (Univ of Padua, Italy; Natl Health Service, Padua, Italy)

N Engl J Med 339:364-369, 1998

5–18

Introduction.—Cardiovascular disease is the most common cause of sudden death in athletes. For athletes older than age 35 years, atherosclerotic coronary artery disease is the most common cause of sudden death. Hypertrophic cardiomyopathy has been implicated as the cause of death in about one third of younger competitive athletes. Early identification of abnormalities by screening before athletes participate in competitive sports may prevent sudden death. Since 1971, Italian law has required that every athlete undergo annual clinical evaluation before participating in competitive sports. The effects of this strategy on the prevention of hypertrophic cardiomyopathy was assessed in athletes in the Veneto region of Italy.

Methods.—Sudden deaths among athletes and nonathletes aged 35 years or younger were prospectively studied in the Veneto region from 1979 to 1996. The causes of death among athletes and nonathletes were assessed and pathologic findings were compared with clinical histories and ECGs. Cardiovascular reasons for disqualification from sports competition were analyzed. A consecutive series of 33,735 young athletes from Padua, Italy, who underwent preparticipation screening during the same period were observed.

Results.—Of 269 young people with sudden death, 49 (18.2%) were competitive athletes, mean age, 23 years (44 males, 5 females). The most

TABLE 2.—Causes of Sudden Death in Athletes and Nonathletes

Cause	Athletes (N=49)	Nonathletes (N=220)	Total (N=269)
		Number (Percent)	
Arrhythmogenic right ventricular cardiomyopathy	11 (22.4)	18 (8.2)*	29 (10.8)
Atherosclerotic coronary artery disease	9 (18.4)	36 (16.4)	45 (16.7)
Anomalous origin of coronary artery	6 (12.2)	1 (0.5)†	7 (2.6)
Disease of conduction system	4 (8.2)	20 (9.1)	24 (8.9)
Mitral-valve prolapse	5 (10.2)	21 (9.5)	26 (9.7)
Hypertrophic cardiomyopathy	1 (2.0)	16 (7.3)	17 (6.3)
Myocarditis	3 (6.1)	19 (8.6)	22 (8.2)
Myocardial bridge	2 (4.1)	5 (2.3)	7 (2.6)
Pulmonary thromboembolism	1 (2.0)	3 (1.4)	4 (1.5)
Dissecting aortic aneurysm	1 (2.0)	11 (5.0)	12 (4.5)
Dilated cardiomyopathy	1 (2.0)	9 (4.1)	10 (3.7)
Other	5 (10.2)	61 (27.7)	66 (24.5)

*$P = 0.008$ for the comparison with the athletes.

†$P < 0.001$ for the comparison with the athletes.

TABLE 4.—Cardiovascular Conditions Causing Disqualification
From Competitive Sports

Condition	No. (%)
Rhythm and conduction abnormalities	238 (38.3)
Systemic hypertension	168 (27.1)
Valvular diseases (including mitral-valve prolapse)	133 (21.4)
Hypertrophic cardiomyopathy	22 (3.5)
Others	60 (9.7)

(Reprinted by permission of *The New England Journal of Medicine* from Corrado D, Basso C, Schiavon M, et al: Screening for hypertrophic cardiomyopathy in young athletes. *N Engl J Med* 339:364-369, copyright 1998, Massachusetts Medical Society. All rights reserved.)

common causes of sudden death in these athletes and percentages affected were as follows: 22.4%, arrhythmogenic right ventricular cardiomyopathy; 18.4%, coronary atherosclerosis; and 12.2%, anomalous origin of a coronary artery (Table 2). One death in young competitive athletes (2%) was caused by hypertrophic cardiomyopathy; in young nonathletes, the rate was 7.3% (16 deaths). Hypertrophic cardiomyopathy was found during preparticipation examination in 22 athletes (0.07%) and accounted for 3.5% of cardiovascular reasons for disqualification (Table 4). None of the athletes who were disqualified because of hypertrophic cardiomyopathy died during a mean follow-up of 8.2 years.

Conclusion.—Hypertrophic cardiomyopathy was a rare cause of death in young competitive athletes in Italy who underwent preparticipation screening. It is possible that sudden death was prevented in athletes who were screened and disqualified before participating in competitive sports.

▶ For the last 20 years, Italy has led the world in having a national program for the systematic screening of all young competitive athletes. The low incidence of death from hypertrophic cardiomyopathy in Italian athletes noted in this report may reflect the successful screening of such individuals. The screening for hypertrophic cardiomyopathy in Italy is primarily based on the ECG. Of interest, only 3,016 (8.9%) of the 33,735 athletes initially screened were referred for echocardiographic evaluation, and only 22 were eventually found to have evidence of hypertrophic cardiomyopathy.

The surprisingly high incidence of arrhythmogenic right ventricular cardiomyopathy may, in part, be unique to Italy, where the condition may occur more frequently than in the United States. In general, these results provide strong support for those who have proposed a similar screening program for young athletes in the United States before participation in competitive sports.

R.C. Schlant, M.D.

Mechanism of Benefit of Negative Inotropes in Obstructive Hypertrophic Cardiomyopathy

Sherrid MV, Pearle G, Gunsburg DZ (Columbia Univ, New York)
Circulation 97:41-47, 1998
5–19

Objective.—Negative inotropes reduce or eliminate obstruction in hypertrophic cardiomyopathy (HCM). Echocardiography is the modality of choice for studying the mechanism of such therapy.

Methods.—M-mode, 2-dimensional, and pulsed Doppler echocardiography was performed on 11 patients with symptomatic obstructive HCM and mitral-septal apposition before and after elimination of obstruction and on 10 normal controls, average age 59. The peak pressure gradient across the left ventricular (LV) outflow tract was calculated.

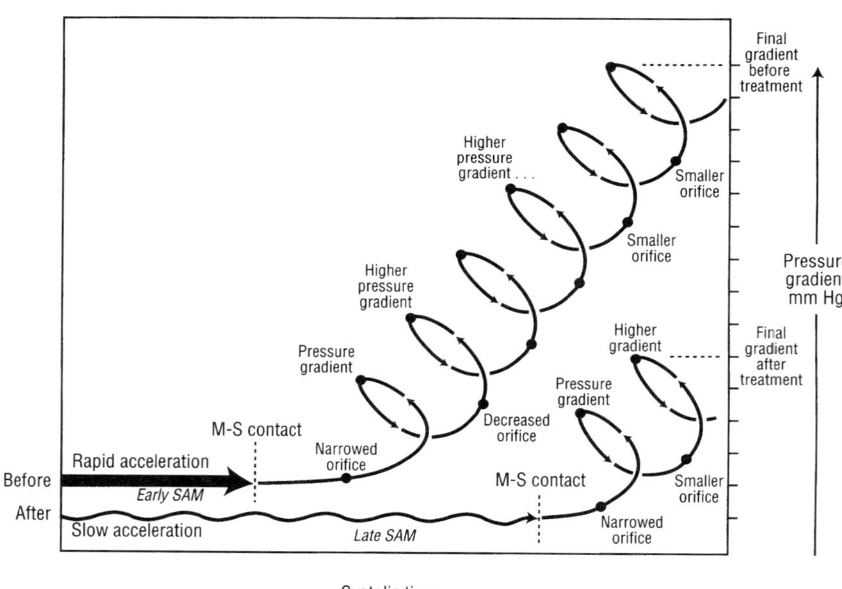

FIGURE 6.—Proposed explanation of pressure gradient development before and after treatment of obstruction. Before treatment (*top tracing*), rapid left ventricular acceleration apical of the mitral valve, shown as a horizontal *thick arrow*, triggers early systolic anterior motion (SAM) and early mitral-septal (M-S) contact. Once M-S contact occurs, a narrowed orifice develops, and a pressure difference results. The pressure difference forces the leaflet against the septum, which decreases the orifice size and further increases the pressure difference. An amplifying feedback loop is established, shown as a rising spiral. The longer the leaflet is in contact with the septum, the higher the pressure gradient. After treatment (*bottom tracing*), negative inotropes slow early SAM (shown as a horizontal *waxy arrow*) and may thereby decrease the force on the mitral leaflet, delaying SAM. Mitral-septal contact would occur later, leaving less time in systole for the feedback loop to narrow the orifice. This would reduce the final pressure difference. Delaying SAM may also allow more time for papillary muscle shortening to provide countertraction. In the figure, for clarity, the "before" arrow is positioned above the "after" arrow, although at the beginning of systole they both actually begin with a pressure gradient of 0 mm Hg. (Courtesy of Sherrid MV, Pearle G, Gunsburg DZ: Mechanism of benefit of negative inotropes in obstructive hypertrophic cardiomyopathy. *Circulation* 97:41-47, 1998.)

Results.—A total of 148 LV Doppler flow velocity tracings at the apical of the mitral valve point were compared before and after treatment. Whereas peak and mean ejection velocities were similar before and after treatment, mean acceleration to peak ejection velocity was significantly decreased from 839 cm/sec before treatment to 557 cm/sec after treatment. Mean acceleration time increased significantly from 137 to 179 msec. Time from ejection onset to a velocity of 60 cm/sec increased significantly from 35 to 67 msec. Whereas before treatment flow velocity peaked in the first half of ejection, after treatment velocity peaked in the second half of ejection. Peak left ventricular ejection velocity was unchanged after treatment. There was less mitral regurgitation after treatment (1.4 vs. 0.6). All parameters measured were significantly higher in patients than in controls. Development of a pressure gradient before and after treatment may explain how the measured decrease in ejection acceleration can lead to a decrease in obstruction (Fig 6).

Conclusion.—Negative inotropes appear to eliminate the hydrodynamic force on the mitral leaflet by decreasing LV ejection acceleration.

▶ This study clearly identifies that negative inotropes decrease left ventricular ejection acceleration. This decreases the obstruction produced by the anterior mitral leaflet, whether it be by a Venturi mechanism or by drag that pushes the anterior mitral leaflet against the septum.

R.C. Schlant, M.D.

Percutaneous Transluminal Septal Myocardial Ablation in Hypertrophic Obstructive Cardiomyopathy: Results With Respect to Intraprocedural Myocardial Contrast Echocardiography
Faber L, Seggewiss H, Gleichmann U (Ruhr-Univ of Bochum, Bad Oeynhausen, Germany)
Circulation 98:2415-2421, 1998   5–20

Introduction.—Alcohol-induced percutaneous transluminal septal myocardial ablation (PTSMA) is an alternative to surgical myectomy for patients with hypertrophic cardiomyopathy (HOCM). The goal of treatment is to reduce the left ventricular outflow tract gradient (LVOTG). The authors have been performing myocardial contrast echocardiography (MCE) during the PTSMA procedure. They report the acute and midterm results in patients undergoing intraprocedural MCE.

Methods.—The analysis included 91 patients with symptomatic HOCM in whom PTSMA was planned. The patients were 46 women and 45 men (mean age, 54 years). The procedure could not be completed in 2 patients. In the first 30 patients, probatory balloon occlusion was used to identify the target vessel. Thereafter, the target vessel was identified using additional intraprocedural MCE. The outcomes and complications of PTSMA with and without intraprocedural MCE were analyzed in the hospital and at 3 months' follow-up.

Results.—The PTSMA procedure reduced mean resting LVOTG from 74 to 17 mm Hg and postextrasystolic LVOTG from 149 to 62 mm Hg. The short-term hemodynamic success rate, defined as complete elimination or a greater than 50% reduction in LVOTG, was 84% overall: 92% in patients with intraprocedural MCE and 70% in those without. Eleven percent of patients required permanent universal pacemaker implantation. One patient with chronic obstructive pulmonary disease died of ventricular fibrillation after 9 days, and a second patient died of fulminant pulmonary embolism after 2 days. The patients' mean New York Heart Association class decreased from 2.8 at baseline to 1.1 at 3 months' follow-up. Mean LVOTG at rest was 15 mm Hg, and mean postextrasystolic LVOTG was 49 mm Hg. Midterm success rates were 94% with intraprocedural MCE and 64% without. Symptoms were completely eliminated in one third of patients.

Conclusions.—For patients with HOCM, PTSMA gives promising immediate and midterm results. It reduces LVOTG while improving symptoms and exercise tolerance. Intraprocedural MCE to provide additional information on target vessel selection may be associated with better results. Large, prospective studies with long-term follow-up are needed to compare PTSMA with established therapies for HOCM.

▶ This technique, which improves the symptoms and hopefully the prognosis of patients with HOCM, was introduced by Sigwart.[1] These authors used MCE to map the vascular beds of the septal perforators to predict the size of the infarct that follows injection of ethanol. The benefits of MCE have also been reported by 2 other groups,[2,3] while a study from Poland reported the many electrocardiographic changes that may occur after alcohol septal ablation in patients with HOCM.[4]

R.C. Schlant, M.D.

References

1. Sigwart U: Non-surgical myocardial reduction for hypertrophic obstructive cardiomyopathy. *Lancet* 346:211-214, 1995.
2. Nagueh SF, Lakkis NM, He Z-X, et al: Role of myocardial contrast echocardiography during nonsurgical septal reduction therapy for hypertrophic obstructive cardiomyopathy. *J Am Coll Cardiol* 32:225-229, 1998.
3. Lakkis MN, Nagueh SF, Kleiman NS, et al: Echocardiography-guided ethanol septal reduction for hypertrophic obstructive cardiomyopathy. *Circulation* 98:1750-1755, 1998.
4. Kazmierczak J, Kornacewicz-Jach Z, Kisly M, et al: Electrocardiographic changes after alcohol septal ablation in hypertrophic obstructive cardiomyopathy. *Heart* 80:257-262, 1998.

Restrictive Cardiomyopathy, Atrioventricular Block and Mild to Subclinical Myopathy in Patients With Desmin-Immunoreactive Material Deposits
Arbustini E, Morbini P, Grasso M, et al (Istituto di Ricovero e Cura a Carattere Scientifico, Policlinico San Matteo, Italy; Fondazione Istituto Neurologico Casimiro Modino, Italy; Centro Medico di Monstescano, Pavia, Italy; et al)
J Am Coll Cardiol 31:645-653, 1998   5–21

Objective.—Granulofilamentous or cytoplasmic inclusion-type desmin accumulation in the heart can lead to disorders of cardiac and skeletal muscle. The clinical, ultrastructural, biochemical, and immunohistochemical findings in 6 Italian patients with desmin deposits in cardiac and skeletal myocytes, cardiomyopathy, atrioventricular (AV) block, and varying degrees of skeletal myopathy are discussed.

Methods.—Between January 1985 and December 1995, of 631 patients with primary cardiomyopathies who underwent endomyocardial biopsy (EMB), 5 of 12 with restrictive cardiomyopathy and 1 who underwent skeletal muscle biopsy were found to have desmin-storage cardiomyopathy as established by histopathologic, electron microscopic, light microscopic, immunocytologic, and Western blot studies.

Results.—All patients had AV block, and 5 had myopathy. Three of the 6 patients were first-degree relatives. Electrophoretic studies revealed 2 isoforms of desmin–one with a normal molecular weight of 55 kd and one with a molecular weight of 53 kd.

Conclusion.—Desmin cardiomyopathy should be considered in patients with restrictive cardiomyopathy and AV block. Desmin accumulation in cardiac and skeletal muscle can be confirmed ultrastructurally and immunohistochemically and distinguished from nonspecific cytoskeletal abnormalities.

▶ Although desmin cardiomyopathy appears to be relatively rare, we should certainly think of it in any patient with a clinical syndrome of restrictive cardiomyopathy, especially in a patient with AV block and either mild or subclinical systemic myopathy.

R.C. Schlant, M.D.

Echocardiographically Guided Pericardiocentesis: Evolution and State-of-the-Art Technique
Tsang TSM, Freeman WK, Sinak LJ, et al (Mayo Clinic Rochester, Minn)
Mayo Clin Proc 73 647-652, 1998   5–22

Introduction.—Percutaneous pericardiocentesis was performed blindly with unacceptably high morbidity and mortality rates before the advent of two-dimensional echocardiography (Fig 1).

General Overview.—The equipment and supplies required are available in any hospital (Table 1). Needle entry is at the site of the largest fluid

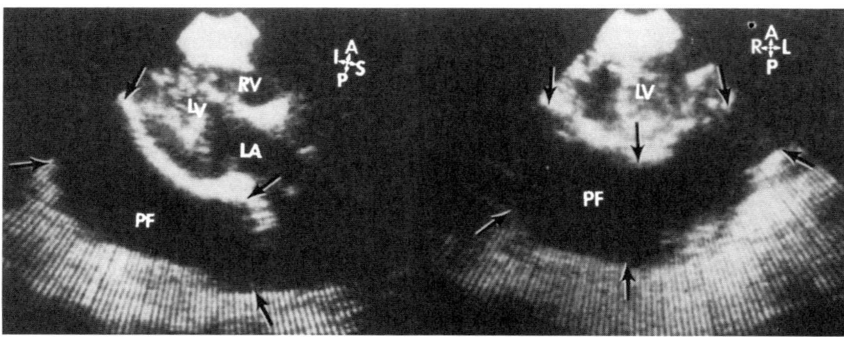

FIGURE 1.—First use of echo-guided pericardiocentesis in 1979. Two-dimensional echocardiographic images show a large loculated posterior pericardial effusion (*arrows*) with compression of heart anteriorly. Effusion was inaccessible from subcostal approach. After multiple blind attempts at pericardiocentesis in the surgical suite, fluid was removed, through entry site on chest wall, by echocardiographic guidance. Fluid 2 cm from chest wall was removed without incident. *Abbreviations: A*, anterior; *I*, inferior; *L*, left; *LA*, left atrium; *LV*, left ventricle; *P*, posterior; *PF*, pericardial fluid; *R*, right; *RV*, right ventricle; *S*, superior. (Courtesy of Tsang TSM, Freeman WK, Sinak LJ, et al: Echocardiographically guided pericardiocentesis: Evolution and state-of-the-art technique. *Mayo Clin Proc* 73:647-652, 1998.)

accumulation and at an angle that avoids vital structures as revealed by the ultrasound beam.

Technique.—The step-by-step approach involves two-dimensional echocardiographic and Doppler examination, echocardio-

---

TABLE 1.—Equipment and Supplies for Echo-Guided Pericardiocentesis

---

Pericardiocentesis tray
  Povidone-iodine solution (skin antiseptic)
  Sterile transparent plastic drape (1030 Drape, Baxter)
  One 20- to 25-gauge needle for local anesthetic infiltration
  1 to 2% lidocaine (local anesthetic)
  Multiple 16- to 18-gauge (5.1- to 8.3-cm) polytef-sheathed venous "intracath" needles (Deseret)
  Syringes (10 to 20 mL and one 60 mL)
  Specimen-collecting tubes for fluid analyses and cultures
  Plastic tubing (30 cm) and three-way stopcock
  Scalpel (No. 11 blade)
  4 by 4 in. gauze dressing

Other supplies
  Sheath introducer set (Cordis)
    Fine-gauge (0.035-mm) polytef-coated, floppy-tipped guidewire
    Dilator and introducer sheath (6 F to 8 F)
  A 65-cm standard pigtail angiocatheter (6 F to 8 F) with multiple side holes (Cordis)
  Fluid receptacle (1 L vacuum bottle)
  Manometer (for pericardial pressure measurement)
  Dressings and antiseptic ointment
  Sterile isotonic saline (for flushing catheter)
  Sterile gloves, mask, and gown

(Courtesy of Tsang TSM, Freeman WK, Sinak LJ, et al: Echocardiographically guided pericardiocentesis: Evolution and state-of-the-art technique. *Mayo Clin Proc* 73:647-652, 1998.)

---

graphic selection of the ideal entry site, sterile preparation, local anesthetic administration, insertion of polytef-sheathed needle, saline echo-contrast medium for confirmation of position, intraperitoneal pressure measurement, diagnostic tap, catheter drainage, dressing, and subsequent catheter drainage and maintenance.

Other Pericardial Drainage Techniques.—Surgical techniques such as subxiphoid pericardiotomy and partial or complete pericardiectomy have been associated with 30-day mortality rates of 20% to 50%. Sclerotherapy was associated with recurrence rates similar to those associated with catheter drainage and surgical decompression. Complication rates after balloon pericardiotomy are as high as 18%.

Conclusion.—Echo-guided pericardiocentesis is simple, safe, effective, and relatively inexpensive. It reduces recurrence rates, uses readily available equipment and supplies, and does not require specialized personnel.

▶ This technique is now widely used throughout the United States because it appears to overcome many of the problems with "blind" pericardiocentesis. For patients who need a histologic examination of the pericardium, we would recommend a pericardial or subxiphoid surgical procedure with direct exposure and biopsy of the pericardium in addition to catheter drainage.

R.C. Schlant, M.D.

Colchicine Treatment for Recurrent Pericarditis: A Decade of Experience
Adler Y, Finkelstein Y, Guindo J, et al (Tel Aviv Univ, Israel; Hosp de Sant Pau, Barcelona; Sheba Med Ctr, Tel Hashomer, Israel; et al)
Circulation 97:2183-2185, 1998   5–23

Objective.—The best way to prevent recurrent acute inflammation of the pericardium has not been established. Nonsteroidal anti-inflammatory drugs, corticosteroids, immunosuppressive drugs, and pericardiectomy are nonspecific. The preventive use of colchicine is discussed.

Discussion.—Colchicine has been used successfully to treat relapses of systemic inflammatory processes in familial Mediterranean fever and recurrences of acute pericarditis in patients in whom nonsteroidal anti-inflammatory drugs and corticosteroids have failed. In a larger study, colchicine prevented relapses of pericarditis in patients who were studied for as long as 10 years. Colchicine inhibits some polymorphonuclear leukocytes, interferes with transcellular movement of collagen, and may reduce immunopathic antifibroblastic properties. Colchicine may be effective in treating initial episodes of pericarditis as well as large pericardial effusions. Colchicine may also have steroid-sparing effects.

Conclusion.—Colchicine appears to be safe and effective for preventing recurrences of pericarditis and is well-tolerated. Long-term treatment with corticosteroids should be limited to very severe cases. Large, controlled, prospective studies are needed to establish the safety and efficacy of colchicine.

▶ This article discusses the management of recurrent pericarditis, which may result from almost any cause, and particularly discusses therapy with colchicine. Recurrent pericarditis (or mediastinitis) can even occur after apparently total pericardiectomy.

Although there are no large, controlled, prospective studies to prove the efficacy and safety of colchicine for recurrent pericarditis, the available data reviewed in this article suggest that most patients can and should be treated with colchicine before they are treated with corticosteroids.

R.C. Schlant, M.D.

Congestive Heart Failure in the Community: A Study of All Incident Cases in Olmsted County, Minnesota, in 1991

Senni M, Tribouilloy CM, Rodeheffer RJ, et al (Mayo Clinic and Mayo Found, Rochester, Minn)
Circulation 98:2282-2289, 1998   5–24

Background.—Congestive heart failure (CHF) is a condition of increasing prevalence and carries high morbidity and mortality. Previous studies of CHF have focused largely on selected referral patients and have excluded very old patients. There is little information about the classification and prognosis of CHF patients in the community. Data from a population-based epidemiologic study were used to analyze the characteristics, treatment, and outcomes of CHF in the community.

Patients.—The authors used data from the Rochester Epidemiology Project to identify all 216 residents of 1 Minnesota county who received an initial diagnosis of CHF during 1991. The patients were 125 men and 91 women (mean age, 77 years); 88% were aged 65 years or older, and 49% were aged 80 years or older. Of 137 patients undergoing echocardiographic assessment of ejection fraction, 43% had preserved systolic function, defined as an ejection fraction of 50% or greater; the remaining 57% had predominantly systolic dysfunction. Women were more likely to have preserved ejection fraction, patients aged 90 years or older were more likely to have normal systolic function, and patients with left bundle branch block or myocardial infarction pattern on ECG were more likely to have a decreased ejection fraction. Analysis of treatments found that patients with heart failure and systolic dysfunction were more likely to be hospitalized. Only 44% of patients received angiotensin-converting enzyme inhibitor therapy.

Outcomes.—Survival decreased from 86% at 3 months after diagnosis to 76% at 1 year and 35% at 3 years. Of patients surviving for 3 months, survival was 88% at 1 year and 41% at 5 years. On multivariate analysis, negative predictors of long-term survival were advanced age and moderate to severe New York Heart Association functional class. After adjustment

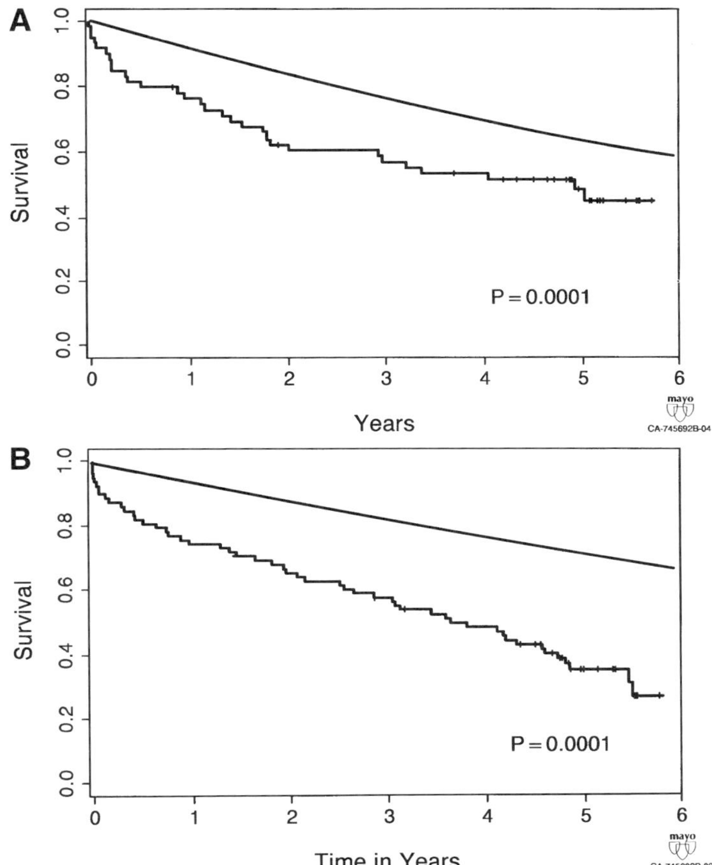

FIGURE 3.—Survival of patients with ejection fraction of 50% or greater (A) and less than 50% (B) compared with that for age- and sex-matched population. (Courtesy of Senni M, Tribouilloy CM, Rodeheffer RJ, et al: Congestive heart failure in the community: A study of all incident cases in Olmsted County, Minnesota, in 1991. *Circulation* 98:2282-2289, 1998.)

for these factors, for sex, and for coronary artery disease, survival was similar for patients with preserved and patients with reduced systolic function (Fig 3).

Conclusions.—The clinical features and natural history of CHF in the community were clarified. Congestive heart failure affects a very elderly population, often with a normal ejection fraction. The prognosis for these patients is poor, even with preserved systolic function. Patients with CHF in the community differ from those enrolled in clinical trials in some important ways. These differences must be considered in assessing the impact of advances in the diagnosis and treatment of CHF.

▶ This important article emphasizes the significance of congestive heart failure in the "very elderly" group, in whom it has a significantly poor prognosis. It is interesting that hypertension remains one of the preexisting conditions most important to the development of heart failure in this county. Somewhat surprising is the fact that the prognosis was poor in the very elderly with heart failure, despite their level of systolic function. Accordingly, even those who had well preserved systolic function had a poor prognosis.

R.C. Schlant, M.D.

Biomechanical Detection of Left-Ventricular Systolic Dysfunction

McDonagh TA, Robb SD, Murdoch DR, et al (Univ of Glasgow, Scotland; Glasgow Royal Infirmary, Scotland)

Lancet 351:9-13, 1998

5–25

Objective.—Chronic heart failure (CHF) is sometimes difficult to diagnose. Natriuretic peptides can be used to distinguish left ventricular systolic dysfunction from the asymptomatic form of left ventricular systolic dysfunction. The utility of the N-terminal atrial natriuretic peptide (NT-ANP) and brain natriuretic peptides (BNP) in the identification of left ventricular systolic dysfunction as a screening method is discussed.

Methods.—Questionnaires were mailed to 2,000 participants, aged 25 to 74, from 30 family physicians' lists in Glasgow, Scotland, soliciting information about previous myocardial infarction, angina, hypertension, diabetes, and drug therapy. Left ventricular systolic function was investigated in 1,653 selected study participants by echocardiography and electrocardiography. Left ventricular systolic dysfunction was defined as an ejection fraction of 30% or less. Plasma NT-ANP and BNP levels were measured by radioimmunoassay.

Results.—Complete data were obtained for 1,252 participants. There were 18 participants with symptomatic and 19 with asymptomatic left ventricular systolic dysfunction. Groups with both symptomatic and asymptomatic left ventricular systolic dysfunction had significantly higher median concentrations of NT-ANP than did those with normal left ventricular function (3.3 and 2.2 vs. 1.3 ng/ml). BNP concentrations were also significantly higher in participants with left ventricular systolic dysfunction than in participants with normal left ventricular function (24.0 vs. 7.7 pg/ml). Ischemic heart disease was the most significant predictor of a reduced left ventricular ejection fraction, according to multivariate analysis. An increase of 50% in BNP or NT-ANP level was a significant predictor of left ventricular systolic dysfunction. Using a cutoff of 17.9 pg/ml, the sensitivity, specificity, and positive and negative predictive values for a BNP concentration in patients aged 25 to 74 were 77%, 87%, 16%, and 97.5%, respectively. Sensitivity and specificity in participants aged 55 or older were 89% and 71%, respectively.

Conclusion.—Measurement of BNP is a sensitive, specific, and cost-effective technique for screening for left ventricular systolic dysfunction in high-risk individuals in the general population.

▶ It would appear that the measurement of BNP is significantly better than the measurement of MT-ANP in predicting which patients will have left ventricular systolic dysfunction. In a related study, Tanaka and co-workers[1] found that BNP levels in pericardial fluid more accurately reflected left ventricular dysfunction than did plasma levels of BNP. In their study, none of the measured hemodynamic variables correlated with ANP levels in either plasma or pericardial fluid. Tsutamoto and co-workers[2] found that increased plasma levels of inter eukin-6 were associated with poor prognosis in patients with congestive heart failure.

R.C. Schlant, M.D.

References

1. Tanaka T, Hasegawa K, Fujita M, et al: Marked elevation of brain natriuretic peptide levels in pericardial fluid is closely associated with left-ventricular dysfunction. *J Am Coll Cardiol* 31:399-403, 1998.
2. Tsutamoto T, Hisanaga T, Wada A, et al: Interleukin-6 spillover in the peripheral circulation increases with the severity of heart failure, and the high plasma level of interleukin-6 is an important prognostic predictor in patients with congestive heart failure. *J Am Coll Cardiol* 31:391-398, 1998.

Pro-inflammatory Cytokines and Endothelium-Dependent Vasodilation in the Forearm: Serial Assessment in Patients With Congestive Heart Failure
Vanderheyden M, Kersschot E, Paulus WJ (OLV Ziekenhuis, Aalst, Belgium)
Eur Heart J 19:747-752, 1998   5–26

Background.—Patients with heart failure have elevated plasma levels of the proinflammatory cytokines interleukin 6 (IL-6) and tumor necrosis factor alpha (TNF-α). Elevated TNF-α levels are known to alter vasomotoricity, and affected patients also have impaired endothelium-dependent vasodilation of the forearm vessels. This study investigated whether the endothelium-dependent vasodilation of the forearm vessels was caused by these increased plasma cytokine levels and compared patients with congestive heart failure during an episode of acute failure and at the time of recompensation.

Methods.—Sixteen patients (13 men and 3 women, with a mean age of 64 years) were hospitalized for an acute episode of congestive heart failure. Hemodynamic parameters and plasma cytokine levels were measured immediately after admission and a mean of 11 days later, after recompensation. During recompensation, all patients received loop diuretics and 4 also received potassium-sparing diuretics. Hemodynamic parameters included the measurement of brachial artery diameters at rest and during hyperemia. Plasma levels of IL-6 and TNF-α were measured by immunoradiometric assay.

Findings.—Mean (± standard deviation) serum concentrations of TNF-α were high in all patients, both at admission (25 ± 23 pg/mL) and after recompensation (26 ± 17 pg/mL), but did not differ significantly between these 2 time points. Similarly, mean serum concentrations of IL-6 were high at admission in 15 patients (27 ± 24 pg/mL) and high in 12 patients after recompensation (20 ± 18 pg/mL). There was a trend toward fewer patients having elevated IL-6 levels at follow-up, but the trend did not reach statistical significance. Reactive hyperemia caused a significant increase in brachial artery diameter during both the acute episode (from 3.7 ± 0.7 to 4.0 ± 0.5 mm) and after recompensation (from 3.7 ± 0.5 to 3.8 ± 0.2 mm). The proportionate increase in diameter with reactive hyperemia, however, did not differ during the acute episode (117% ± 14%) and after recompensation (112% ± 6%). During the acute episode, there was no correlation between the TNF-α level and the percentage change in brachial artery diameter induced by reactive hyperemia. After recompensation, however, TNF-α levels significantly correlated with flow-mediated brachial artery vasodilation (r = 0.75).

Conclusions.—During an acute episode of congestive heart failure, the elevated levels of TNF-α had no correlation with changes in the brachial artery diameter induced by reactive hyperemia. After recompensation, however, this correlation was restored.

▶ It is now well established that levels of proinflammatory cytokines may be increased in patients with chronic heart failure. This article documents a positive correlation between flow-mediated endothelium-dependent vasodilatation and circulating levels of TNF-α following recompensation. Several other articles have reviewed the role of cytokines in heart failure.[1-3]

R.C. Schlant, M.D.

References

1. Blum A, Miller H: Role of cytokines in heart failure. *Am Heart J* 135:181-186, 1998.
2. Bristow MR: Tumor necrosis factor-α and cardiomyopathy (editorial). *Circulation* 97:1340-1341, 1998.
3. Ferrari R: Tumor necrosis factor in CHF: A double facet cytokine. *Cardiovasc Res* 37:554-559, 1998.

The Effects of Diuresis on the Pharmacokinetics of the Loop Diuretics Furosemide and Torsemide in Patients With Heart Failure
Gottlieb SS, Khatta M, Wentworth D, et al (Univ of Maryland, Baltimore; Boehringer Mannheim Corp, Gaithersburg, Md)
Am J Med 104:533-538, 1998

5–27

Introduction.—IV diuretics are commonly administered to patients with decompensated heart failure, on the assumption that oral diuretics will be ineffective. However, IV diuretics are expensive, and their use in this situation is based on 1 small study suggesting that absorption and peak concentrations of loop diuretics are reduced in patients with fluid overload. Patients with marked fluid overload were studied to examine the pharmacokinetics of furosemide and torsemide before and after diuresis.

Methods.—The study included 44 patients with confirmed congestive heart failure, in New York Heart Association class III or IV, and having an ejection fraction of 40% or less. All patients had massive edema, with an estimated excess fluid body weight of 6.8 kg or greater. Patients were randomized to receive oral furosemide or torsemide (mean dose, 127 and 65 mg, respectively) before and after diuresis. The pharmacokinetics of the 2 drugs were assessed at both times. Rescue treatment with IV diuretics was permitted if sufficient diuresis did not begin within a reasonable period.

Results.—Peak plasma drug concentration increased from 11.0 before to 13.9 µg/mL after diuresis in the torsemide group and from 3.1 to 3.9 µg/mL in the furosemide group. The increase exceeded 30% in one third of patients. As calculated by the area under the curve method, the increase in total absorption was 6% in the torsemide group and 7% in the furosemide group. An increase of greater than 30% was achieved in only 5% and 11% of patients, respectively. Time to peak concentration decreased by more than 30% in 68% of patients receiving torsemide and in 50% of those receiving furosemide. The 2 groups showed no differences in the effects of edema on absorption or in weight loss.

Conclusions.—In patients with marked fluid overload, marked diuresis alters the pharmacokinetics of furosemide or torsemide in a small percentage of cases. These results question the commonly held notion that such patients should receive IV therapy to achieve adequate diuresis. If given adequate doses of oral diuretics, these patients can be successfully managed at home, lowering the cost of therapy. The doses given may need to be higher than those used for maintenance therapy.

▶ As the population of patients with heart failure increases in future years, it will be more and more important to utilize diuretics. In this study, most patients with significant congestive heart failure and massive fluid overload were still able to absorb loop diuretics and to have an effective diuresis. The recent review of diuretics by Brater is also very thoughtful and useful.[1]

R.C. Schlant, M.D.

Reference

1. Brater DC: Diuretic therapy. *N Engl J Med* 339:387-395, 1998.

Experience From Controlled Trials of Physical Training in Chronic Heart Failure: Protocol and Patient Factors in Effectiveness in the Improvement in Exercise Tolerance
Piepoli M, for the European Heart Failure Training Group (Royal Brompton Natl Heart & Lung Hosp, London)
Eur Heart J 19:466-475, 1998   5–28

Background.—Numerous studies have shown that physical training can have beneficial effects on exercise tolerance, muscle function, and limb blood flow in patients with chronic heart failure (CHF). Cardiac rehabilitation is expensive, however, and it does involve risks. Therefore, a method to determine which patients are most likely to benefit from or be harmed by a physical training program would help in allocating resources and in avoiding danger to these patients. These authors examined the characteristics of patients with CHF who were most likely to benefit from physical training and of those who were most likely not to benefit.

Methods.—The participants were 134 patients (126 men and 8 women; mean age, 60.5 years) with CHF (New York Heart Association functional class I, II, or III). Before entering the training program, all patients underwent clinical, cardiopulmonary, and autonomic nervous system measurements; training-induced changes in these parameters were also measured. The training program included exercise on a cycle ergometer for 20 minutes 4 or 5 days per week (all patients) and calisthenics with stationary running (40% of patients). Training lasted from 6 to 16 weeks, and patients trained at home (69.4%), in the hospital (19.4%), or at both locations (11.2%).

Findings.—None of the patients experienced adverse effects related to training, but 8 dropped out of the exercise program. Men and women had similar beneficial effects from physical training. New York Heart Association classification improved significantly (by 0.45) with training. Peak heart rate increased with training, and there was a significant (38.5%) increase in the chronotropic response. Peak oxygen consumption improved significantly overall (13%), and it improved by more than 10% in 68 patients (53.9%). The longer the training, the better the improvement in oxygen consumption (2.6 ± 3.0 mL/kg/minute at 16 weeks vs. 0.3 ± 3.1 mL/kg/minute at 6 weeks). Also, the combination of a cycle ergometer with calisthenics improved oxygen consumption significantly more than did using the cycle ergometer alone (2.7 ± 4.2 vs. 1.2 ± 2.0 mg/kg/minute). With exercise, resting levels of epinephrine, norepinephrine, aldosterone, atrial natriuretic peptide, plasma renin activity, and aldosterone decreased (although the decrease was significant only for norepinephrine). None of the clinical, ventilatory, hemodynamic, or autonomic factors analyzed was a significant predictor of outcome. Even patients with nonsustained ventricular tachycardia were able to benefit from training, as were those aged more than 70 years (although these benefited less than younger patients). The location of the training (home/hospital/both) had no effect on exercise outcome.

Conclusion.—Physical rehabilitation had positive effects on oxygen consumption and autonomic factors in these patients with CHF. No baseline patient characteristic was a significant predictor of outcome. A moderate, home-based exercise training program that combines the use of a cycle ergometer with calisthenics can be beneficial in many patients with CHF.

▶ This article clearly shows the beneficial effects of physical training as part of rehabilitation in patients with chronic stable heart failure. Other studies of physical exercise in patients with chronic heart failure have documented correction of endothelial dysfunction.[1] Studies from Japan[2] indicate that the exercise capacity of patients with chronic heart failure is limited by skeletal muscle metabolism.

R.C. Schlant, M.D.

References

1. Hambrecht R, Fiehn E, Weigl C, et al: Regular physical exercise corrects endothelial dysfunction and improves exercise capacity in patients with chronic heart failure. *Circulation* 98:2709-2715, 1998.
2. Okita K, Yonezawa K, Nishijima H, et al: Skeletal muscle metabolism limits exercise capacity in patients with chronic heart failure. *Circulation* 98:1886-1891, 1998.

Plasma Brain Natriuretic Peptide as a Biochemical Marker of High Left Ventricular End-Diastolic Pressure in Patients With Symptomatic Left Ventricular Dysfunction

Maeda K, Tsutamoto T, Wada A, et al (Shiga Univ, Otsu, Japan)
Am Heart J 135:825-832, 1998   5–29

Background.—Many neurohumoral factors are elevated in patients with chronic congestive heart failure (CHF). Elevated plasma levels of atrial natriuretic peptide (ANP) are an independent predictor of CHF. These authors examined ANP and other neurohumoral factors to determine if any is a significant predictor of increased left ventricular end-diastolic pressure (LVEDP) in patients with left ventricular dysfunction.

Methods.—The patients were 72 adults (53 men and 19 women; mean age, 61 years) with a left ventricular ejection fraction less than 50%. Fifteen patients (21%) had severe CHF (New York Heart Association functional classes II and IV) and 57 had mild CHF (New York Heart Association functional classes I and II). Cardiac catheterization was performed and LVEDP was measured. Blood samples were drawn from the femoral artery for measuring levels of ANP, brain natriuretic peptide (BNP), norepinephrine (NE), and endothelin-1 (ET-1). Eight patients with severe CHF repeated these tests more than 4 weeks after the initial measurements, to assess the effects of angiotensin-converting enzyme (ACE) inhibitor therapy.

Findings.—Patients with severe CHF had significantly higher plasma ANP (152.7 ± 96.9 vs. 67.1 ± 48.3 pg/mL), BNP (690.6 ± 491.1 vs. 86.8 ± 82.6 pg/mL), NE (1032 ± 1042 vs. 260 ± 218 pg/mL), and ET-1 (3.56 ± 1.67 vs. 2.21 ± 0.67 mg/mL) levels than patients with mild CHF. In multivariate analysis, both plasma ANP and BNP levels correlated significantly with ET-1 levels and with LVEDP; BNP levels also correlated with NE levels. However, stepwise multivariate analysis indicated that only plasma BNP level was a significant independent predictor of LVEDP. In all 8 patients who were retested after more than 4 weeks of ACE inhibitor therapy, LVEDP decreased. BNP levels also decreased in all 8 patients. However, ANP levels did not change in 1 patient and actually increased in 1 patient, NE levels increased in 1 patient, and ET-1 levels increased in 3 patients.

Conclusions.—The plasma BNP level was the best predictor of increased LVEDP in these patients with left ventricular dysfunction. BNP levels also paralleled the decrease in LVEDP in patients treated with ACE inhibitors, whereas in some patients ANP, NE, and ET-1 levels increased despite the decrease in LVEDP. Thus, plasma levels of BNP, which are secreted primarily by the ventricle, appear to be a useful marker of left ventricular dysfunction.

▶ Brain natriuretic peptide is an indigenous polypeptide hormone that has vasodilating and natriuretic properties. Plasma BNP levels are elevated in CHF and are also elevated in pericardial fluid.[1,2] It is possible that BNP may prove useful in treating patients with acute pulmonary edema or unresponsive chronic decompensated heart failure (see next article).

R.C. Schlant, M.D.

References

1. Nagaya N, Nishikimi T, Okano Y, et al: Plasma brain natriuretic peptide levels increase in proportion to the extent of right ventricular dysfunction in pulmonary hypertension. *J Am Coll Cardiol* 31:202-208, 1998.
2. Tanaka T, Hasegawa K, Fujita M, et al: Marked elevation of brain natriuretic peptide levels in pericardial fluid is closely associated with left ventricular dysfunction. *J Am Coll Cardiol* 31:399-403, 1998.

Systemic Hemodynamic, Neurohormonal, and Renal Effects of a Steady-State Infusion of Human Brain Natriuretic Peptide in Patients With Hemodynamically Decompensated Heart Failure

Abraham WT, Lowes BD, Ferguson DA, et al (Univ of Colorado, Denver)
J Card Fail 4:37-44, 1998   5–30

Background.—Better pharmacologic therapies are needed to treat hemodynamically decompensated chronic heart failure. Human brain natriuretic peptide (hBNP) has been shown to retain its vasodilatory and natriuretic properties in heart failure. To determine whether hBNP might be a promising treatment for this condition, these authors administered hBNP to patients with decompensated heart failure and studied its systemic hemodynamic, neurohormonal, and renal effects.

Methods.—The participants were 16 adults (15 men and 1 woman, with a mean age of 57 years) with decompensated chronic heart failure. They were randomized to receive either placebo (n = 4) or hBNP, 0.025 µg/kg/minute (n = 8) or 0.05 µg/kg/minute (n = 8). The experiment consisted of 3 4-hour periods: baseline, continuous infusion of drug, and posttreatment. Hemodynamic, neurohormonal, and renal effects were assessed during each period, and urinary losses were replaced each hour with saline (to separate the vasodilatory and natriuretic effects of hBNP).

Findings.—Two patients taking hBNP experienced adverse events (excessive pharmacologic response, a febrile event caused by staphylococcal bacteremia) and their data were excluded from analysis. Most of the hemodynamic parameters were significantly affected by hBNP. There were significant decreases in mean arterial pressure (from 88 ± 4 to 73 ± 4 mm Hg), right arterial pressure (from 13 ± 2 to 9 ± 1 mm Hg), pulmonary capillary wedge pressure (from 27 ± 3 to 16 ± 2 mm Hg), and systemic vascular resistance (from 1,722 ± 139 to 1,101 ± 83 dynes×sec/cm⁵). These unloading effects of hBNP improved cardiac performance (cardiac index increased from 1.84 ± 0.15 to 2.35 ± 0.14 L/minute/m²), yet no reflex increase in heart rate occurred. hBNP also had significant effects on neurohormonal responses, with an increase in the cyclic guanosine monophosphate level and decreases in levels of norepinephrine and aldosterone. Plasma renin activity and arginine vasopressin levels did not change during hBNP infusion. hBNP had little effect on renal parameters (renal blood flow, glomerular filtration rate).

Conclusions.—A continuous 4-hour infusion of hBNP had favorable hemodynamic effects (primarily a decrease in cardiac preload and systemic vascular resistance) and neurohormonal effects (primarily a decrease in plasma norepinephrine and aldosterone levels), and maintained renal function in these patients with hemodynamically decompensated heart failure. Furthermore, despite the hemodynamic changes, heart rate was not increased by hBNP. Thus, exogenous hBNP infusion warrants further examination as a potential therapy for patients with decompensated heart failure.

▶ Although hBNP was given for only a 4-hour steady-state infusion, it resulted in significantly improved hemodynamics in patients with decompensated heart failure. Thus, this agent may be of significant clinical value in patients with acute pulmonary edema. It is particularly noteworthy that its infusion appeared to be associated with preservation of renal function, despite decreases in systemic vascular resistance and in renal and mean arterial pressure.

R.C. Schlant, M.D.

Vitamin C Improves Endothelial Function of Conduit Arteries in Patients With Chronic Heart Failure

Hornig B, Arakawa N, Kohler C, et al (Medizinische Hochschule Hannover, Germany)
Circulation 97:363-368, 1998

5–31

Introduction.—Systemic vasoconstriction and a reduced peripheral perfusion are seen in patients with chronic heart failure. In these patients, recent studies have shown endothelial dysfunction of peripheral resistance arteries and an impaired flow-dependent, endothelium-mediated dilation of conduit arteries. In patients with chronic heart failure, the portion of flow-dependent dilation mediated by nitric oxide is reduced in comparison with normal subjects. A reduced synthesis of nitric oxide, possibly caused by a reduced nitric oxide-synthase gene expression, may be the cause of endothelial dysfunction in chronic heart failure. Radical formation may be increased in patients with chronic heart failure as the result of inactivation of nitric oxide by oxygen free radicals. The inactivation of nitric oxide–mediated vasodilation has been prevented by antioxidants such as vitamin C. The effect of vitamin C on nitric oxide–mediated flow-dependent dilation in patients with chronic heart failure was determined.

Methods.—In 15 patients with chronic heart failure and 8 healthy volunteers, high-resolution ultrasound and Doppler were used to measure radial artery diameter and blood flow. At rest and during reactive hyper-

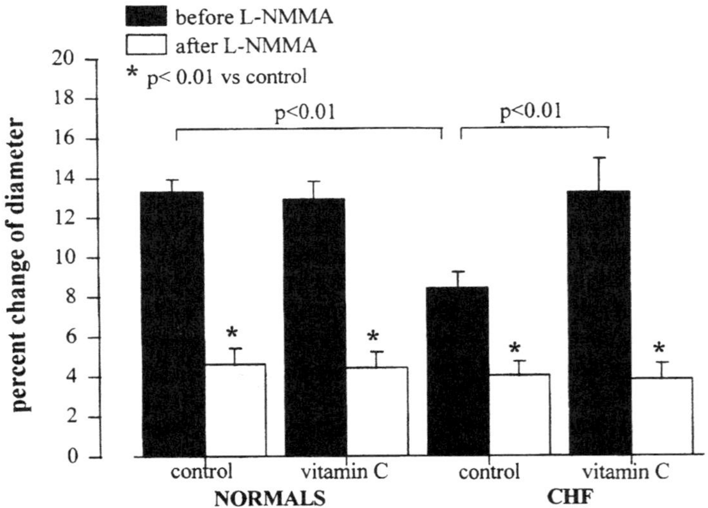

FIGURE 1.—Change in radial artery diameter (percentage) during reactive hyperemia (flow-dependent dilation) after wrist occlusion in normal individuals (N = 8) and patients with chronic heart failure (N = 10) before (*black bars*) and after (*open bars*) intra-arterial infusion of N-monomethyl-L-arginine (*L=NMMA*); effect of intra-arterial infusion of vitamin C. (Courtesy of Hornig B, Arakawa N, Kohler C, et al: Vitamin C improves endothelial function of conduit arteries in patients with chronic heart failure. *Circulation* 97:363-368. Reproduced with permission of *Circulation*. Copyright 1998, American Heart Association.)

emia (causing endothelium-mediated dilation) vascular effects of vitamin C administered at 25 mg/min intra-arterially and placebo were determined, as well as before and after intra-arterial infusion of N-mono-methyl-L-arginine to inhibit endothelial synthesis of nitric oxide.

Results.—In patients with heart failure, after acute intra-arterial administration, vitamin C restored flow-dependent dilation (13.2 ± 1.7% vs. 8.2 ± 1.0% for placebo) and after 4 weeks of oral therapy (11.9 ± 0.9% vs. 8.2 ± 1.0%). After acute as well as after chronic treatment, the portion of flow-dependent dilation mediated by nitric oxide (inhibited by intra-arterial infusion of N-monomethyl-L-arginine) was increased. The chronic heart failure baseline was 4.2 ± 0.7%; acute was 9.1 ± 1.3%, chronic was 7.3 ± 1.2%, and for normal controls it was 8.9 ± 0.8%. A significant increase in radial arterial diameter was seen after wrist occlusion, representing flow-dependent dilation, which was impaired in patients with chronic heart failure in comparison with normal individuals (Fig 1).

Conclusion.—In patients with chronic heart failure, vitamin C improves flow-dependent dilation as the result of increased availability of nitric oxide. Endothelial dysfunction in patients with chronic heart failure is, at least in part, caused by accelerated degradation of nitric oxide by radicals.

▶ This intriguing study needs confirmation in a larger number of patients. It is also of interest that vitamin C has been reported to decrease the development of nitrate tolerance in patients with congestive heart failure.[1]

R.C. Schlant, M.D.

Reference

1. Watanabe H, Kakihana M, Ohtsuka S, et al: Randomized, double-blind, placebo-controlled study of ascorbate on the preventive effect of nitrate tolerance in patients with congestive heart failure. *Circulation* 97:886-891, 1998.

Randomized, Double-blind, Placebo-controlled Study of Ascorbate on the Preventive Effect of Nitrate Tolerance in Patients With Congestive Heart Failure
Watanabe H, Kakihana M, Ohtsuka S, et al (KINU Med Assoc Hosp, Mitsu-kaido, Ibaraki, Japan; Univ of Health Science, Ami, Ibaraki, Japan; Univ of Tsukuba, Ibaraki, Japan)
Circulation 97:886-891, 1998   5–32

Objective.—Tolerance to nitrates can develop in patients taking nitrate therapy, probably as a result of an increased vascular production of superoxide anions. Whether ascorbate can prevent tolerance during the continuous administration of nitroglycerine in patients with congestive heart failure was investigated in a randomized, double-blind, placebo-controlled study.

Methods.—Nitroglycerin (0.5 γ/kg/min) and either ascorbate (55 γ/kg/min) (n = 10) or placebo (n = 10) were intravenously infused into 20 patients (5 females), with congestive heart failure. The infusion rate was doubled every 15 minutes until a pulmonary capillary wedge pressure (PCWP) had been reduced 30%. Platelet cGMP assays were performed, plasma vitamin E was measured, and heart rate and blood pressure were measured at 0, 6, 12, 18, and 24 hours after titration.

Results.—Whereas heart rate was unchanged in both groups, systolic blood pressure, pulmonary artery pressure, and PCWP decreased significantly in both groups. Pressures remained decreased for 24 hours in the ascorbate group but began to increase after 18 hours in the placebo group. Platelet cGMP levels increased significantly in both groups during titration but remained elevated in only the ascorbate group at 24 hours. Plasma vitamin E levels decreased significantly at 18 hours in the placebo group but remained unchanged throughout the study period in the ascorbate group.

Conclusion.—Combining ascorbate therapy with continuous nitrate therapy may prevent nitrate intolerance in patients with congestive heart failure.

▶ It has previously been shown by Hornig et al.[1] that vitamin C improves endothelial function in patients with chronic heart failure. This study adds additional data supporting the value of ascorbate in patients with congestive heart failure, in whom it may prevent or decrease the development of nitrate tolerance during continuous nitrate therapy. One wonders whether other antioxidants would also prevent the development of nitrate tolerance.

R.C. Schlant, M.D.

Reference

1. Hornig B, Arakawa N, Kohler C, et al: Vitamin C improves endothelial function of conduit arteries in patients with chronic heart failure. *Circulation* 97:363-368, 1998.

Current Status of Cardiac Transplantation
Hunt SA (Stanford Univ, Calif)
JAMA 280:1692-1698, 1998

5–33

Background.—The first human-to-human heart transplantation was successfully performed 30 years ago. This article summarizes the advances since then, and it projects the advances we can expect to see in the next 30 years.

Current Status of Heart Transplantation.—Approximately 2,500 heart transplantations are performed each year in the United States, and this number has been fairly constant for the past decade. The indications for heart transplantation also have remained the same: end-stage heart disease that cannot be managed by more conventional treatment and the absence of contraindications that would limit the patient's survival. However, these indications have been interpreted differently at different centers, and efforts are currently under way to devise guidelines that ensure the selection of the patient who is most likely to benefit from the procedure. As more effective methods to treat heart failure have been developed, surgeons have enjoyed more leeway in determining the timing of the transplantation.

In the 1980s, cyclosporine use became widespread and significantly improved survival rates after heart transplantation. The combination of cyclosporine, azathioprine, and corticosteroids for long-term immunosuppression remains a mainstay of treatment. Newer immunosuppressive drugs, including tacrolimus and mycophenolate mofetil, have also been introduced. However, overall 1-year survival rates are still 80%, and have not changed since the 1980s. The youngest (aged less than 1 year) and oldest (aged more than 65 years) patients have the worst probability of survival (5-year survival rates of 60% or less vs. more than 65% in the other age groups). The main limitations to heart transplantation remain infection, rejection, and coronary artery disease or malignancy in the graft.

Future Alternatives.—Numerous new immunosuppressive drugs are in clinical trials; eventually, we may be able to induce a state of tolerance that will obviate the need for long-term immunosuppression. Despite advances in immunosuppression, more and more transplant candidates will be turned away unless more donors become available. Currently, cardiac allografts are available for perhaps only 1 of 10 needy candidates. Alternative donor materials under development include nonbiologic or mechanical heart replacements and xenografts. The first clinical trial of a left ventricular assist device is currently underway. Perhaps the biggest advantage of this device is that it will not require immunosuppression. Attempts to create an optimum xenograft are progressing, but are hampered by serious ethical issues. Given the great disparity between the number of available allografts and the number of needy patients, alternatives to allografts for heart transplantation are urgently needed.

▶ This excellent article summarizes the current status of cardiac transplantation. It is noteworthy that the number of transplants in the United States has reached a plateau at an annual rate of approximately 2,500 per year. Since the donor supply will probably always be limited, we must look to the development of permanent mechanical support systems or xenotransplantation. I would think that permanent mechanical support systems will ultimately be developed, although they are likely to be initially very expensive.

R.C. Schlant, M.D.

Short-term Oral Endothelin-Receptor Antagonist Therapy in Conventionally Treated Patients With Symptomatic Severe Chronic Heart Failure

Sütsch G, Kiowski W, Yan X-W, et al (Univ Hosp Zürich, Switzerland; Triemli Hosp Zürich, Switzerland; Univ Hosp Basel, Switzerland)
Circulation 98:2262-2268, 1998

5–34

Purpose.—Endothelin-1 is believed to play an important role in regulating vascular tone in patients with chronic heart failure. Treatment with an endothelin-receptor antagonist might improve hemodynamic status and reduce symptoms in these patients. However, the effects of endothelin-receptor blockade in addition to conventional triple therapy have not been studied. The hemodynamic and clinical effects of oral bosentan in symptomatic patients with severe chronic heart failure were investigated.

Methods.—The analysis included 36 men (mean age, 55 years) who had clinically stable but symptomatic congestive heart failure. All patients were in New York Heart Association functional class III; the mean left ventricular ejection fraction was 22%. The patients remained symptomatic despite conventional therapy with diuretics, digoxin, and angiotensin-converting enzyme inhibitors. While continuing treatment, they were randomized to receive 2 weeks of therapy with oral bosentan, 1 g twice a day, or placebo. Before and at the start and end of bosentan therapy, 24-hour hemodynamic and hormonal measurements were taken.

Results.—After the first day of bosentan treatment, mean arterial pressure was reduced by 14%, pulmonary artery mean pressure by 13%, pulmonary artery capillary wedge pressure by 14.5%, and right atrial pressure by 20%. Bosentan was associated with a 15% increase in cardiac output, but no change in heart rate. The bosentan group had a 24% reduction in systemic vascular resistance and a 20% reduction in pulmonary vascular resistance. By the end of the second week of bosentan treatment, cardiac output had increased by an additional 15%, whereas systemic vascular resistance had decreased by 9% and pulmonary vascular resistance had decreased by 10%. There was still no change in heart rate. The only hormonal change with bosentan was an increase in plasma endothelin-1; norepinephrine, renin activity, and angiotensin II were unchanged.

Conclusions.—In patients with symptomatic congestive heart failure, adding the oral endothelin receptor antagonist bosentan to conventional therapy can improve systemic and pulmonary hemodynamics, at least in the short term. These improvements are achieved without neurohormonal activation or volume retention. Further studies are needed to assess the safety and efficacy of endothelin-receptor antagonist therapy, including its effects on symptom status, morbidity, and mortality.

▶ These 36 men with symptomatic heart failure who were in New York Heart Association class III despite therapy with diuretics, digoxin, and angiotensin-coverting enzyme inhibitors, appeared to tolerate the addition of the endothelin-receptor antagonist (oral bosentan) well and to improve in hemodynamics. Although bosentan was given for only 2 weeks, it holds promise as an effective addition to the long-term therapy of patients with heart failure. We await further investigations with great eagerness.

R.C. Schlant, M.D.

Combined Oral Positive Inotropic and Beta-Blocker Therapy for Treatment of Refractory Class IV Heart Failure
Shakar SF, Abraham WT, Gilbert EM, et al (Univ of Colorado, Denver; Univ of Utah, Salt Lake City)
J Am Coll Cardiol 31:1336-1340, 1998   5–35

Objective.—For patients with class IV heart failure, mortality is high despite standard treatments, and β-blocker therapy is not well tolerated. Long-term therapy with phosphodiesterase inhibitors and other positive inotropes carries high mortality in these patients. This problem might be overcome by the addition of a β-blocker, or long-term oral inotropic therapy might serve as a bridge to β-blocker treatment. Combination therapy with the β-blocker metoprolol and the phosphodiesterase inhibitor enoximone was evaluated in patients with severe, refractory heart failure.

Methods.—The study included 30 patients at 2 centers who had functional class IV heart failure caused by left ventricular systolic dysfunction. The patients had a mean left ventricular ejection fraction of 17.2%, with a cardiac index of 1.6 L/minute/m^2. The patients were first stabilized with enoximone, at a dose of 1 mg/kg or less 3 times daily. After optimization of outpatient heart failure therapy, metoprolol was added, starting at 6.25 mg twice daily and gradually increasing to a target dosage of 100 to 200 mg/day. If the patient remained stable on combination therapy for 2 to 4 months, withdrawal of enoximone was attempted. Depending on their response, patients remained on metoprolol alone or with enoximone. Mean follow-up was 21 months.

Results.—Long-term oral enoximone therapy was tolerated by 96% of patients, and the combination of enoximone and metoprolol by 80%. Twenty-three of 30 patients received combination therapy, which continued for a mean of 9 months. Mean enoximone dosage was 189 mg/day, and mean metoprolol dosage was 113 mg/day. Forty-eight percent of patients receiving combination therapy were eventually weaned off enoximone. Mean left ventricular ejection fraction increased from 17.7% to 27.6%. Twenty-five patients improved to at least New York Heart Association functional class III, and 9 improved to class II or I. Treatment reduced the number of hospitalizations. Estimated survival was 96% at 6 months, 81% at 1 year, and 69% at 2 years, and was significantly better for patients treated with enalapril (Fig 2). Nine patients underwent successful heart transplantation.

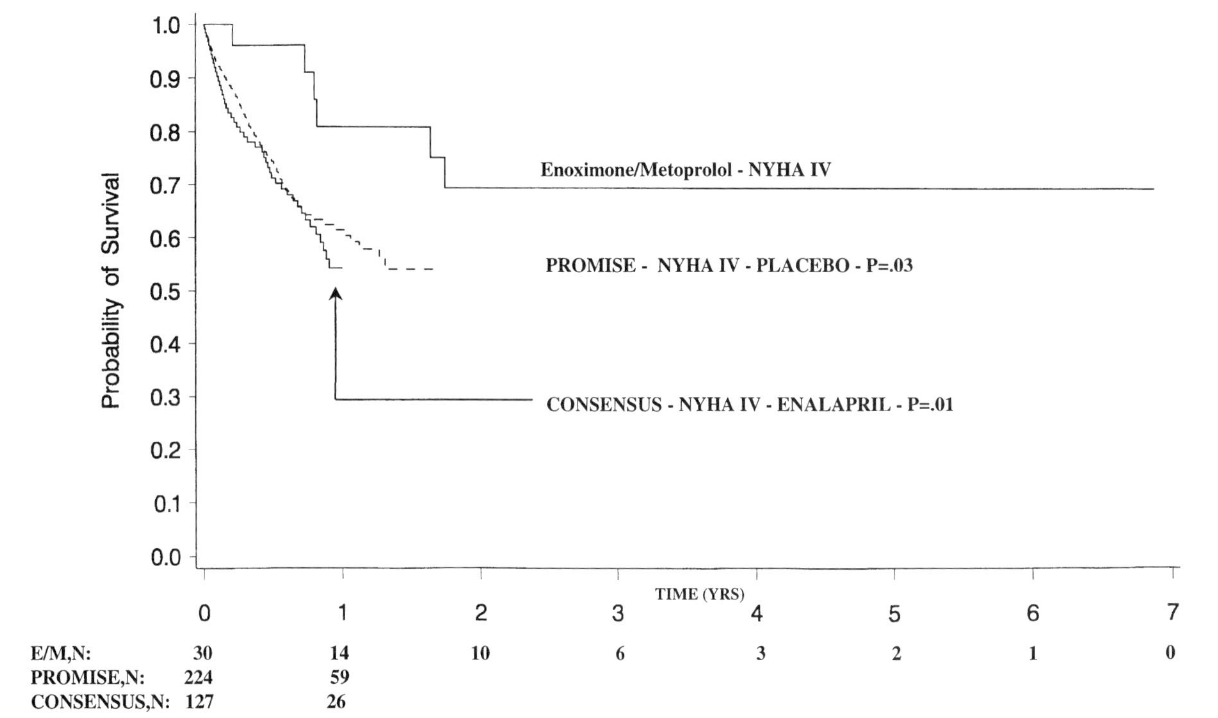

FIGURE 2.—Comparison of the survival probability curves of our patients treated with enoximone (E) and metoprolol (M) with curves of placebo-treated patients in New York Heart Assocation functional class IV in the PROMISE trial and enalapril-treated patients in the CONSENSUS trial. (Courtesy of Shakar SF, Abraham WT, Gilbert EM, et al: Combined oral positive inotropic and beta-blocker therapy for treatment of refractory class IV heart failure. *J Am Coll Cardiol* 31:1336-1340, 1998. Reprinted with permission from the American College of Cardiology.)

Conclusions.—For patients with class IV heart failure, the combination of a positive inotrope and a β-blocker appears to be a useful and well-tolerated therapy. Combination therapy may provide a valuable bridge to heart transplantation, or an option for palliative therapy if transplantation is not an option. If validated by future studies, this approach would provide a cost-effective means of reducing or delaying the need for heart transplantation.

▶ This is one of the few studies of therapy in patients with advanced, refractory class IV heart failure. In 30 such patients, the very cautious combination of an oral inotropic agent (enoximone) was used together with oral metroprolol. It is noteworthy that the metoprolol was initiated at 6.25 mg twice a day and very slowly titrate to a target dose of 100 to 200 mg/day. Of the 23 patients who received the combination therapy, 48% were weaned off enoximone over the long-term. There was a tendency for the number of hospital admissions to decrease and for the survival to be somewhat higher than expected. This promising combined therapy for this advanced stage of heart failure appears to be useful both as a bridge to heart transplantation and when heart transplantation is not an option.

R.C. Schlant, M.D.

Structural Alterations in the Latissimus Dorsi Muscles in Three Patients More Than 2 Years After a Cardiomyoplasty Procedure
Davidse JHL, van der Veen FH, Lucas CMHB, et al (Univ Hosp Maastricht, The Netherlands)
Eur Heart J 19:310-318, 1998

5–36

Objective.—Whether the skeletal muscle adaptation of the latissimus dorsi muscle after cardiomyoplasty occurs in humans the way it occurs in experimental animals is not known. The muscle structure's appearance was examined in 3 male patients (New York Heart Association functional class IV at surgery) more than 2 years after cardiomyoplasty.

Methods.—According to protocol, 2 weeks after cardiomyoplasty, the left latissimus dorsi muscle was stimulated with 30-Hz bursts in a 2:1 ratio with an upper stimulation rate of 50 pulses per minute. Density of arteries and arterial wall integrity were evaluated from biopsy specimens.

Results.—The 3 patients, aged 57, 57, and 66 at surgery, died 2 years, 5 years, and 2 years, respectively, after cardiomyoplasty. Preoperatively, the left latissimus dorsi muscle was composed mainly of type II fibers (70% to 83%) with a small amount of fatty tissue (3% to 9%) and 17% to 30% of type I fibers. After more than 2 years of electrical stimulation, muscle structure was lost and a large random amount of fatty tissue (10% to 50%) had built up. Contribution of type I fibers made up 68%, 76%, and 80% in the 3 patients and decreased gradually from the proximal to the distal region (Fig 3). The number of arteries was almost 4 times higher in stimulated than in unstimulated muscles.

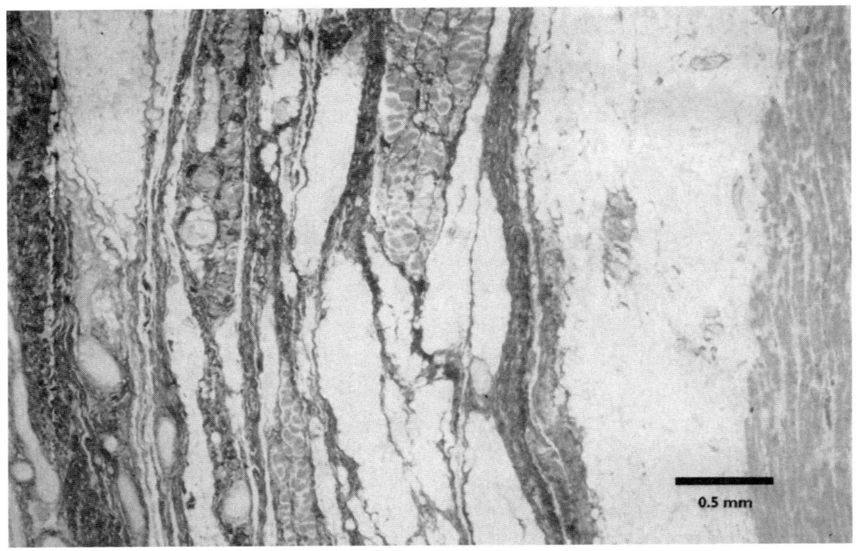

FIGURE 3.—Postmortem specimen from the distal part of the left latissimus dorsi muscle and part of the subepicardium of patient C. Sirius red staining. (Bar 0.5 mm.) (Courtesy of Davidse JHL, van der Veen FH, Lucas CMHB, et al: Structural alterations in the latissimus dorsi muscles in three patients more than 2 years after a cardiomyoplasty procedure. *Eur Heart J* 19:310-318, 1998. Reprinted by permission of the publisher, WB Saunders Company Ltd, London.)

Conclusion.—Skeletal muscle adaptation appears to be less complete in humans than in animals. Type I fibers decreased significantly, and muscle structure was lost and randomly replaced with fatty tissue in 3 patients more than 2 years after cardiomyoplasty.

▶ It will be important to determine how frequently the transformations reported in this article occur in patients treated with dynamic cardiomyoplasty. It is hoped that, with adjustment of the conditioning protocol, the development of fatty changes in the muscle can be reduced. If these structural alterations cannot be reduced, such changes could mean the death knoll for this procedure.

R.C. Schlant, M.D.

Warfarin Anticoagulation and Survival: A Cohort Analysis From the Studies of Left Ventricular Dysfunction

Al-Khadra AS, Salem DN, Rand WM, et al (Tufts Univ, Boston)
J Am Coll Cardiol 31:749-753, 1998

5–37

Objective.—The use of anticoagulants in patients with heart failure (HF) is controversial. Because warfarin is known to reduce the likelihood of nonfatal myocardial infarction (MI) in patients with coronary artery disease and to reduce the risk of thromboembolic strokes in patients

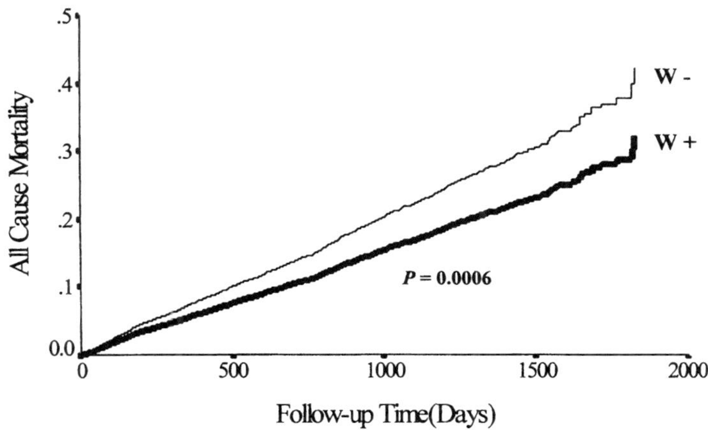

FIGURE 1.—Adjusted all-cause mortality in warfarin users (W+) and nonusers (W−) in the combined SOLVD trial. (Reprinted by permission of the American College of Cardiology from Al-Khadra AS, Salem DN, Rand WM, et al: Warfarin anticoagulation and survival: A cohort analysis from the studies of left ventricular dysfunction. *J Am Coll Cardiol* 31:749-753, 1998.)

recovering from MI, the relation between warfarin use and survival and cardiovascular morbidity in patients with left ventricular systolic dysfunction was evaluated in the multicenter, randomized, double-blind, placebo-controlled Studies of Left Ventricular Dysfunction (SOLVD) trial.

Methods.—All-cause mortality, death from or hospital admission for HF, death due to HF, fatal MI, and noncardiac vascular causes of death were assessed and related to use of warfarin in 6,797 patients enrolled in the SOLVD study.

Results.—There were 210 deaths among the 2,569 warfarin users and 1,334 deaths among the 4,228 placebo users, with 177 and 1,181 deaths, respectively, resulting from cardiovascular disease. Warfarin use was a significant predictor (hazard ratio [HR] 0.76 for all-cause mortality) of favorable outcome and significantly reduced mortality from cardiovascular disease (HR 0.72) (Fig 1). There were 306 deaths or hospital admissions attributed to HF in the warfarin group and 1,910 deaths in the placebo group. Warfarin use significantly reduced deaths and hospital admissions (HR 0.82) and significantly reduced hospital admissions for nonfatal MI by 44%. Results were the same, whether the study was analyzed as a whole or both trials were analyzed separately.

Conclusion.—Warfarin use in patients with HF decreases morbidity and mortality. Atrial fibrillation, age, ejection fraction, sex, New York Heart Association functional class, and etiology did not alter the results.

▶ In an excellent review of anticoagulation and dilated cardiomyopathy immediately preceding this article in the *Journal of the American College of Cardiology*, Koniaris and Goldhaber[1] conclude that the only clearcut indications for anticoagulations in most patients with dilated cardiomyopathy are atrial fibrillation, a previous thromboembolic event or left ventricular thrombus. They also note that low-dose aspirin may be quite useful in preventing thromboembolism in such patients. Al-Khadra and co-workers have also recently documented the value of antiplatelet agents and survival in patients with heart failure.[2]

R.C. Schlant, M.D.

References

1. Koniaris L, Goldhaber S: Anticoagulation in dilated cardiomyopathy. *J Am Coll Cardiol* 31:745-748, 1998.
2. Al-Khadra A, Salen D, Rand W, et al: Antiplatelet agents and survival: A cohort analysis from the studies of left ventricular dysfunction. *J Am Coll Cardiol* 31:419-425, 1998.

A Clinical Trial of Vena Caval Filters in the Prevention of Pulmonary Embolism in Patients With Proximal Deep-Vein Thrombosis
Decousus H, for the Prévention Du Risque D'Embolie Pulmonaire Par Interruption Cave Study Group (Bellevue Hosp, Saint-Etienne, France; Cardiological Hosp, Lyons, France; Antoine Béclère Hosp, Clamart, France; et al)
N Engl J Med 338:409-415, 1998   5–38

Background.—The safety and efficacy of vena caval filters in preventing pulmonary embolism in patients with proximal deep-vein thrombosis have not been definitively established. These issues were further investigated.

Methods.—In a 2-by-2 factorial design, 400 patients with proximal deep-vein thrombosis at risk for pulmonary embolism were randomly assigned to receive a vena caval filter or no filter and to receive low–molecular weight heparin or unfractionated heparin. On day 12 and at 2 years, the rates of recurrent venous thromboembolism, death, and major bleeding were determined.

Findings.—By day 12, symptomatic or asymptomatic pulmonary embolism had occurred in 1.1% of the patients with filters and in 4.8% of those with no filters. By 2 years, 20.8% and 11.6%, respectively, had had recurrent deep-vein thrombosis. Mortality and other outcomes did not differ significantly between groups. By day 12, 1.6% of the patients receiving low–molecular weight heparin and 4.2% given unfractionated heparin had had symptomatic or asymptomatic pulmonary embolism.

Conclusions.—The initial benefits of vena caval filter use for preventing pulmonary embolism in high-risk patients with proximal deep-vein thrombosis is counterbalanced by an excess of recurrent deep-vein thrombosis, with no difference in mortality. Low–molecular weight heparin is as safe and effective as unfractionated heparin for preventing pulmonary embolism.

▶ This important study documents that vena caval filters are effective for the prevention of pulmonary embolism but that they are associated with an increase in recurrent deep-vein thrombosis. Because significant collaterals can develop around the filter, a good percentage of which thrombose, it is probably wise to cont nue most patients with vena caval filters on chronic warfarin anticoagulant therapy indefinitely. Once again, there is a need for appropriately designed large clinical trials to better define the clinical usefulness of vena caval filters.

R.C. Schlant, M.D.

Reduction in Pulmonary Vascular Resistance With Long-term Epoprostenol (Prostacyclin) Therapy in Primary Pulmonary Hypertension

McLaughlin VV, Gerthner DE, Panella MM, et al (Rush-Presbyterian-St Luke's Med Ctr, Chicago)
N Engl J Med 338:273-277, 1998   5–39

Introduction.—As a treatment for advanced primary pulmonary hypertension, IV epoprostenol, also known as prostacyclin, was recently introduced. Epoprostenol has antithrombotic properties related to its effects on platelets and is a potent vasodilator of systemic and pulmonary arteries. Because epoprostenol has been shown to produce vasodilation more consistently than calcium-channel blockers in the short-term, it has become the preferred long-term treatment for patients with primary pulmonary hypertension who continue to have symptoms in spite of conventional therapy. In patients with primary pulmonary hypertension, the effectiveness and potential mechanisms of action of epoprostenol given according to an aggressive dosing strategy for longer than 1 year were evaluated.

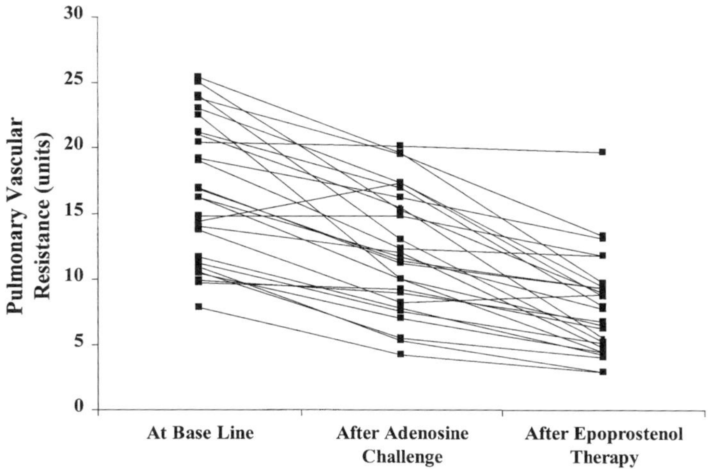

FIGURE 1.—Pulmonary vascular resistance at base line, after administration of IV adenosine to test pulmonary vasoreactivity, and after long-term epoprostenol therapy. In all but 1 patient, the long-term effects of epoprostenol in lowering pulmonary vascular resistance exceeded the short-term pulmonary vasodilator response to adenosine. (Reprinted by permission of *The New England Journal of Medicine* courtesy of McLaughlin VV, Genthner DE, Panella MM, et al: Reduction in pulmonary vascular resistance with long-term epoprostenol (prostacyclin) therapy in primary pulmonary hypertension. *N Engl J Med* 338: 273-277, copyright 1998, Massachusetts Medical Society.)

Methods.—An assessment of pulmonary vascular dilation in response to IV adenosine was the base-line evaluation. There was a monthly increase of the epoprostenol dose to the maximum tolerated. Measurements of improvement in symptoms, exercise capacity, and hemodynamic variables were used to evaluate long-term therapy. Over a mean of 16.7 ± 5.2 months, 27 patients with primary pulmonary hypertension were evaluated.

Results.—There was a mean reduction of 27% in pulmonary vascular resistance with IV adenosine. The rate of infusion of epoprostenol therapy was increased by an average of 2.4 ng/kilogram of body weight/minute each month. Improvement in symptoms and hemodynamic measurements were seen in 26 of 27 patients. There was a 53% decline in pulmonary vascular resistance to 7.9 ± 3.8 resistance units at the time of restudy. In all but 1 patient, the long-term effects of epoprostenol exceeded the short-term pulmonary vasodilator response to adenosine (Fig 1). There was still a significant reduction in pulmonary vascular resistance after treatment with epoprostenol in 6 of the 8 patients who had minimal pulmonary vasodilation in response to adenosine (mean reduction in resistance units, less than 20%).

Conclusion.—Long-term therapy with epoprostenol lowers pulmonary vascular resistance beyond the level achieved in the short term with IV adenosine in primary pulmonary hypertension. In this disorder, epoprostenol appears to have sustained efficacy.

▶ Epoprostenol is a potent systemic and pulmonary vascular vasodilator. In addition, it has platelet effects that are generally antithrombotic. Because of these effects, it has evolved as a useful means of producing vasodilatation in patients with primary pulmonary hypertension.

It should be noted that the continuous IV infusion used in this study requires the insertion of a Hickman catheter into a subclavian vein and a portable infusion pump. All 27 patients appeared to have had an improvement in their symptoms. It is noteworthy that the major problems encountered with this therapy were the serious infections related to the delivery system. This might limit its applicability for many patients. At present, the technique is perhaps primarily useful as a bridge for patients waiting for lung transplants. It may be particularly useful for those patients who do not respond to a calcium-channel blocker. Although tolerance to epoprostenol develops with long-term treatment, it is unclear whether the infusion rate should be increased, even if the patient improves clinically, or whether one should wait for a return of symptoms before increasing the infusion rate.

R.C. Schlant, M.D.

Long Term Intravenous Prostaglandin (Epoprostenol or Iloprost) for Treatment of Severe Pulmonary Hypertension
Higenbottam T, Butt AY, McMahon A, et al (Univ of Sheffield, England; Papworth Hosp, Cambridge, England; Inst of Public Health, Cambridge, England)
Heart 80:151-155, 1998

5–40

Introduction.—Many patients with primary pulmonary hypertension do not receive treatment. Selection criteria for patients who may benefit from therapy with intravenous prostaglandin are difficult to discern. The relationship between severity of pulmonary hypertension and outcome of medical treatment was examined retrospectively in a series of 98 patients with pulmonary hypertension.

Methods.—Of 146 patients evaluated between 1982 and 1995, 9 (6%) had systemic disease and pulmonary hypertension and 39 (27%) had thromboembolic pulmonary hypertension. These patients received long-term intravenous prostaglandin treatment: 61 received epoprostenol, 13 received iloprost, and the remaining patients received conventional treatment with oral anticoagulants (with or without calcium channel blockers). Event-free survival was monitored until death, transplant surgery, or pulmonary thromboendarterectomy.

Results.—At final follow-up, 20 patients (14%) had undergone heart-lung transplantation, 2 (1%) underwent a pulmonary thromboendarterectomy, and 72 (49%) had died. Median survival was 695 days (range, 426 to 964 days) for 22 patients who underwent surgery and it was 345 days (240 to 456 days) in the 72 patients who died. Prognosis was influenced by New York Heart Association grade, mixed venous oxygen saturation, cardiac index, mean right atrial pressure, and pulmonary vascular resistance. Median event-free survival in patients with Svo_2 below 60% was 239 days (range, 0 to 502 days) for 22 patients who received conventional treatment and 585 days (range, 300 to 870 days) for 42 patients on prostaglandin treatment. For patients with Svo_2 60% or above, there were no significant between-group differences in survival (mean, 1,275 days for conventional treatment and 986 days for prostaglandin treatment).

Conclusion.—In patients with right heart failure, continuous intravenous treatment with prostaglandins was more effective than anticoagulants, with or without calcium channel blockers, in prolonging survival. A capacity to vasodilate was not predictive of treatment outcome in either group.

▶ This article about 98 patients with primary pulmonary hypertension, studied in the United Kingdom between 1982 and 1995, clearly shows that intravenous prostaglandins were more effective than anticoagulants, with or without calcium channel blockers, in prolonging survival in patients with right heart failure. Intravenous prostaglandins have now become the treatment of choice in patients with severe primary pulmonary hypertension. The progress made in diagnosis and treatment of primary pulmonary hypertension over the past 20 years has recently been reviewed.[1]

R.C. Schlant, M.D.

Reference

1. Gaine SP, Rubin LJ: Primary pulmonary hypertension. *Lancet* 352:719-725, 1998.

Effects of the Intracoronary Infusion of Cocaine on Left Ventricular Systolic and Diastolic Function in Humans

Pitts WR, Vongpatanasin W, Cigarroa JE, et al (Univ of Texas, Dallas; Parkland Mem Hosp, Dallas)
Circulation 97:1270-1273, 1998
5–41

Objective.—In dogs, a large amount of cocaine results in a worsening of left ventricular function. But studies have shown that intracoronary infusion in humans is safe. The effects of a direct intracoronary infusion of cocaine on left ventricular (LV) systolic and diastolic performance in human beings was investigated using a high intracoronary cocaine concentration.

Methods.—Either a 15-minute intracoronary infusion of saline (n = 10) or cocaine hydrochloride (10% solution at 1 mg/min) (n = 10) was administered to 20 patients (6 women), aged 39 to 72, who were undergoing cardiac catheterization for the evaluation of chest pain. Heart rate, systemic arterial pressure, LV pressure, the first derivative of LV pressure,

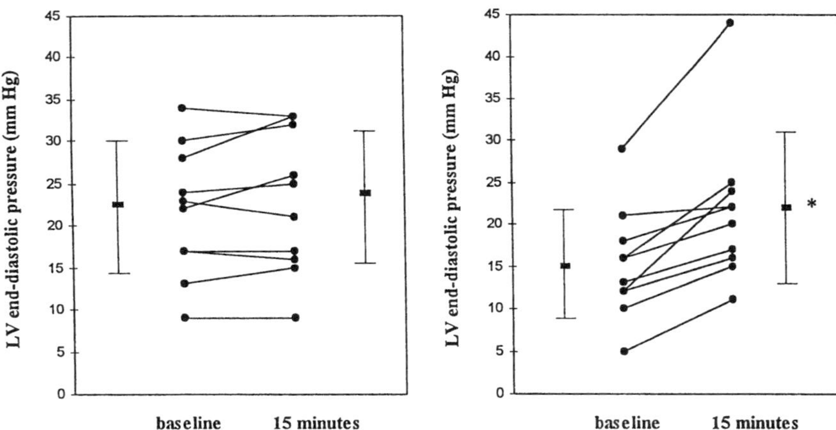

FIGURE 1.—Left ventricular (*LV*) end-diastolic pressure before and after an intracoronary saline (**left**) or cocaine (**right**) infusion. Each *line* represents the data from 1 patient, and mean±1 standard deviation values are shown on either side of each set of lines. LV end-diastolic pressure increased with intracoronary cocaine (*P=.001 compared with baseline). (Courtesy of Pitts WR, Vongpatanasin W, Cigarroa JE, et al: Effects of the intracoronary infusion of cocaine on left ventricular systolic and diastolic function in humans. *Circulation* 97:1270-1273, 1998.)

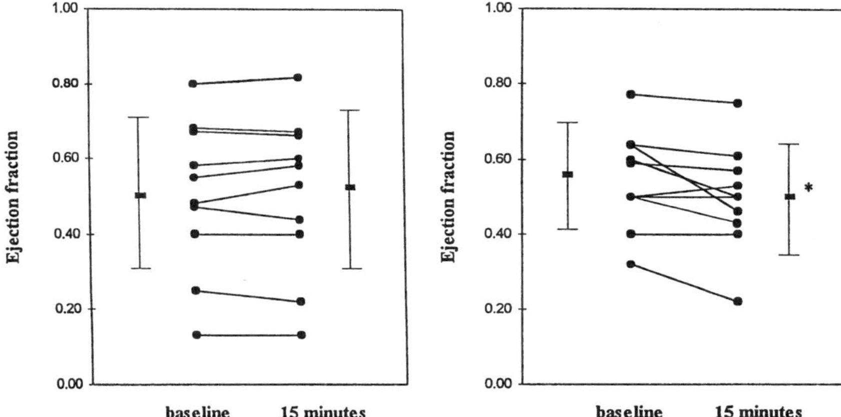

FIGURE 2.—Left ventricular (*LV*) end-diastolic pressure before and after an intracoronary saline (**left**) or cocaine (**right**) infusion. Each *line* represents the data from 1 patient, and mean±1 standard deviation values are shown on either side of each set of lines. Left ventricular ejection fraction decreased with intracoronary cocaine (*P=.03 compared with baseline). (Courtesy of Pitts WR, Vongpatanasin W, Cigarroa JE, et al: Effects of the intracoronary infusion of cocaine on left ventricular systolic and diastolic function in humans. *Circulation* 97:1270-1273, 1998.)

and ejection fraction were measured at baseline and during the final 2 to 3 minutes of the infusion. Results were compared statistically.

Results.—The average cocaine concentration in coronary sinus blood was 3.0 mg/L and in systemic blood was 0.17 mg/L. Although intracoronary cocaine exerted a deleterious effect on LV systolic and diastolic blood pressure and LV end-systolic volume, it did not change heart rate, the first derivative of LV pressure, or LV end-diastolic volume (Fig 1 and Fig 2).

Conclusion.—Intracoronary infusion of cocaine resulted in a deterioration of LV systolic and diastolic function.

▶ This elegant article from Dallas demonstrates that intracoronary cocaine (1mg/min for 15 minutes) causes an increase in systolic and mean arterial pressure together with a direct, deleterious decrease in LV systolic and diastolic function, an increase in LV end-diastolic pressure and LV end-systolic volume, and a decrease in LV ejection fraction. When the cocaine is administered intranasally, it has been noted to increase LV performance.[1]

R.C. Schlant, M.D.

Reference

1. Boehrer JD, Moliterno DJ, Willard JE, et al: Hemodynamic effects of intranasal cocaine in humans. *J Am Coll Cardiol* 20:90-93, 1992.

6   Cardiac Arrhythmias, Conduction Disturbances, and Electrophysiology

Introduction

A few areas really stand out this year. One, at least for me, is the difficulty achieving warfarin therapy for patients with atrial fibrillation. The message seems to be getting out, but there appears to be a reluctance on the part of physicians to use warfarin in some patient groups, particularly the elderly. The selected articles abstracted this year again overwhelmingly emphasize the need for such therapy and the fact that aspirin really provides little, if any, benefit. We have also acquired more useful data on the epidemiology of atrial fibrillation.

The biggest advance in catheter ablation therapy of cardiac arrhythmias is the identification of patients (a subset as yet incompletely characterized) who have a single focus firing rapidly, principally in one of the pulmonary veins, that is responsible for generating atrial fibrillation. Identifying such patients and the focus permits cure by ablation of the focus. This exciting area will undoubtedly continue to be a focus (no pun intended) of our interest in the coming year. We also have continued to learn more of help from ablative therapy for this and other arrhythmias.

There is not too much new in drug therapy, although there are useful articles dealing with drug therapy (flecainide and propafenone) for cardioversion. Other selections help give us a better understanding of the use of such drugs as sotalol and amiodarone in patients with atrial fibrillation.

Device therapy continues to be important for both bradyarrhythmia and tachyarrhythmia. We continue to learn more about the implantable cardioverter defibrillator and its increasing role in primary and secondary prevention of sudden cardiac death. The implantable atrial defibrillator is here, and the initial reports about it are encouraging. There is also a new and exciting area in the use of pacing techniques to treat heart failure. Initial reports are favorable, and we look forward to further systematic studies.

Basic science continues to make strides, and in some areas the gap between the transfer of data from basic science to the clinic has been considerably narrowed, especially with new insights into mechanism. This includes our finally understanding the U wave, the importance of the midventricular myocardium in repolarization abnormalities—including the long QT syndrome—and T-wave alternans as a clinical tool.

However, the big player this year is still atrial fibrillation.

Albert L. Waldo, M.D.

Anticoagulation: Atrial Fibrillation and Atrial Flutter

Underutilization of Warfarin in Older Persons With Chronic Nonvalvular Atrial Fibrillation at High Risk for Developing Stroke
Mendelson G, Aronow WS (Mount Sinai School of Medicine, New York)
J Am Geriatr Soc 46:1423-1424, 1998   6–1

Introduction.—Increased age is accompanied by a rise in the incidence of chronic atrial fibrillation (AF). Treatment with warfarin varies in this patient cohort. The prevalence of use of warfarin to maintain an international normalized ratio (INR) between 2.0 and 3.0 was assessed in older patients with chronic nonvalvular AF at high risk for having new thromboembolic (TE) stroke develop.

Methods.—Medical charts of all older patients seen in 1997 at an academic hospital-based geriatrics practice were reviewed for chronic nonvalvular AF documented by ECG. Patients were considered at high risk for TE stroke if they had a previous thromboembolism, congestive heart failure, or echocardiographic evidence of abnormal left ventricular systolic function, systolic blood pressure of greater that 160 mm Hg, or were women older than 75 years.

Results.—Of 1,563 charts of older persons reviewed, 1,183 were female and 280 were male with a mean age of 80 years (range, 59-103 years). Nine percent (141 patients) had chronic nonvalvular AF. Of these, 127 (90%) were at high risk for TE stroke. Only 3 (2%) had contraindications to warfarin therapy. Of the 124 patients with AF at high risk for TE stroke, only 61 (49%) were receiving warfarin in a dose to maintain an INR between 2.0 and 3.0. Forty-five patients (36%) received aspirin (325 mg daily) and 18 (15%) received neither. In 14 persons with AF at low risk of TE stroke, only 1 (7%) was treated with warfarin to maintain an INR between 2.0 and 3.0; 6 (43%) were treated with 325 mg of aspirin daily and 7 (50%) received neither.

Conclusion.—Warfarin is underused as a treatment to maintain an INR between 2.0 and 3.0 in older patients (with no contraindications to warfarin) with chronic nonvalvular AF at high risk for TE stroke.

▶ This important, simple retrospective review of patients with AF at high risk for TE stroke per the Stroke Prevention in Atrial Fibrillation (SPAF III) criteria shows that physicians are still not using warfarin anticoagulation properly. It is a double whammy because warfarin is not being used when it should be used; and aspirin, which doesn't have any efficacy in patients older than 75 years (per SPAF I), and whose inefficacy was confirmed by SPAF III, is still being used. Only 3 patients in this study had contraindications to Coumadin (2%). And increased age is an increased risk for stroke. So the message is that warfarin should be used whenever possible when indicated in patients, regardless of age.

A.L. Waldo, M.D.

Prevalence of Atrial Fibrillation and Eligibility for Anticoagulants in the Community
Sudlow M, Thomson R, Thwaites B, et al (Univ of Newcastle upon Tyne, England; Wansbeck Gen Hosp, Ashington, England)
Lancet 352:1167-1171, 1998   6–2

Background.—The risk of stroke in patients with atrial fibrillation or flutter (AF) can be reduced by anticoagulation. But how many people in the community have AF? And how many of these people could benefit from anticoagulants? A large group of community-living elderly people were screened for the prevalence of AF and the use of anticoagulants was evaluated in this group.

Methods.—Electrocardiography was used to screen a random sample of 3,678 people 65 years and older living in the community. Subjects with AF were evaluated further with interviews, echocardiography, and laboratory tests (including coagulation screening) to determine their risk for stroke. Three different sets of criteria were used to determine stroke risk and contraindications to anticoagulation: a pooled analysis of 5 clinical trials of anticoagulants in AF, an analysis of stroke risk in patients receiving placebo in the Stroke Prevention in Atrial Fibrillation (SPAF) trial, and the inclusion criteria in SPAF III (which selects for high-risk patients). Additionally, medical records of 1,795 patients in 10 practices were reviewed to determine how many records noted AF.

Findings.—ECGs revealed AF in 207 of the 3,678 subjects (5.6%). Record review indicated that the prevalence of AF in elderly people was 4.7%; for subjects 75 years and older, the prevalence increased (10.0% for men and 5.6% for women). Based on the different inclusion criteria, from 41% to 61% of these people would have benefited from anticoagulation. However, only 23% of the subjects were receiving warfarin. And many patients with no irreversible contraindications and no clinical risk factors had echocardiographic risk factors, which suggested anticoagulation would be beneficial. Warfarin use was greatest in men 65 to 74 years old (41%) and least in women 75 years and older (12%). Virtually all subjects with AF who were 75 years and older had at least 1 risk factor for stroke.

Conclusions.—According to the selection criteria applied, anticoagulation in elderly patients with AF seems to be dramatically underused. A greater use of anticoagulants among these patients would be expected to decrease the incidence of stroke in this age group. Also, because virtually all the oldest subjects had at least 1 risk factor for stroke, echocardiographic results would add little to the clinical picture. Thus, echocardiography can be best used to assess patients 75 years old and younger who have no clinical risk factors for stroke and no contraindications to anticoagulation.

▶ This community-based analysis emphasizes that most patients with AF and identifiable risks for stroke infrequently have an irreversible indication for warfarin therapy, yet are clearly undertreated with warfarin despite the indication. The contraindication criteria used were those of the SPAF trial: gastrointestinal or genitourinary bleeding in the past 6 months; history of more than 3 falls in the past year or recurrent or injurious falls; inability to comply with anticoagulants; excessive use of alcohol; uncontrolled hypertension; and daily use of nonsteroidal anti-inflammatory agents. Those criteria remain useful as a relative contraindication to warfarin therapy. Yet, by those indications, very few patients are ineligible for warfarin therapy despite older age.

A.L. Waldo, M.D.

The Effect of Age and Quality of Life on Doctors' Decisions to Anticoagulate Patients With Atrial Fibrillation

Sudlow M, Thomson R, Rodgers H, et al (Univ of Newcastle upon Tyne, England)
Age Ageing 27:285-289, 1998

6–3

Introduction.—As is widely recognized, several trials have shown that treating appropriately selected patients who have nonvalvular atrial fibrillation (NVAF) with anticoagulants decreases their risk of stroke. Despite this, large numbers of patients who meet medical criteria and may be appropriate for treatment are not receiving anticoagulation therapy. A physician questionnaire was used to determine whether age or medicosocial factors influence the clinical decisions of general practitioners or consultants with regard to anticoagulation of patients with NVAF, and whether these factors influence general practitioners and consultants to differing extents.

Methods.—A 50% random sample of 824 general practitioners and all 207 hospital consultants with a commitment to general practice in the former Northern Region in the United Kingdom were mailed a questionnaire asking about their views on the use of anticoagulants in patients with atrial fibrillation.

Results.—Overall response rates for general practitioners and consultants were 56% and 79%, respectively. A large proportion of clinicians in both groups reported that they felt it was inappropriate to treat patients above a certain age: 43% and 46% of general practitioners and consultants, respectively, reported that they felt no patient above the age of 84 years should be treated. Also, a small minority felt it inappropriate to treat those between 65 and 74 years (7.9% and 2%, respectively) and between 75 and 84 years (19.4% and 9.17%). Physicians in both groups felt that a patient's quality of life was an important medico-social factor affecting treatment decisions: 38.4% of general practitioners and 45.8% of consultants believed it would be inappropriate to treat patients with severely impaired quality of life. Very few physicians in either group (6.1% of general practitioners and 5.2% of consultants) felt that a mild impairment should prevent patients from being treated with warfarin. Handicap and place of residence were not important factors in the decision to use anticoagulants.

Conclusion.—A clinician's decision to treat NVAF with anticoagulants is influenced by a patient's age and quality of life. However, nonuse of anticoagulants based on patient age is unfounded and is likely to lead to inadequate treatment of elderly patients. A substantial number of strokes could be prevented with appropriate use of anticoagulants in the elderly population.

▶ This article by the same group as Abstract 6–2 confirms our overall impression that many physicians use age as an important consideration in denying warfarin therapy to patients with atrial fibrillation when the therapy is otherwise indicated. As emphasized by this article, there are no good data to support that contention.[1] Careful use of the Stroke Prevention in Atrial Fibrillation criteria for contraindication to warfarin therapy is recommended, but every effort should be made to provide patients who have atrial fibrillation with warfarin therapy when the latter is indicated.

A.L. Waldo, M.D.

Reference

1. Landefeld CF, Beyth RJ: Anticoagulant related bleeding: Clinical epidemiology, prediction and prevention. *Am J Med* 95:315-328, 1993.

Thromboembolic Prophylaxis in 3575 Hospitalized Patients With Atrial Fibrillation

Teo KK, for the Clinical Quality Improvement Network (CQIN) Investigators (Univ of Alberta, Edmonton, Canada)
Can J Cardiol 14:695-702, 1998

6–4

Introduction.—Atrial fibrillation (AF) will become more prevalent as the population gets older. This clinically important arrhythmia is already the major contributing factor in 15% of strokes overall and in 36% of strokes in persons over age 80. Even in the presence of overwhelming evidence that prophylactic anticoagulation is efficacious in patients with AF, this therapy is used less than optimally, particularly in the elderly population at greatest risk. One of the primary reasons for underuse of anticoagulants is concern about bleeding. It is not known to what extent these conflicting concerns influence clinicians' practice patterns in the treatment of AF. Contemporary utilization patterns of anticoagulant and antiplatelet therapy for thromboembolic prophylaxis in AF were assessed in a large cohort of patients from 12 Canadian hospitals.

Methods.—Of 3,375 consecutive patients with AF, 1,570 were females and 2,005 were males, with a mean age of 72 years. There were 1,353 patients who were younger than age 70 and 2,222 who were age 70 or older. Patients were monitored for use of warfarin or acetylsalicylic acid (ASA) at any time during hospitalization or upon discharge.

Results.—Thirty-three percent (1,188) of patients did not receive prophylaxis. Of those treated, 852 (24%) received warfarin alone, 1,247 received ASA alone, and 288 (8%) received both drugs. Thirteen percent and 6% of patients with AF had specific contraindications to warfarin therapy and ASA, respectively. Twenty percent (65) of patients with documented valvular AF not related to recent cardiac surgery and with no contraindications to warfarin or ASA did not receive any therapy, 55% (181) received warfarin alone, 14% (46) received ASA alone, and 12% (39) received a combination of warfarin and ASA. Thirty-seven percent (823) of patients with nonvalvular heart disease and no contraindications received no therapy, 31% (677) received ASA alone, 23% (504) received warfarin alone, and 9% (195) received both drugs. Warfarin use was less likely in patients aged 70 or older, in patients with nonvalvular associated abnormalities, with postcardiac surgery, and in sinus rhythm at discharge. Patient sex was not significantly associated with warfarin use. There was an increased likelihood of ASA treatment in patients with postcardiac surgery, with admission for AF or thromboembolic or other cardiac events, in sinus rhythm at discharge, aged 70 years or older, with duration of AF less than 1 month, with paroxysmal AF, and of male sex. Valvular causes of AF were correlated with a lower likelihood of receiving ASA.

Conclusion.—Anticoagulation and antiplatelet prophylaxis may be less than optimal in patients with AF. Concerns about bleeding seem to be partially responsible for the uneven and incomplete use of thromboembolic prophylaxis in patients with AF. It is important to determine the reasons for suboptimal treatment and to develop effective strategies to enhance patients' care and treatment outcomes.

▶ In this very large retrospective study, once again, we find that one third of patients were receiving no anticoagulant therapy, and another one third were receiving aspirin alone. Thus, two thirds of the patients in this study were getting either no or insufficient anticoagulation therapy. Moreover, those who need it most, patients over age 70, were more likely not to receive any thromboembolic prophylaxis. Ironically, older patients were more likely to receive aspirin than warfarin, presumably because of the fear of bleeding. But aspirin is clearly not effective in this group. Women were also less likely to receive warfarin therapy. The data are clear: give warfarin when indicated unless it is contraindicated.

A.L. Waldo, M.D.

Prospective Evaluation of an Index for Predicting the Risk of Major Bleeding in Outpatients Treated With Warfarin

Beyth RJ, Quinn LM, Landefeld CS (Case Western Univ, Cleveland, Ohio; Cleveland Veterans Affairs Med Ctr, Ohio; Univ Hosps of Cleveland, Ohio)
Am J Med 105:91-99, 1998   6–5

Introduction.—Anticoagulant-related bleeding reduces the net benefit of therapy. Concerns about bleeding may influence physicians to avoid warfarin therapy in patients who might otherwise be helped. The accuracy and clinical utility of the Outpatient Bleeding Risk Index and its ability to estimate the probability of major bleeding, defined as overt bleeding that led to the loss of 2 units or more in 7 days or less or bleeding that was otherwise life-threatening, were assessed.

Methods.—Warfarin was initiated in 264 outpatients to validate the index prospectively. Data regarding potential predictors of outpatient bleeding were gathered at the beginning of warfarin therapy. Bleeding was classified according to amount, rate, and consequences. Physicians made estimates of the probability of major bleeding.

Results.—The rate of major bleeding was 6.5% per year (87 of 820). The index provided 4 independent risk factors for major bleeding: age 65 years or older, history of gastrointestinal bleeding, history of stroke, and 1 or more of 4 specific co-morbid conditions. The index predicted major bleeding better than did physicians, who estimated the probability of major bleeding no better than expected by chance. The cumulative rate of major bleeding at 48 months was: 3% in 80 patients at low risk (i.e., no risk factors), 12% in 166 patients at intermediate risk (i.e., 1-2 risk factors), and 53% in 18 patients at high risk (i.e., 3-11 risk factors). Seventeen of the 18 episodes of major bleeding were potentially preventable.

Conclusion.—The Outpatient Bleeding Risk Index performed better than physician estimates and prospectively classified patients into 3 groups with different cumulative risks of major bleeding. The index was able to discriminate between patients who developed major bleeding and those who did not. Avoiding overanticoagulation and nonsteroidal anti-inflammatory agents may prevent major bleeding in most high-risk patients.

▶ For those concerned about an objective way to identify patients at greatest risk for major bleeding, this study provides a useful screen. But even so, a major problem is that, even in this high-risk cohort, bleeding could have been prevented in almost all patients. Thus, 11 of 18 patients had excessive warfarin therapy (the international normalized ratio mean was 12.2; range, 4.8-56). Four of 18 patients had bleeding secondary to aspirin therapy, which is largely ineffective anyway. In short, even in high-risk patients, careful patient follow-up and patient education should minimize this bleeding risk.

A.L. Waldo, M.D.

Transesophageal Echocardiographic Correlates of Clinical Risk of Thromboembolism in Nonvalvular Atrial Fibrillation

Zabalgoitia M, for the Stroke Prevention in Atrial Fibrillation III Investigators (Univ of Texas, San Antonio; Mt Sinai Med Ctr, New York; Statistics and Epidemiology Research Corp, Seattle; et al)
J Am Coll Cardiol 31:1622-1666, 1998

6–6

Background.—Patients with nonvalvular atrial fibrillation (AF) are at increased risk of arterial thromboembolic events. These authors used transesophageal echocardiography (TEE) to identify factors associated with thromboembolic risk in these patients.

Methods.—Patients with nonvalvular AF who were receiving aspirin therapy were stratified into groups at low, moderate, or high risk of thromboembolism. Four risk factors for thromboembolism were examined: female sex and age older than 75 years, systolic blood pressure greater than 160 mm Hg, congestive heart failure or fractional shortening (as shown by precordial echocardiography), and previous thromboembolism. Patients who had none of these risk factors and no history of hypertension were classified as low risk (n = 234). Patients who had none of these risk factors but a history of hypertension were classified as moderate risk (n = 170). Patients with 1 or more of these risk factors were classified as high risk (n = 382). Within 3 months after study enrollment, patients underwent TEE to image the left atrium and its appendages and the thoracic aorta. Then the TEE features correlating with thromboembolic risk were analyzed.

Findings.—Compared with the low-risk group, patients in the moderate- and high-risk groups were significantly more likely to have dense spontaneous echo contrast (relative risk [RR], 3.7), thrombi of the left atrial appendage (RR, 2.5), complex aortic plaque (RR, 2.1), and a peak flow velocity in the left atrial appendage less than 20 cm/sec (RR, 1.7). Compared with the moderate-risk group, those in the high-risk group had significantly higher risks for complex aortic plaque (RR, 2.9) and dense spontaneous echo contrast (RR, 2.7). Compared with group 1 (no hypertension), patients in group 2 (hypertension) were significantly more likely to have thrombi in the left atrial appendage (RR, 2.7) or reduced peak flow velocity through the left atrial appendage (RR, 1.8). Among patients in the high-risk group, no single risk factor conferred a higher risk of thromboembolism than any of the others. Among patients in the low-risk group, TEE findings did not differ based on the nature of the AF (intermittent vs. constant).

Conclusions.—TEE of patients with nonvalvular AF identified left atrial stasis/thrombosis and aortic atheroma as independent predictors of a moderate to high risk of thromboembolism. Left atrial stasis/thrombosis also helps to explain the increased risk of stroke in patients with AF who have hypertension. In particular, the presence of complex aortic plaque confers a high risk of thromboembolism in patients with AF.

▶ This study confirms that risk stratification does indeed reliably identify those patients at increased risk for thromboembolism associated with AF. Two other points are worth emphasis. First, the authors once again confirm that aspirin has little efficacy in this patient population. Second, even the low-risk patients had an incidence of positive echocardiographic correlates of thromboembolic risk: 4% had dense systolic echo contrast, 3% had left atrial appendage thrombus, and 19% had left atrial appendage peak flow velocity (20 cm/sec). One wonders if there isn't a role for a transesophageal echocardiogram in low-risk patients (e.g., when they are first seen to suggest which low-risk patients might benefit from warfarin therapy).

A.L. Waldo, M.D.

Atrial Fibrillation and Cognitive Function: Case-Control Study
O'Connell JE, Gray CS, French JM, et al (Univ of Newcastle upon Tyne, England; Addenbrooke's Hosp, Cambridge, England)
J Neurol Neurosurg Psychiatry 65:386-389, 1998   6–7

Introduction.—The most important potentially preventable form of dementia is cerebrovascular disease. A major and independent risk factor for cerebrovascular disease at all ages is atrial fibrillation, which increases in prevalence with increasing age, reaching up to 13% in those older than 85 years. It was previously hypothesized that people with nonvalvular atrial fibrillation are at increased risk of progressive cognitive impairment as a result of silent cerebral infarction. This was a community-based pilot study to determine whether this hypothesis could be tested in a prospective controlled study design and to discover which subtests in the selected psychometric test battery were most applicable to patients without prior stroke or transient ischemic attack.

Methods.—There were 27 patients with nonvalvular atrial fibrillation (median duration, 2 years; range, 1-23 years) without a history of transient ischemic attack, dementia, thyrotoxicosis, or stroke, who were compared with 54 age- and sex-matched controls in sinus rhythm. No patient was taking warfarin. Clinical examination, ECG, and psychological assessment using a battery of 9 neuropsychological tests, administered in 60 minutes, were performed on all patients and included a Mini-Mental State Examination, general cognitive function test, national adult reading test, control for premorbid intelligence, Wechsler logical memory test, verbal long-term memory test, Rey complex figure test and non-verbal memory test, digit span subtest of the Wechsler Adult Intelligence Scale, short-term memory test, paced auditory serial addition test, map search subtest of the test of everyday attention, and telephone search task test. The 2 groups were compared.

Results.—Poorer performances on all the subtests of the neuropsychological battery were consistently associated with the presence of atrial fibrillation. However, performance was not associated with duration of atrial fibrillation. There was a significant difference in the paced auditory serial addition test, in speed of information processing, and in the attention test.

Conclusion.—Further prospective studies should be conducted on a larger scale to determine whether patients at maximal risk of silent cerebral ischemia and associated cognitive decline can be protected by antithrombotic therapy.

▶ This is an important pilot study, because it clearly shows, using objective testing, that atrial fibrillation in the absence of warfarin therapy is associated with cognitive loss, particularly memory. This article serves once again to reinforce the need to anticoagulate patients with atrial fibrillation who have indications for anticoagulation, particularly the elderly.

A.L. Waldo, M.D.

Acute Changes in Spontaneous Echo Contrast and Atrial Function After Cardioversion of Persistent Atrial Flutter

Weiss R, Marcovitz P, Knight BP, et al (Univ of Michigan, Ann Arbor)
Am J Cardiol 82:1052-1055, 1998
6–8

Introduction.—After conversion of atrial fibrillation to sinus rhythm, a transient decrease in atrial mechanical function occurs known as atrial stunning. This phenomenon may be responsible for the heightened risk of thromboembolic complications associated with cardioversion of atrial fibrillation. Transesophageal echocardiography has rarely been used to evaluate atrial function or spontaneous echo contrast after conversion of atrial flutter. The short-term effects of transthoracic electrical cardioversion of atrial flutter on atrial mechanical function and the incidence of spontaneous echo contrast was determined with transesophageal echocardiography.

Methods.—Transthoracic cardioversion was performed on 30 patients who had atrial flutter for a mean of 6.4 ± 12.2 months. Immediately before cardioversion, a transesophageal echocardiogram was recorded. In 28 patients, the left atrial appendage–emptying velocity and spontaneous contrast were assessed at 1, 3, and 5 minutes after cardioversion. In a subgroup of 13 patients, a similar assessment was made at 8, 10, and 15 minutes after cardioversion. Because a thrombus was found in the left atrial appendage, cardioversion was deferred in 2 patients (7%).

Results.—In 7 (25%) of 28 patients who had cardioversion, spontaneous echo contrast was present in the left atrium before cardioversion. At 1 minute after restoration of sinus rhythm, the mean left atrial appendage–emptying velocity of 54 ± 22 cm/sec before cardioversion fell by 26% to 40 ± 25 cm/sec. Between 1 and 15 minutes after cardioversion, there were no significant changes in the mean left atrial appendage–emptying velocity. Left atrial spontaneous echo contrast developed de novo or worsened in 12 (43%) of the 28 patients within 5 minutes after conversion to sinus rhythm.

Conclusion.—Left atrial thrombi may be associated with persistent atrial flutter before cardioversion, and a significant degree of atrial stunning and formation of spontaneous echo contrast is associated with cardioversion of atrial flutter.

▶ The implications of this study are important. They confirm that the risk of clot formation and potential for embolic stroke associated with atrial fibrillation is also present with atrial flutter. The fact that 2 of the patients in this study were found with a left atrial thrombus that led to deferral of cardioversion is very important because it again says that even though the atria may be "contracting" during atrial flutter, the atrial myopathy that is associated with clot formation is still present. Therefore, the same rules that apply to anticoagulation of atrial fibrillation should apply to atrial flutter.

A.L. Waldo, M.D.

Risk of Thromboembolic Events in Patients With Atrial Flutter
Seidl K, Hauer B, Schwick NG, et al (Herzzentrum Ludwigshafen, Germany)
Am J Cardiol 82:580-583, 1998   6–9

Introduction.—Patients with atrial fibrillation are treated with anticoagulation for up to several weeks before and after cardioversion to inhibit thromboembolism. The value of this treatment approach has not been established in patients with atrial flutter. The frequency and risk of thromboembolism was evaluated in 191 consecutive unselected patients hospitalized with atrial flutter.

Methods.—All patients underwent transthoracic echocardiography. Forty-four selected patients with a history of thromboembolism or with expected increased risk for embolism underwent transesophageal echocardiography. Evaluated risk factors included: age, sex, duration of atrial flutter, presence of atrial fibrillation, organic heart disease, systemic hypertension, diabetes mellitus, left ventricular function, left atrial size, left ventricular wall thickness, and spontaneous echo contrast.

Results.—There were 11 patients with a history of embolic events. Four patients had acute embolism of less than 48 hours. Of these, 3 were after direct current cardioversion and 1 was after catheter ablation. Nine patients had thromboembolic events during an 18-month follow-up period. The overall thrombolic rate was 7% and included acute embolism and thromboembolic events during follow-up. Univariate analysis revealed risk factors for an embolic event were organic heart disease, depressed left ventricular function, history of systemic hypertension, and diabetes mellitus. For multivariate analyses, history of hypertension was the only independent predictor of elevated risk.

Conclusion.—Thrombolic risk is higher than previously believed in patients with atrial flutter. Anticoagulants may diminish the risk of thrombolic events in these patients.

▶ This paper serves, once again, to emphasize that atrial flutter has similar risks for systemic embolism and stroke, as does atrial fibrillation. It requires the same sort of approach with anticoagulation treatment. Although there has been no long-term study in doing that in atrial flutter, it is clear that the results would be the same as those already demonstrated in atrial fibrillation.

A.L. Waldo, M.D.

Epidemiology of Atrial Fibrillation

Impact of Atrial Fibrillation on the Risk of Death: The Framingham Heart Study
Benjamin EJ, Wolf PA, D'Agostino RB, et al (NIH, Framingham, Mass; Boston Univ; Beth Israel Hosp, Boston; et al)
Circulation 98:946-952, 1998   6–10

Introduction.—The morbidity of atrial fibrillation (AF) is well established. However, it is not known if AF per se results in excess mortality. The mortality associated with AF was assessed using data from the original Framingham Heart Study.

Findings.—Of 5,209 original participants in the Framingham Heart Study, 296 males and 325 females (with mean ages of 74 and 76 years, respectively) experienced AF. The mortality of participants aged 55 to 94 years who developed AF during the 40 years of follow-up was recorded.

Results.—After adjusting for age, hypertension, smoking, diabetes, left ventricular hypertrophy, myocardial infarction, congestive heart failure, valvular heart disease, and stroke or transient ischemic attack, AF was correlated with an odds ratio for death: 1.5 in males and 1.9 in females.

Conclusion.—AF was independently associated with a 50% to 90% rise in the risk of death. Increased mortality was observed in both males and females with AF, across the 4 decades of age evaluated. These findings support early reports regarding an association between AF and excessive mortality, an association that persists after adjusting for coexisting cardiovascular conditions.

▶ This study confirms earlier data that indicate an almost doubling of the risk of mortality associated with AF. However, when one looks at the curves, one notices that most of them are pretty parallel except for an initial difference. One wonders if that difference is associated with some acute co-morbid event. The investigators carefully separated and carefully adjusted for age, hypertension, smoking, diabetes, left ventricular hypertrophy, myocardial infarction, congestive heart failure, valvular heart disease, and stroke or transient ischemic attack. That doesn't leave much to explain the apparent early risk. Nonetheless, it is troublesome. Clearly, AF is an important clinical problem. But trials such as the AFFIRM trial are more likely to tell us whether that risk really is twofold, because they are comparing strategies for maintenance of sinus rhythm vs. maintenance of rate control, with both strategies including warfarin therapy. We await the results of the several such trials in the United States and abroad.

A.L. Waldo, M.D.

Predictors of Primary Atrial Fibrillation and Concomitant Clinical and Hemodynamic Changes in Patients With Chronic Heart Failure: A Prospective Study in 344 Patients With Baseline Sinus Rhythm
Pozzoli M, Cioffi G, Traversi E, et al (Montescano Med Ctr, Pavia, Italy; Rehabilitation Ctr Eremo, Arco di Trento, Italy; Inst of Care and Research, Pavia, Italy)
J Am Coll Cardiol 32:197-204, 1998   6–11

Introduction.—Structural cardiac diseases are present in a high percentage of patients with atrial fibrillation (AF); congestive heart failure (CHF) is one of AF's most common precursors. However, the factors that predispose patients with CHF to onset of AF are not known. The incidence, predisposing factors, and significance of the onset of AF were assessed in 344 patients with CHF and sinus rhythm.

Methods.—All patients had more than 2 episodes of CHF requiring hospitalization in the 6 months before undergoing evaluation for heart transplantation. Serial clinical, laboratory, ergometric, hemodynamic, and echocardiographic evaluations were conducted every 6 months. Patients were contacted by telephone between visits. No patients were lost to follow-up. Patients were monitored for the development of chronic AF and major and minor cardiac events. Twenty-eight patients developed AF; of these, 18 were treated with low-dose amiodarone.

Results.—There were no between-group differences in any clinical or hemodynamic variables in patients who did and did not develop chronic AF. Reversible AF and lower mitral flow velocity at atrial contraction were independent predictors of subsequent development of chronic AF. The New York Association functional class deteriorated when AF occurred: peak exercise oxygen consumption declined from 16 to 11 mL/kg per minute; cardiac index was reduced from 2.2 to 1.8; and mitral and tricuspid regurgitation rose from grade 1.8 to 2.4 and from grade 1.0 to 1.9, respectively. Three of the 18 patients with chronic AF developed systemic thromboembolism. Nine patients died after AF. AF was a predictor of major cardiac events.

Conclusion.—Reversible AF and diminished left atrial contribution to left ventricular filling were predictive of subsequent development of AF. Numerous clinical trials have demonstrated that the onset of AF is associated with clinical and hemodynamic deterioration and that AF may predispose patients to systemic thromboembolism and a poorer prognosis.

▶ This is an important study because it prospectively investigated a very large group of patients with CHF failure who had sinus rhythm at the time of entry into the study. The results showed that, in these patients, the occurrence of AF could not be predicted by any baseline variable, whereas previous episodes of reversible AF, reduced left atrial contribution to filling, and reduced atrial-emptying fraction, observed during follow-up, were significantly associated with a later occurrence of AF. Furthermore, the study demonstrates that the occurrence of AF is associated with clinical and hemodynamic deterioration, and may predispose to systemic thromboembolism. The latter 2 conclusions may not be a surprise, but these data are important because previous studies investigated patients with AF already present, not those with sinus rhythm already present. Thus, although this study confirms what has already been widely accepted, it is a very solid and definitive proof of this concept.

A.L. Waldo, M.D.

Atrial Fibrillation Is Associated With an Increased Risk for Mortality and Heart Failure Progression in Patients With Asymptomatic and Symptomatic Left Ventricular Systolic Dysfunction: A Retrospective Analysis of the SOLVD Trials

Dries DL, Exner DV, Gersh BJ, et al (Natl Heart, Lung and Blood Inst, Bethesda, Md; Georgetown Univ, Washington, DC; Brigham and Women's Hosp, Boston)

J Am Coll Cardiol 32:695-703, 1998   6–12

Introduction.—In patients with heart failure, atrial fibrillation occurs in up to 30% during the course of their disease. The prognostic implications of atrial fibrillation in heart failure remain unclear despite the potentially adverse hemodynamic and electrophysiologic consequences of this common dysrhythmia. To evaluate the association of atrial fibrillation with all-cause mortality, death from progressive pump failure, and arrhythmic death, a retrospective analysis was conducted on patients with atrial fibrillation and those in sinus rhythm.

Methods.—There were 2,569 patients with symptomatic heart failure who were randomly assigned to receive either placebo or enalapril at doses of 2.5 to 20 mg/day in a double-blind manner. Each patient had a baseline ECG before randomization, and this was used to determine which patients had atrial fibrillation and which had sinus rhythm for the retrospective review. All patients had an ejection fraction of 35% or less. Total mortality was the primary end point in both trials. Patients were followed up for an average of 33.4 ± 14.3 months.

Results.—Greater all-cause mortality was found among patients with atrial fibrillation at baseline compared with those in sinus rhythm (34% vs. 23%). Patients with atrial fibrillation had more deaths attributed to pump failure (16.7% vs. 9.4%) and were more likely to reach the composite end point of death or hospitalization for heart failure (45% vs. 33%) than those with sinus rhythm. Regarding arrhythmic deaths, there was no significant difference between the groups.

Conclusion.—An increased risk for all-cause mortality is associated with the presence of atrial fibrillation in patients with asymptomatic and symptomatic left ventricular systolic dysfunction. An increased risk for pump failure death is largely explained by this phenomenon. Progression of left ventricular systolic dysfunction is associated with atrial fibrillation according to these data. The presence of atrial fibrillation may be a marker for more severe underlying disease. The optimal treatment strategy for patients with atrial fibrillation is still unknown. With regard to the adequacy of their medical regimen and the frequency of follow-up, patients with atrial fibrillation appear to warrant particular vigilance.

▶ The importance of this study is that the analysis of the SOLVD trials demonstrates that atrial fibrillation is associated with an increased mortality risk largely explained by an increased risk for death from pump failure. The data differ from some other studies in that they demonstrate no association with the risk of arrhythmic death. This may have been caused by the fact that the population was not quite as sick as in some of the previous trials, and they speculate there is a significant decreased use of class I antiarrhythmic agents. What is particularly interesting is that the adverse prognostic impact of atrial fibrillation in the SOLVD trials was apparent even in patients with atrial fibrillation reporting no use of antiarrhythmic drugs at baseline and subsequently randomly assigned to receive treatment with enalapril.

A.L. Waldo, M.D.

Atrial Fibrillation After Radiofrequency Ablation of Type I Atrial Flutter: Time to Onset, Determinants, and Clinical Course

Paydak H, Kall JG, Burke MC, et al (Univ of Chicago)
Circulation 98:315-322, 1998   6–13

Introduction.—Even with technical refinements and improved long-term efficacy of the ablation procedure, the subsequent occurrence of atrial fibrillation (AF) continues to be a significant clinical problem in up to 30% of ablation procedures. Time to onset of AF, determinants, and clinical course of AF after ablation of type I flutter were assessed in a large patient cohort to enhance knowledge of the pathogenesis and significance of postablation AF.

Methods.—One hundred ten consecutive patients underwent radiofrequency catheter ablation for recurrent type I atrial flutter between July 1994 and June 1997. Patients underwent at least 24 hours of continuous ECG before hospital discharge. Only 6 patients who were taking amiodarone before ablation were treated with antiarrhythmic drugs after ablation. Patients underwent ECG at 1-, 4-, and 6-month intervals. Patients with palpation underwent Holter monitor or transtelephonic ambulatory

ECG monitoring. A number of clinical and procedural variables were examined.

Results.—AF was documented in 28 (25%) patients during a mean follow-up of 20.1 months. Significant and independent predictors of subsequent AF were a history of spontaneous AF and a left ventricular ejection fraction less than 50%. The presence of both of these factors identified a high-risk patient group with a 74% occurrence of AF. Patients with only 1 of these factors were at intermediate risk (20%); those with neither factor were at 10% risk. Early or late onset of AF had no effect on determinants or clinical course. Eighteen patients had persistent and recurrent AF that required long-term therapy, including 12 of 19 (63%) patients with prior AF and left ventricular dysfunction.

Conclusion.—A small subset of patients with both left ventricular dysfunction and a history of AF (17% of the population) were responsible for 67% of all postablation AF needing long-term treatment. This does not mean that these patients are inappropriate candidates for catheter ablation of type I flutter. The ongoing risk of AF suggests a potentially important role for AF as a trigger rather than a consequence of type I atrial flutter.

▶ This article indicates that patients with both left ventricular dysfunction and a history of AF should be advised of the risk of recurrence. Continuation or initiation of systematic anticoagulation may be appropriate, as may continuation of suppressive antiarrhythmic drug therapy. In patients without both of these risk factors, it seems reasonable to suggest a follow-up without additional treatment unless warranted.

A.L. Waldo, M.D.

Mechanical Dysfunction of the Left Atrium and the Left Atrial Appendage Following Cardioversion of Atrial Fibrillation and Its Relation to Total Electrical Energy Used for Cardioversion

Harjai K, Mobarek S, Abi-Samra F, et al (Ochsner Med Institutions, New Orleans, La)
Am J Cardiol 81:1125-1129, 1998   6–14

Purpose.—Cardioversion of atrial fibrillation (AF) may be followed by impairment of mechanical atrial function, as well as decreased left atrial (LA) appendage filling. Some patients with AF may require multiple shocks and receive high doses of electrical energy for cardioversion. This study assessed the effects of total electrical energy used for cardioversion on the subsequent mechanical function of the left atrium and LA appendage.

Methods.—The randomized study included 39 hemodynamically stable patients undergoing electrical cardioversion for AF. Patients were assigned to receive an initial shock of 1.5 J/kg, based on body weight; 2.5, 3.5, or 5.0 J/kg; or 360 J, followed by increasingly greater shock intensities until they achieved sinus rhythm. Within 24 hours, the patients underwent transthoracic echocardiography to assess the effects of total cardioversion energy on postcardioversion peak LA rapid-filling velocity and atrial-emptying fraction, and recovery of LA effective mechanical atrial function. In addition, 27 patients had transesophageal echocardiography before and after cardioversion to examine relationships between total electrical energy, LA appendage–filling and –emptying velocities, and spontaneous echo contrast.

Results.—Left atrial appendage–filling and –emptying velocities were significantly decreased in association with conversion to sinus rhythm: 0.42 vs. 0.29 m/sec for filling velocity and 0.40 vs. 0.29 m/sec for emptying velocity. However, spontaneous echo contrast was unaffected (61% vs. 70%). Dividing the patients according to quartiles of total energy required for cardioversion showed no differences in LA appendage–filling or –emptying velocities, incidence of spontaneous echo contrast, or worsening of spontaneous echo contrast. Neither were there any differences in change in LA appendage–filling and –emptying velocities, nor in postcardioversion peak A velocity, atrial-emptying function, or recovery of effective mechanical atrial function.

Conclusions.—Total electrical energy required for cardioversion of AF has no impact on the postcardioversion mechanical function of the left atrium or LA appendage. Most patients regain effective mechanical atrial function within 7 days after cardioversion.

▶ The importance of this study is that it confirms that cardioversion per se is not what affects atrial contractility. Rather, it is the remodeling due to the AF itself. Once again, the recommendation is for anticoagulation therapy in this group of patients, to help prevent clot formation in the period following cardioversion during sinus rhythm.

A.L. Waldo, M.D.

New Insights Into Radiofrequency Ablation for Treatment of Atrial Fibrillation, Atrial Flutter, and Ventricular Tachycardia

Spontaneous Initiation of Atrial Fibrillation by Ectopic Beats Originating in the Pulmonary Veins
Haïssaguerre M, Jaïs P, Shah DC, et al (Hôpital Cardiologique du Haut-Lévêque, Bordeaux-Pessac, France)
N Engl J Med 339:659-666, 1998   6–15

Introduction.—Experimental and human surgical mapping trials have demonstrated that atrial fibrillation (AF) is perpetuated by re-entrant wavelets reproducing in an abnormal atrial-tissue substrate. There are few data regarding the spontaneous initiation of AF. The mode of initiation of spontaneous paroxysms of human AF by atrial ectopic beats, characteristics of these triggering beats, and effects of local ablation with radiofrequency energy were assessed in 45 patients with frequent episodes of AF.

Methods.—All patients had frequent AF that was resistant to more than 2 drugs, were on oral anticoagulants, had at least 1 episode of AF every 2 days, and had over 700 isolated atrial ectopic beats per 24 hours. The spontaneous initiation of AF was mapped, using a multielectrode catheter to record the earliest electrical activity preceding the onset of AF and associated ectopic beats. Accuracy of mapping was substantiated by the abrupt disappearance of triggering atrial ectopic beats after ablation with local radiofrequency energy.

Results.—Sixty-nine ectopic foci were identified in this patient cohort: 29 patients, single point of origin of atrial ectopic beats; 9 patients, 2 points of origin; and 7 patients, 3 to 4 points of origin. Location of the foci: 3 right atrium, 1 posterior left atrium, and 65 (94%) pulmonary veins (31 left superior, 17 right superior, 11 left inferior, and 6 right inferior). When located in a pulmonary vein, the earliest activation occurred 2 to 4 cm inside the main pulmonary vein or 1 of its proximal branches. Depolarization was marked by a spike that preceded the atrial ectopic beats on the surface ECG by 106 msec (range, 40-160 msec). Atrial fibrillation was induced by a sudden burst of rapid depolarization (340 per minute). A local depolarization was also observed during sinus rhythm and was abolished by radiofrequency ablation. Twenty-eight (62%) patients had no recurrence of AF during a follow-up period of 8 months.

Conclusion.—In this patient cohort, atrial premature beats that generate frequent paroxysms of AF most often originated in the pulmonary veins. These foci trigger AF with a burst of rapid discharges. AF caused by this mechanism can be cured by local application of radiofrequency energy using catheter ablation techniques.

▶ This is a seminal study. It holds hope for cure of at least a subset of patients with paroxysmal AF. It also emphasizes that when the mechanism is understood, we can be much smarter about directed therapy, such as radiofrequency ablation to cure AF. We should begin to look for appropriate AF patients systematically to identify patients who might benefit from this therapeutic procedure. Twenty-four–hour ambulatory (Holter) monitor ECGs seem to be our best screen at this time. We await further maturation of this field, but it is most exciting.

A.L. Waldo, M.D.

Assessment of Atrioventricular Junction Ablation and VVIR Pacemaker Versus Pharmacological Treatment in Patients With Heart Failure and Chronic Atrial Fibrillation: A Randomized, Controlled Study

Brignole M, Menozzi C, Gianfranchi L, et al (Ospedali Riuniti, Lavagna, Italy; Ospedale S Maria Nuova, Reggio Emilia, Italy; Ospedale Civile, Imperia, Italy)
Circulation 98:953-960, 1998   6–16

Introduction.—Patients receiving ablation and pacemaker treatment of chronic atrial fibrillation (AF) have not been assessed in comparison with a control group of patients treated medically during a long follow-up. The clinical effects of atrioventricular junctional ablation and a VVIR pacemaker (Abl+Pm) were compared with those of pharmacologic treatment in 66 patients with chronic AF in a multicenter, controlled, randomized trial.

Methods.—Patients had AF of greater than 6 months duration, with clinically manifest heart failure and heart rate of over 90 beats per minute on 3 standard ECGs, recorded at rest during stable conditions on different days. Patients were randomized to either Abl+Pm or conventional drug therapy. Follow-up was 12 months. Primary end points were quality of life and specific symptoms.

Results.—Eight patients in the drug group and 4 patients in the Abl+Pm group did not complete the trial. Twenty-eight patients treated by Abl+Pm had significantly lower scores for palpation and effort dyspnea than the 26 patients in the drug group. Though the difference was not significant, patients in the Abl+Pm group had lower scores in exercise intolerance, easy fatigue, and chest discomfort, and on the Living with Heart Failure Questionnaire, New York Heart Association functional classification, and Activity scale. An intrapatient comparison between enrollment and 12-month evaluation revealed that all variables except easy fatigue improved significantly, from 14% to 82%, in the Abl+Pm group. Patients in the drug group also improved in these variables. Differences between the 2 groups for the intrapatient comparison were significant only for palpitation, effort dyspnea, exercise intolerance, easy fatigue, and chest discomfort. Patients in both groups had similar findings in cardiac performance that remained stable over time, as determined by standard echocardiography and exercise testing.

Conclusion.—Treatment with Abl+Pm was superior to drug therapy in controlling specific symptoms. Its efficacy was lower than that seen in the intrapatient comparison, since some improvement was also observed in the drug group. Improvement was greater for specific disease symptoms than for health-related quality-of-life variables. Cardiac performance and disease progression were similar in the 2 groups.

▶ This study is of interest because it shows that although ablation and pacemaker treatment was superior to drug therapy in controlling symptoms of AF, its efficacy appears to be less than that observed in uncontrolled studies, because improvement occurred in the medically treated patients as well. In addition, contrary to previous studies, the present study did not show significant modifications of echocardiographic parameters and exercise stress testing either in intergroup or intrapatient comparisons. Thus, increases in the ejection fraction seen after 12 months were present in both groups. This improvement was likely due to control of the ventricular rate rather than to the method of control of the ventricular rate. This suggests to this editor that a clinical trial first of drug therapy to control ventricular rate is quite reasonable. One can always cross over to "ablate and pace" if it seems necessary, and as happened in several patients in the present study.

A.L. Waldo, M.D.

Uncommon Atrial Flutter: Characteristics, Mechanisms, and Results of Ablative Therapy

Gomes JA, Santoni-Rugiu F, Mehta D, et al (Mt Sinai Med Ctr, New York)
PACE 21:2029-2042, 1998   6–17

Background.—Uncommon atrial flutter (AF) is defined by the presence of predominantly positive f waves in leads II, III, and aVF. The activation sequence in the uncommon type proceeds in a clockwise fashion, in contrast to the counterclockwise direction seen with the common type. Data also suggest that the uncommon type is less responsive to radiofrequency ablation (RFA). These authors examined patients with uncommon AF and identified features associated with RFA failure.

Methods.—Thirty-seven patients (31 men and 6 women; mean age, 62 years) with AF underwent RFA through endoscopic mapping. Twenty of the patients (54%) had uncommon AF, and 2 patterns were noted. The AF made a single clockwise circuit in 15 patients (group 1). In 5 patients, however, there was ≥ 1 circuit, with both common and uncommon AF (group 2). The electrophysiologic characteristics and outcomes of these 2 groups were determined and compared over a mean follow-up period of 13 ± 10 months.

Findings.—In group 2, tachycardia cycle lengths for the common AF circuits were significantly longer than those for the uncommon AF circuits (247 ± 36 vs. 223 ± 40 msec, respectively). However, the mean tachycardia cycle lengths did not differ significantly between groups 1 and 2. Similarly, the echocardiographic parameters measured did not differ between the groups. However, the success rates of RFA did differ: acute success rates with RFA were 93% in group 1 (14 of 15 patients) and only 40% (2 of 5 patients in group 2. Furthermore, during follow-up, 12 of the 14 successfully treated patients in group 1 remained free of AF recurrences (86%), but only 1 of the 2 patients in group 2 remained recurrence free (20%).

Conclusions.—One or more re-entrant circuits seem to be involved in uncommon AF. Results of RFA in patients with a single uncommon AF circuit were excellent. However, RFA had only limited success in patients with at least 1 uncommon AF circuit. Thus, a patient who has multiple uncommon AF circuits may not be suitable for RFA.

▶ This interesting paper suggests 2 important points. First, one cannot take for granted that all AF circuits will be classical. Second, there is still more to learn about AF. The notion of figure-of-eight re-entry in AF has been confirmed in an animal model by our laboratory. Although it is not exactly the same as suggested by this article, it nevertheless points to the fact that systematic studies of AF still should be done in connection with ablation procedures to cure AF to be sure of what the re-entrant circuit comprises.

A.L. Waldo, M.D.

Radiofrequency Catheter Ablation of Ventricular Tachycardia After Myocardial Infarction

Stevenson WG, Friedman PL, Kocovic D, et al (Harvard Med School, Boston; Univ of California, Los Angeles; Univ of Pennsylvania, Philadelphia)
Circulation 98:308-314, 1998   6–18

Introduction.—Catheter ablation of ventricular tachycardia (VT) after myocardial infarction (MI) is frequently more problematic than supraventricular tachycardia. The presence of multiple morphologies of inducible monomorphic VT is often a complicating factor. Attempting to determine and target a single "clinical" VT is frequently limited by the inability to obtain 12-lead ECGs of VTs that are terminated emergently or by DC cardioversion. The feasibility of ablation in patients selected without regard to the presence of multiple VT was evaluated by targeting all VT that allowed mapping.

Methods.—Mapping and radiofrequency catheter ablation were undertaken in 52 patients with sustained monomorphic VT late after MI. All inducible monomorphic VTs that allowed mapping were targeted by radiofrequency catheter ablation. Forty-one patients (79%) had unsuccessful antiarrhythmic drug therapy, including 36 (69%) patients taking amiodarone.

Results.—There was an average of 3.6 morphologies of VT induced per patient. More than 1 ablation session was needed in 16 patients (31%). Five patients (10%) had complications, including 1 (2%) death caused by acute MI. During follow-up, 59% and 45% of patients, respectively, continued to receive amiodarone or had a cardioverter-defibrillator implanted. At a mean follow-up of 18 months (range, 0-51 months), 1 patient died suddenly, 2 died of uncontrollable VT, and 5 died of heart failure. Three-year survival rate and rate for risk of VT recurrence were 70% and 33%, respectively.

Conclusion.—Radiofrequency catheter ablation of VT after MI was able to eliminate spontaneous episodes of VT in two thirds of patients, regardless of the presence of multiple morphologies of inducible VT. It offered excellent palliation for many patients with repeated episodes of spontaneous VT. This treatment approach was largely adjunctive to amiodarone therapy and placement of a cardioverter-defibrillator.

▶ This report emphasizes that radiofrequency ablation techniques to treat VT is possible as an adjunct to drug therapy and the implantable cardioverter-defibrillator. It requires that the VT be stable enough to map, often possible enough during drug therapy. It is not clear that one can avoid an implantable cardioverter-defibrillator despite noninducibility of VT after the ablation because most patients will have been taking antiarrhythmic agents, especially amiodarone.

A.L. Waldo, M.D.

Ventricular Tachycardia in Valvular Heart Disease: Facilitation of Sustained Bundle-Branch Reentry by Valve Surgery

Narasimhan C, Jazayeri MR, Sra J, et al (Univ of Wisconsin, Milwaukee)
Circulation 96:4307-4313, 1997
6–19

Background.—Patients with severe valvular heart disease who undergo valve replacement continue to be at increased risk for untoward events, including sudden cardiac death. Previous studies have indicated that one of the risk factors associated with cardiac death in these patients is ventricular tachycardia (VT). These authors examined the clinical and electrophysiological findings associated with sustained monomorphic VT (SMVT) as well as the prevalence of bundle-branch re-entry (BBR) in patients who had undergone valve replacement.

Methods.—Chart review identified 31 patients (30 men and 1 woman, with a mean age of 64 years) who had undergone valvular surgery, had documented or suspected ventricular arrhythmias, and had inducible SMVT. None of the patients had acute mitral regurgitation caused by myocardial infarction. The patients were grouped according to the mechanism of the inducible SMVT: either BBR VT (n = 9, or 29%), non-BBR (myocardial) VT (n = 20, or 65%), or both (n = 2, or 6%). The extent of valvular disease, coronary artery disease, and left ventricular function was assessed by cardiac catheterization and Doppler echocardiography. Electrophysiologic parameters were assessed with catheters in the right atrium, right ventricle, and across the tricuspid valve.

Findings.—Patients with BBR VT were significantly less likely than patients with non-BBR VT to have coronary artery disease (2 of 9, or 22% vs. 15 of 20, or 75%). Patients with BBR VT were also significantly more likely to have normal left ventricular function (ejection fraction, 55% or greater; 44% vs. 5%). The tachycardia cycle did not differ appreciably between the groups, but the interval from His bundle to ventricular activation was significantly longer in the patients with non-BBR VT (82 ± 13 vs. 51 ± 15 msec). Eight of nine patients with BBR were treated with radiofrequency ablation of the right bundle branch; the ninth patient received an implantable cardiac defibrillator (ICD). All but 2 patients were alive after a mean follow-up of 30 ± 29 months. Nineteen of the 20 patients with non-BBR were treated with an ICD; the remaining patient was treated with amiodarone. Thirteen patients were alive after a mean follow-up of 38 ± 28 months. The 2 patients who had both BBR and non-BBR VT received ICDs, and both patients were alive at follow-up. Patients with BBR VT were significantly more likely to develop the SMVT within 1 month after surgery (89%; median, 10 days) than patients with non-BBR VT (15%; median, 72 months).

Conclusions.—Cases of non-BBR VT were more frequent and were associated with coronary artery disease, abnormal left ventricular function, and a longer period between valvular replacement and the development of the VT. In contrast, BBR VT accounted for about 30% of the cases, and the SMVT developed soon after surgery. For patients without coronary artery disease who experience a VT in the early postoperative period after valvular surgery, ablation of the appropriate bundle branch should be considered.

▶ This is quite a useful article, as it identifies a very treatable, in fact curable etiology for SMVT occurring after open-heart surgery for valvular heart disease. The presence of BBR as the etiology of SMVT in these patients seems likely to be due to trauma to the specialized atrioventricular conduction system associated with the surgery. This should not be a surprise, as both the aortic and mitral valves are in very close proximity to the His bundle and left bundle branch. What is surprising is that SMVT due to BBR in these patients was often associated with a normal left ventricular ejection fraction. Usually, we expect SMVT due to BBR to be associated with a dilated cardiomyopathy and poor left ventricular ejection fraction.

A.L. Waldo, M.D.

Antiarrhythmic Drug Therapy for Atrial Fibrillation

Selective Versus Non-selective Antiarrhythmic Approach for Prevention of Atrial Fibrillation After Coronary Surgery: Is There a Need for Preoperative Risk Stratification? A Prospective Placebo-controlled Study Using Low-Dose Sotalol
Weber UK, Osswald S, Huber M, et al (Univ Hosp, Basel, Switzerland; Statistics and Software Solutions Inc, Zurich, Switzerland)
Eur Heart J 19:794-800, 1998   6–20

Introduction.—Up to 50% of patients who undergo coronary bypass grafting experience atrial fibrillation (AF). The peak incidence occurs on the second or third postoperative day. Prophylactic use of antiarrhythmic drugs for prevention of AF exposes 60% to 70% of patients without postoperative AF to increased cost and possible side effects. Data from a cohort of patients with sinus rhythm undergoing elective coronary artery bypass grafting were retrospectively analyzed to develop an appropriate risk prediction algorithm based on clinical, electrocardiographic, and hemodynamic variables. This algorithm was tested in a second independent population receiving antiarrhythmic drugs to prevent postoperative AF after coronary surgery.

Methods.—A model for risk prevention was developed, based on clinical data of a control group of 107 patients (group A). This model was tested in a second group of 107 patients who were treated with low-dose sotalol. Using this algorithm, the effect of a "selective" antiarrhythmic treatment approach to patients at high risk for development of AF was compared to a "nonselective" group in which all patients received prophylactic sotalol.

Results.—Seventy-five (35%) patients developed AF. Fourteen (7%) patients had side effects that necessitated discontinuation of sotalol. Thirty-six percent of group A patients were classified as high risk. The incidence of AF in high-risk patients was 76%, compared to 26% in a low-risk group (a significant difference). With the selective approach, the incidence of AF decreased from 76% to 50%, compared to a reduction from 44% to 26% using a nonselective approach. All patients in the nonselective group were exposed to the possible side effects of sotalol and its costs, compared to 24% of patients in the selective approach group (a significant difference).

Conclusion.—The cost-effectiveness and safety of low-dose sotalol in the prevention of AF after coronary artery bypass surgery should improve with the use of a selective approach based on a clinical risk prediction algorithm.

▶ In addition to previously published predictors of postoperative AF (age, left ventricular ejection fraction, no β-blocker therapy, and a history of AF), prolonged P-wave duration in the normal 12-lead ECG was identified by the present investigators as the strongest predictor of postoperative development of AF. Incorporation of these independent parameters into a risk prediction algorithm proved to be a powerful tool for the prospective identification of high-risk patients, with a 3-fold increased incidence of postoperative AF. The other interesting thing about this study is that it demonstrated that low-dose (80 mg twice daily) sotalol for 3 months proved to be quite effective. Eighty mg twice daily is largely a β-blocker effect. There is some antiarrhythmic action of sotalol at this dose, but it is thought that the best therapeutic dose of sotalol is 120 mg twice daily. One wonders whether if this dose were used, the drug therapy in this study might have been still more effective.

A.L. Waldo, M.D.

Spontaneous Conversion and Maintenance of Sinus Rhythm by Amiodarone in Patients With Heart Failure and Atrial Fibrillation: Observations From the Veterans Affairs Congestive Heart Failure Survival Trial of Antiarrhythmic Therapy (CHF-STAT)
Deedwania PC, for the Department of Veterans Affairs CHF-STAT Investigators (Univ of California, Fresno; Stanford Univ, Calif; Veterans Affairs Med Ctr, Fresno, Calif; et al)
Circulation 98:2574-2579, 1998   6–21

Introduction.—The most common cardiac arrhythmia requiring treatment for significant morbidity and possibly death is atrial fibrillation. Restoration and maintenance of sinus rhythm and anticoagulation to reduce thromboembolism and control ventricular rate are the 2 fundamental therapeutic approaches used to alleviate symptoms. Amiodarone is a class III agent that has been shown to exhibit the lowest proarrhythmic potential without exerting a potent negative inotropic effect in heart failure. Little is known, however, about the potential of the drug for controlling atrial fibrillation in patients with congestive heart failure. Long-term treatment with amiodarone was compared with placebo in patients with congestive heart failure and atrial fibrillation.

Methods.—There were 667 patients with congestive heart failure and 103 (15%) with atrial fibrillation at baseline. Placebo was given to 52 patients, and 51 received amiodarone. Atrial fibirillation was found to be more common in patients with nonischemic vs. ischemic cardiomyoapthy compared with patients in sinus rhythm (41% vs. 27%).

Results.—At 2 weeks, the mean ventricular response during atrial fibrillation over a 24-hour period was reduced by amiodarone by 20%. At 6 months, it was reduced by 18%, and at 12 months, it was reduced by 16%. There was a reduction of 22% at 2 weeks of maximal ventricular response, 19% at 6 months, and 14% at 12 months. During the study, 16 of 51 patients taking amiodarone and 4 of 52 taking placebo converted to sinus rhythm. Atrial fibrillation developed in 11 of 268 patients in sinus rhythm taking amiodarone at baseline and in 22 of the 263 patients in sinus rhythm taking placebo, demonstrating a significant difference during follow-up. Patients in atrial fibrillation at baseline who subsequently converted to sinus rhytm with amiodarone showed a significantly lower mortality rate than those who did not convert to sinus rhythm on the drug.

Conclusion.—Amiodarone has a significant potential to spontaneously convert atrial fibrillation to sinus rhythm in patients with congestive heart failure. Those who are converted to sinus rhythm have a lower mortality rate than those who are not. The development of new-onset atrial fibrillation was prevented by the drug, and in those patients with persistent atrial fibrillation there was a significant reduction of ventricular response with the drug.

▶ This is the first report of a blinded, placebo-controlled study in which spontaneous conversion of atrial fibrillation to sinus rhythm and the prevention of new-onset atrial fibrillation while receiving amiodarone in patients with heart failure has been documented during prolonged follow-up. These clinical effects, combined with the drug's propensity to help control ventricular rate effectively. was also found in this study and is clearly of therapeutic relevance because it reduces the need for negative inotropic drugs used to control ventricular response rate. These data support the notion that chronic amiodarone therapy either alone or in combination with digoxin is the first line of therapy in patients with atrial fibrillation and heart failure.

A.L. Waldo, M.D.

Conversion of Recent-Onset Atrial Fibrillation to Sinus Rhythm: Effects of Different Drug Protocols
Boriani G, Biffi M, Capucci A, et al (Univ of Bologna, Italy; S Orsola Hosp, Bologna, Italy)
PACE 21:2470-2474, 1998   6–22

Background.—Many different antiarrhythmic drugs are used to treat atrial fibrillation (AF) of recent onset, but there are few data on their comparative efficacies. These authors compared the efficacy and safety of

4 antiarrhythmic dosing regimens against placebo in converting AF of recent onset to sinus rhythm.

Methods.—The subjects were 417 hospitalized patients who had AF of recent onset (≤7 days). None of the patients had heart failure, and all were in New York Heart Association class ≤II. Patients were randomly assigned to 1 of 5 treatment groups. The first group (n = 212) received placebo. The IV amiodarone group (n = 51) received a 5-mg/kg bolus, then an infusion of 1.8 g/24 hr. The IV propafenone group (n = 57) received a 2-mg/kg bolus, then an infusion at 0.0078 mg/kg/min. The oral propafenone group (n = 119) received a single dose of 600 mg. The oral flecainide group (n = 69) received a single dose of 300 mg. Mean patient ages in the 5 groups ranged from 57 to 59 years, and men accounted for 55% to 59% of the patients (no significant differences between groups). Blood pressure and ECGs were monitored through the study, and at 1, 3, and 8 hours after dosing, the number of conversions to sinus rhythm was noted. A stable sinus rhythm that lasted at least 1 hour was considered conversion.

Findings.—All comparisons are against placebo. At 1 hour, IV propafenone was the only regimen to have a significant effect on the conversion rate (39%). At 3 hours, both IV and oral propafenone and oral flecainide had significant effects on conversion (58%, 45%, and 57%, respectively). At 8 hours, all 4 regimens had a significantly higher conversion rate than placebo (37%): rates for IV amidarone, IV propafenone, oral propafenone, and oral flecainide were 57%, 75%, 76%, and 75%, respectively. No patient died during the study, but there were 6 cases of severe adverse effects. Atrial flutter with a rapid ventricular response in the absence of structural heart disease occurred in 3 patients (1 taking placebo, 2 taking oral flecainide), left ventricular decompensation in the presence of structural heart disease occurred in 2 patients taking oral flecainide, and hypotension and pulmonary edema in the presence of mildly dilated cardiomyopathy occurred in 1 patient receiving IV propafenone.

Conclusions.—In these selected patients with recent-onset AF, a single oral dose of propafenone or flecainide produced a significant response at 3 hours that grew stronger over time (conversion rates 76% and 75%, respectively). IV amidarone took the longest time to affect conversion rates significantly. Oral flecainide was associated with 4 of the 6 severe adverse effects that occurred, whereas there were no serious adverse effects with oral propafenone. By 8 hours, more than one third of the patients in the placebo group had converted to sinus rhythm. This finding underscores the need to measure the effectiveness of antiarrhythmic drugs against placebo in the management of recent-onset AF.

▶ This study underlines the value of the "pill of the pocket" approach to conversion of atrial fibrillation to sinus rhythm in the patient who doesn't get frequent episodes and in whom the medication is used early after the development of atrial fibrillation. Importantly, there are several caveats that the data also emphasize: (1) class 1C agents (propafenone or flecainide) should not be used without concomitant use of a drug to block conduction at the atrioventricular (AV) node. This is because the rhythm may convert from atrial fibrillation to atrial flutter with a slow atrial rate (200 ± 20 beats/min). Therefore, it is critical that there be adequate block at the AV node. This usually can be obtained by first administering an oral agent such as a calcium channel blocker or a β-blocker, and then allowing enough time for it to have effect. (2) It also emphasizes that class 1C agents are important negative inotropic agents, and these drugs should be used warily, if at all, in patients with structural heart disease, particularly with left ventricular dysfunction.

A.L. Waldo, M.D.

Is Hospital Admission for Initiation of Antiarrhythmic Therapy With Sotalol for Atrial Arrhythmias Required? Yield of In-Hospital Monitoring and Prediction of Risk for Significant Arrhythmia Complications
Chung MK, Schweikert RA, Wilkoff BL, et al (Cleveland Clinic Found, Ohio; Ischemia Research and Education Found, San Francisco)
J Am Coll Cardiol 32:169-176, 1998   6–23

Introduction.—Hospital admission for monitoring during initiation of antiarrhythmic drugs continues to be controversial, including admission for monitoring sotalol. Patients undergoing in-hospital induction of sotalol for treatment of atrial arrhythmias were evaluated to determine the yield of monitoring in detection of significant arrhythmic complications and to determine factors that could predict safe outpatient initiation.

Methods.—Medical records of 120 patients admitted for initiation of sotalol therapy were examined retrospectively regarding the incidence of significant arrhythmia complications (new or increased ventricular arrhythmias, significant bradycardia, or excessive QTc interval prolongation).

Results.—Twenty-five (20.8%) patients had 35 complications that required treatment changes; of these complications, 21 (17.8%) occurred during hospitalization. Complications included 7 (5.8%) new or increased ventricular arrhythmias (torsades de pointes in 2), 20 (16.7%) significant bradycardia, and 8 (6.7%) excessively prolonged QTc intervals. Mean time to earliest detected complication was 2.1 days after initiation of sotalol. Twenty-two of 25 patients met criteria for complications within 3 days of monitoring. It was not possible to identify a low-risk group by using baseline ECG intervals or absence of heart disease. Absence of a pacemaker was the only significant predictor of arrhythmic complications.

Conclusion.—Initiation of sotalol therapy should be undertaken on an inpatient basis only. Twenty percent of patients who started sotalol therapy experienced clinically significant complications. Without a pacemaker, patients are at an even higher risk for complications.

▶ A careful review of this article leads this editor to a very different conclusion from that of the authors. First, it is widely accepted that patients with underlying structural heart disease should undergo inpatient initiation of any antiarrhythmic drug therapy. That includes 80% of the patients in this study. Second, only 3 patients without underlying structural heart disease had a "significant arrhythmic complication": 2 patients developed important bradycardia (37 and 30 beats/min, respectively) and 1 patient developed increased ectopic ventricular beats, including some nonsustained ventricular tachycardia (not further characterized). This is not, per se, a reason not to initiate sotalol as an outpatient. In fact, recent studies of sotalol as a treatment for atrial fibrillation support selected outpatient initiation of therapy. For this editor, there are a few rules to follow: First, don't give the drug during atrial fibrillation, but rather during sinus rhythm. Second, be sure the baseline QTc in men is 0.46 second and in women less than 0.44 second. Third, be sure the serum potassium is normal and no lower than 4 mEq/L. Fourth, do not initiate sotalol in outpatients receiving a diuretic. Fifth, be sure the creatinine clearance is normal. Sixth, obtain a 12-lead ECG 48 hours after initiating therapy, and if the QTc is greater than 0.52 second, or if the sinus rate is too slow, strongly consider decreasing the dose or stopping the drug. Seventh, provide an ECG event monitor for the patient to use, should there be any symptoms potentially related to the heart rhythm. In fact, have the patient transmit a rhythm strip at least once each day, even if no symptoms are present.

A.L. Waldo, M.D.

Devices for the Treatment of Atrial Fibrillation, Sinus Node Dysfunction, Heart Failure, and Life-Threatening Ventricular Arrhythmia

Atrioverter: An Implantable Device for the Treatment of Atrial Fibrillation

Wellens HJJ, for the METRIX Investigators (Academic Hosp, Maastricht, The Netherlands; Queen Mary Hosp, Hong Kong; Univ of Bonn, Germany; et al)
Circulation 98:1651-1656, 1998   6–24

Introduction.—The safety, efficacy, and complications of an implanted device (InControl METRIX Atrioverter) able to recognize atrial fibrillation and convert the arrhythmia to sinus rhythm by delivery of an appropriately timed low-energy shock (<6 J) were prospectively assessed in 51 patients with recurrent atrial fibrillation refractory to antiarrhythmic drugs.

Methods.—All patients were in New York Heart Association heart failure class I or II and were at low risk for ventricular arrhythmias. Enrolled patients were from 19 centers in 9 different countries. The required atrial defibrillation threshold was 240 V or lower during preimplant testing. Atrial fibrillation detection, R-wave shock synchronization, and defibrillation threshold were evaluated at implantation and during follow-up. Patients underwent termination of spontaneous episodes of atrial fibrillation under physician observation.

Results.—During a mean follow-up of 259 days (range, 72-613 days), 96% of 227 spontaneous episodes of atrial fibrillation were successfully converted to sinus rhythm in 41 patients. Several shocks were necessary because of early recurrence of atrial fibrillation in 27% of episodes. Patients varied markedly in tolerance of shock. Antiarrhythmic medication was administered to most patients during follow-up. Removal of the Atrioverter in 4 patients was because of infection, cardiac tamponade, or frequent episodes of atrial fibrillation requiring His bundle ablation. The right atrial lead had to be repositioned in 4 patients: 1 because of lead dislocation and 3 because of an acute rise in the atrial defibrillation threshold. Shocks (n = 3,719) were delivered without any ventricular pro-arrhythmia. All 47 patients who did not have the device removed were in sinus rhythm at follow-up.

Conclusion.—The Atrioverter recognizes atrial fibrillation with high specificity and can deliver low-energy defibrillation shocks safely and effectively with prompt restoration of sinus rhythm.

▶ This is the first reported clinical experience with this implanted atrial defibrillator. In this reviewer's judgment, this device is still finding its niche but will have one of consequence, particularly in combination with atrial pacing. Most importantly, this study shows that the device is safe, highly effective, and remarkably well tolerated. Ongoing studies are still in progress with the device, but it is important now to recognize that more than 10,000 shocks have been given safely with the device without any ventricular proarrhythmia. Furthermore, increasing numbers of patients are now using the device at home to convert atrial fibrillation to sinus rhythm. Most patients will tolerate up to 2 to 3 shocks. The biggest problem with the device has been early recurrence of atrial fibrillation. The reason for early recurrence is unclear, but it is an important clinical bugaboo because about half of the patients have had it at one time or another. We await further studies with this device, but in this editor's judgment, this device, when wedded to standard cardiac pacing technology will continue to provide a useful form of therapy for selected patients with atrial fibrillation.

A.L. Waldo, M.D.

Safety of Transvenous Low Energy Cardioversion of Atrial Fibrillation in Patients With a History of Ventricular Tachycardia: Effects of Rate and Repolarization Time on Proarrhythmic Risk
Simons GR, Newby KH, Kearney MM, et al (Duke Univ, Durham, NC; Durham Veterans Affairs Med Ctr, Durham, NC)
PACE 21:430-437, 1998   6–25

Background.—Atrial fibrillation is the most common cardiac arrhythmia that requires hospital admission. Although it is usually treated with antiarrhythmic medications, their use is limited by side effects. Alternative nonpharmacologic therapies would be helpful. It has recently been reported that low-energy, R-wave synchronized, direct current shocks applied between catheters in the coronary sinus and the right atrium may be used to treat atrial fibrillation. The safety of transvenous low-energy cardioversion of atrial fibrillation was examined in a large group of patients with a history of ventricular tachycardia.

Study Design.—Thirty-two patients with a history of sustained atrial fibrillation and monomorphic ventricular tachycardia with reduced ejection fraction (group A) and 29 patients with a history of sustained atrial fibrillation, without evidence of structural heart disease or ventricular arrhythmias (group B), had electrophysiologic study at the Durham Veterans Affairs Medical Center. Patients were sedated. Under fluoroscopic guidance, catheters were advanced into position. After diagnostic electophysiologic study, atrial fibrillation was induced by a 60-Hz alternating current. After 30 seconds, atrial defibrillation was performed with an external defibrillator with a biphasic waveform and a 65% fixed tilt. Shock strength was increased from 0.4 to 0.5 J by 0.2- to 0.5-J increments until defibrillation was achieved. Atrial defibrillation was repeated during isoproterenol infusion. In 16 group A patients, ventricular tachycardia was induced with burst pacing during atrial fibrillation and defibrillation. In 20 group A patients, atrial defibrillation was attempted during right ventricular pacing at a cycle length of 280 msec.

Findings.—A total of 932 baseline shocks were administered during atrial fibrillation. No ventricular proarrhythmia was detected after well-synchronized baseline shocks, although ventricular fibrillation did occur after inappropriate T-wave sensing. Shocks administered during wide-complex rhythms often induced ventricular arrythmias, but shocks administered during atrial pacing at identical ventricular rates did not cause proarrhythmia.

Conclusions.—The risk of ventricular proarrhythmia from transvenous low-energy cardioversion of atrial fibrillation appears to be related not to ventricular cycle length, but to the repolarization time. Therefore, the risk is probably not increased in patients with ventricular tachycardia. At identical heart rates, wide QRS rhythms are more likely than narrow QRS rhythms to be associated with shock-induced ventricular proarrhythmia.

▶ These data confirm the safety of low-energy shocks and also confirm studies in animal models. What is important is that sufficient time after the T wave of the previous beat be given before delivering the low-energy shock to the atrium. This technique remains useful in patients who cannot be defibrillated using standard external techniques and in whom the indication to restore sinus rhythm is present. These results also can be extrapolated to the use of the implantable atrial defibrillator.

A.L. Waldo, M.D.

Prevention of Atrial Arrhythmias During DDD Pacing by Atrial Overdrive
Garrigue S, Barold SS, Cazeau S, et al (Univ of Bordeaux, Pessac, France; Univ of Rochester, NY; Centre Chirurgical du Val d'Or, Saint-Cloud, France)
PACE 21:1751-1759, 1998   6–26

Introduction.—Because the diagnosis of atrial arrhythmia depends on symptoms and ECGs, its incidence in patients with dual-chamber pacemakers is underestimated. A previous study found that the incidence of atrial arrhythmia in a large unselected population of patients with DDD pacemakers was close to 50%. These data suggested that a reduced incidence of atrial arrhythmia episodes was correlated with higher percentages of atrial pacing. To evaluate the effect of atrial overdrive in pacemaker patients with frequent atrial arrhythmia, a prospective study was conducted.

Methods.—There were 22 patients with Chorus 6,234 DDD pacemakers who were 67 ± 9 years old. Atrial overdrive was defined as a programmed paced rate 10 pm faster than the mean ventricular rate stored for the last 24-hour period in the pacemaker memory. For the first month, patients were observed after discontinuation of antiarrhythmic therapy. For the second month, arrhythmia was analyzed with the pacemaker memory after programming the lower rate to 55 pm. To document the number and maximal duration of atrial arrhythmia episodes and the total atrial arrhythmia time in a month, the fallback function and histogram data were used. During the third month, atrial overdrive was examined.

Results.—Before atrial overdrive, the mean ventricular heart rate was 65 ± 4 beats/min vs. 75 ± 5 with atrial overdrive. All patients had atrial arrhythmic episodes during the end of the second month, with the mean number per patient being 42 ± 78 per month. No recorded atrial arrhythmias were seen in 14 (64.6%) of patients during atrial overdrive. A significant reduction in the number of atrial arrhythmias was seen in the other 8 patients with persistent atrial arrhythmia episodes (90 ± 106 in the second month vs. 38 ± 87 during atrial overdrive). In the second month, the total duration was 166 ± 115 hours in the second month vs. 92 ± 134 hours during atrial overdrive. The maximum duration was 121 ± 103 minutes in the second month vs. 85 ± 89 minutes during atrial overdrive.

Conclusion.—Atrial arrhythmia episodes are prevented or reduced by atrial overdrive. Long-term studies should be conducted to determine whether this benefit is sustained.

▶ This study provides further evidence that atrial pacing at rates significantly above the spontaneous rate but in the reasonable clinical realm (75-80 beats/min) seem to diminish the number of atrial arrhythmias. Other data have suggested that, in combination with antiarrhythmic drug therapy, this provides very effective therapy. But, as the article emphasizes, prospective studies are really needed.

A.L. Waldo, M.D.

Randomized Prospective Pilot Study of Long-term Dual-Site Atrial Pacing for Prevention of Atrial Fibrillation

Friedman PA, Hill MRS, Hammill SC, et al (Mayo Clinic, Rochester, Minn)
Mayo Clin Proc 73:848-854, 1998   6–27

Introduction.—The limitations of pharmacologic therapy in the treatment of atrial fibrillation (AF) have stimulated increasing interest in non-pharmacologic treatment options for this major health problem. Dual-site atrial pacing was assessed for its ability to prevent the onset of AF in the absence of membrane-active antiarrhythmic drugs during a prospective, randomized, single-blind crossover pilot investigation.

Methods.—Nine research participants with at least 2 episodes per month of symptomatic paroxysmal AF participated in randomly ordered 3-month trials of single-site atrial pacing, dual-site atrial pacing, and control (support-only) pacing.

Results.—Shorter P-wave duration and fewer premature atrial complexes on Holter monitoring were observed with dual-site pacing than with single-site pacing or control sinus rhythm. Dual-site pacing afforded a longer arrhythmia-free interval than single-site or control pacing (67, 62, and 49 days, respectively).

Conclusion.—Dual-site right atrial pacing is feasible and safe. It shortens P-wave duration and tends to diminish premature atrial complexes on Holter monitoring. Too few patients were enrolled in this pilot study for the investigators to determine a significant difference in pacing modes.

▶ This article presents another aspect of the device approach to treatment of AF alone or in combination with antiarrhythmic drug therapy. Although the results are drawn from a pilot study, they are consistent with the notion that pacing at sufficiently rapid rates that are clinically acceptable may provide important therapy in the control of AF.

A.L. Waldo, M.D.

Atrioventricular Conduction During Long-term Follow-up of Patients With Sick Sinus Syndrome

Andersen HR, Nielsen JC, Thomsen PEB, et al (Aarhus Univ Hosp, Denmark)
Circulation 98:1315-1321, 1998   6–28

Introduction.—In patients with sick sinus syndrome, single-chamber atrial pacing was found to be superior to single-chamber ventricular pacing because of lower overall and cardiovascular mortality rates. Later studies suggested that there was an increased risk of developing atrioventricular (AV) block after the implantation of an atrial pacemaker among patients with sick sinus syndrome. There have been no prospective data to document the risk of (AV) block, nor any studies to document the superiority of dual-chamber pacing over single-chamber atrial or ventricular pacing. AV conduction and the risk of developing AV block were evaluated during long-term follow-up of patients with sick sinus syndrome.

Methods.—There were 225 patients with sick sinus syndrome and intact AV conduction who received either single-chamber atrial pacing (110 patients) or single-chamber ventricular pacing (115 patients). Measurement of the PQ interval was conducted at 3 months and yearly thereafter. Determination of the atrial stimulus-Q intervals at pacing rates of 100 and 120 beats/min were evaluated in patients with pacemakers at 3 months and yearly thereafter. Follow-up was 5.5 ± 2.4 years.

Results.—Neither group had any change in PQ interval during follow-up. The atrial pacemaker group had no change in atrial stimulus-Q intervals or AV nodal Wenckebach block point. Grade 2 to 3 AV block that required upgrading of the pacemaker developed in 4 of 110 patients in the atrial pacemaker group (0.6% per year). Right bundle-branch block at pacemaker implantation was seen in 2 of these 4 patients.

Conclusion.—During long-term follow-up, AV conduction, estimated as PQ interval and atrial stimulus-Q interval at atrial pacing rates of 100 and 120 beats/min, and the Wenckebach block point remain stable. Treatment with single-chamber atrial pacing was safe and can be recommended in patients with sick sinus syndrome without bundle-branch block.

▶ This editor certainly accepts the data. However, for several reasons, I am not moved to place a single-chamber atrial pacing device instead of a dual-chamber device in patients with sinus node dysfunction. There is the potential for subsequent development of atrial fibrillation with bradycardia. There is the possibility that development of atrial fibrillation will be associated with ventricular rates that are too rapid, despite drug therapy, so that one might wish to perform His bundle ablation. There is the possibility that, in the presence of AV nodal blocking crugs administered for other reasons, the PR interval will be too long. And if these drugs are administered to control ventricular response to atrial fibrillation, they might not be well tolerated. There probably are a few additional reasons I just haven't thought of. This editor votes for dual-chamber pacing as prediction of the future is difficult. In this study, 2 of the 4 patients who developed significant AV conduction block presented with syncope. That is undesirable, may even be very dangerous, and could easily have been avcided with dual-chamber pacing.

A.L. Waldo, M.D.

Indications, Effectiveness, and Long-term Dependency in Permanent Pacing After Cardiac Surgery
Glikson M, Dearani JA, Hyberger LK, et al (Mayo Clinic and Mayo Found, Rochester, Minn; Sheba Med Ctr, Tel Hashomer, Israel)
Am J Cardiol 80:1309-1313, 1997   6–29

Background.—As many as 4% of patients undergoing cardiac surgery will experience postoperative bradyarrhythmias and require permanent pacing. These authors examined the clinical features of patients with permanent pacing and the short- and long-term results, including survival.

Methods.—Chart review identified 120 adult patients (57 men and 63 women, with a median age at operation of 72 years) who had received a permanent pacemaker because of postoperative bradyarrhythmia within 40 days of cardiac surgery. Patients who had previously undergone surgery for arrhythmia or heart transplantation were excluded, as were those who had preoperative indications for permanent pacing. ECG monitor strips and other standard sources were examined to evaluate the patient's dependency status. Dependency status was either pacemaker-nondependent (n = 35), pacemaker-dependent (any occurrence of continuous ventricular or atrial pacing at a pacing rate of less than 50 beats/min, any occurrence of tracking when the atrioventricular delay was 220 msec or greater, or if programming down the pacemaker caused an abnormal rhythm or decreased heart rate to less than 50 beats/min; n = 51), or indeterminate dependency (n = 34). Median follow-up was 41.2 months (range, 4 days to 13.3 years).

Findings.—The acute complication rate was 0.8% and included pneumothorax, acute lead dislodgment, severe ventricular arrhythmias, and pocket hematoma. The chronic complication rate was 16.7% and consisted mostly of complications related to leads. Of 20 patients with chronic complications, 14 required reoperation. During follow-up, 41% of patients became pacemaker-nondependent. Four patients (3%) died suddenly and 42 (35%) died of noncardiac causes; 74 patients (64%) were alive at the end of follow-up. Aortic valve replacement was more common in the paced population than in the rest of the surgical population. Multivariate analysis identified 1 significant independent predictor of long-term pacemaker dependency: complete atrioventricular block (either narrow- or wide-complex escape) as the indication for pacing. In patients with complete atrioventricular block and narrow-complex escape, the pacemaker was inserted a mean of 9.9 ± 7.8 days after cardiac surgery. In patients with complete atrioventricular block and wide-complex escape, the pacemaker was inserted a mean of 6.4 ± 3.7 days after surgery. Overall, the mean time of permanent pacemaker implantation was 10.7 ± 7.7 days after cardiac surgery.

Conclusions.—Complication rates in these patients were similar to those in the general population of patients with pacemakers. Additionally, about 40% of these patients became pacemaker-nondependent during follow-up. Postoperative patients who develop complete atrioventricular block are at significantly increased risk of being permanently pacemaker-dependent. For these patients, the implantation of a permanent pacemaker should occur by 6 (with wide-complex escapes) or 9 (with narrow-complex escapes) days after cardiac surgery.

▶ These data are most interesting. They reinforce the value of temporary epicardial wire electrodes to treat patients in the postoperative period. If the economics of postoperative care permit, such temporary pacing may permit resolution of transient problems that require only temporary rather than permanent pacing. That 41% of these patients subsequently became non–pacemaker-dependent reinforces this.

A.L. Waldo, M.D.

Transient Sinus Node Dysfunction After the Cox-Maze III Procedure in Patients With Organic Heart Disease and Chronic Fixed Atrial Fibrillation

Pasic M, Musci M, Siniawski H, et al (Deutsches Herzzentrum Berlin)
J Am Coll Cardiol 32:1040-1047, 1998   6–30

Introduction.—Several surgical approaches have been used to treat atrial fibrillation (AF). Among them is the Cox-maze procedure. The original maze procedure has been modified twice to decrease the high incidence of sinus node dysfunction and occasional left atrial dysfunction. Even with these modifications, the postoperative disturbance of sinus node function can occur frequently. The types, frequency, and time dependency of the electrophysiologic manifestations of sinus node dysfunction after the Cox-maze III procedure was prospectively assessed in a series of 15 adult patients with organic heart disease, chronic fixed atrial fibrillation, and no preoperatively overt dysfunction of the sinus node.

Methods.—Patients underwent standard ECG, 24-hour Holter monitoring, power spectral analysis of heart variability, Vasalva maneuver, and rapid positional changes at 3, 6, and 12 months after Cox-maze III procedure and mitral valve surgery or closure of atrial septal defect.

Results.—ECG manifestations of sinus node dysfunction were seen in 12 patients at 3 months, in 6 patients at 6 months, and no patients at 12 months after undergoing the Cox-maze III procedure. Heart rate response to exercise in the first 6 months was diminished in the maze group and was fully normal at 12-month follow-up. Power spectral analysis of heart rate variability revealed exceptionally low-power values at 1-month follow-up with inhibited cardiac autonomic activity and no response on sympathetic stress. A potential of recovery of cardiac autonomic activity was substantiated 12 months after surgery.

Conclusion.—The frequency and intensity of sinus node dysfunction progressively diminished and disappeared within 12 months after patients underwent the Cox-maze III procedure. Permanent pacemaker implantation for sinus node dysfunction in these patients should be used with caution because of the transient nature of this disorder.

▶ This is an encouraging study because of the previously well-recognized problem of sinus node dysfunction after the surgical maze procedure. Unfortunately, it is not clear that one can always wait for a year for return of normal sinus node function; one may have to implant a pacemaker early on for clinical indications. Nevertheless, long-term implications for sinus node function are encouraging.

A.L. Waldo, M.D.

Multisite Pacing as a Supplemental Treatment of Congestive Heart Failure: Preliminary Results of the Medtronic Inc. InSync Study
Gras D, Mabo P, Tang T, et al (Centre Chirurgical du Val d'Or, Saint-Cloud, France)
PACE 21:2249-2255, 1998   6–31

Introduction.—Drugs are the main therapeutic armamentarium available to fight chronic congestive heart failure. Many patients are limited in their daily activities, despite optimal medical management. Multisite pacing has been proposed as an alternative treatment to drugs and surgery. A new pacemaker that offers 3 pacing channels, one each for the right atrium, right ventricle, and left ventricle, is being tested. Its initial results were discussed. Medtronic InSync has a Y adaptor in the connector that allows for the 3 pacing channels as well as leads specially designed to pace the left ventricle from a cardiac vein.

Methods.—There were 81 patients enrolled in the multisite study. and 68 patients (84%) had the pacemaker implanted successfully over a 10-month period. The patients were 66 ± 10 years old and had a mean left ventricular ejection fraction of 21% ± 9%. Thirty-seven percent of the patients were in New York Heart Association function class IV, and 63% were in class III.

Results.—No complication related to system implant occurred. Ten patients left the study during follow-up, and 7 died. Four of these patients died suddenly. Among surviving patients, there was a clinical benefit. A significant improvement in New York Heart Association functional class and the Minnesota Living with Heart Failure Quality of Life questionnaire score were seen. Patients also covered a longer distance during a 6-minute walk test. During biventricular pacing, there was a significant narrowing of the paced QRS. In the interventricular mechanical delay, there was a significant decrease. In the duration of ventricular filling, there was a trend toward an increase.

Conclusion.—In the management of dilated cardiomyopathy, the feasibility and reliability of this new multisite pacing system has been confirmed with these encouraging preliminary results. Further evaluations of this complementary treatment of refractory congestive heart failure should be conducted.

▶ This preliminary report is encouraging, both for safety and efficacy in this patient population. This approach to treatment of heart failure is new, important, and promising. We should follow these and other similar studies carefully and with hopeful anticipation.

A.L. Waldo, M.D.

Evolving Indications for Permanent Cardiac Pacing: An Appraisal of the 1998 American College of Cardiology/American Heart Association Guidelines
Hayes DL, Barold SS, Camm AJ, et al (Mayo Clinic and Mayo Found, Rochester, Minn; Mt Sinai Med Ctr, Cleveland, Ohio; St George's Hosp, London; et al)
Am J Cardiol 82:1082-1086, 1998   6–32

Introduction.—The third revision of the American College of Cardiology/American Heart Association guidelines for implantation of cardiac pacemakers has recently been published. However, there is some disparity between common clinical practice and recommendations based on the availability of high-quality clinical trial data. It is difficult to develop guidelines that achieve unanimity in decision making. It is important to realize the guidelines have limitations and shortcomings, because third-party payors and government agencies tend to look to such guidelines for the basis of their reimbursement decisions.

Definitions.—The guidelines are still unclear regarding common terms such as "asymptomatic" and "persistent" and clinical ambiguities. Thus, these terms must be weighed carefully. Clear definitions of arrhythmias and their classification by ECG pattern and by symptoms are crucial.

Acquired Atrioventricular Block.—The current guidelines have several inconsistencies regarding acquired atrioventricular block. The designation of asymptomatic complete heart block with ventricular escape rates of more than 40 beats/min as a class II indication for pacing is not based on clinical trials, and it is not clear which tests should be performed to determine whether symptoms exist. The rate definition of more than 40 beats/min is unnecessary and arbitrary. There is controversy regarding the timing of including pacing in patients with neuromuscular disease, yet the guidelines suggest waiting for third-degree atrioventricular block. By waiting this long, patients may be exposed to substantial risk of syncope or even sudden death. There is no discussion on 2:1 atrioventricular block, and terms are confusing with the use of advanced atrioventricular block.

Other Conditions.—Excercise-induced atrioventricular block is not discussed in the guidelines. Thus, pacing is recommended for these patients even if they are asymptomatic. Reversible causes of atrioventricular block not discussed are related sleep disorders and sleep apnea. The guidelines for pacing after myocardial infarction are still confusing. Syncope of unknown origin is also not considered in the guidelines.

▶ I recommend that this short article and the revised guidelines (*J Am Coll Cardiol* 31:1175-1206, 1998) be read. It's worth the small effort.
A.L. Waldo, M.D.

Hypertrophic Cardiomyopathy: Role of the Implantable Cardioverter-Defibrillator

Primo J, Geelen P, Brugada J, et al (Onze Lieve Vrouw Hosp, Aalst, Belgium; Univ of Barcelona)
J Am Coll Cardiol 31:1081-1085, 1998   6–33

Background.—Patients with hypertrophic cardiomyopathy (HCM) are at risk of sudden cardiac death. For those patients who survive a near-death episode, preventing the recurrence of sudden death is a challenge. Whether an implantable cardioverter-defibrillator (ICD) would help prevent subsequent sudden cardiac death in these patients is not known. These authors addressed this question by comparing the occurrence of cardiac events in patients with HCM and ICDs who had survived an episode of sudden cardiac death, in patients with structural heart disease and ICDs, and in patients with a structurally normal heart.

Methods.—Thirteen patients (8 men and 5 women; mean age, 48 years) with HCM who had received an ICD constituted group 1. The indications for the ICD were aborted sudden death in 10 patients and sustained ventricular tachyarrhythmia in 3 patients. Group 2 consisted of 215 patients and was divided into 2 subgroups. Group 2a included 196 patients (88% men; mean age, 63 years) with structural heart disease (non-HCM) who had received an ICD for aborted sudden death (41%), syncopal ventricular tachycardia (34%), or refractory ventricular tachyarrhythmias (22%). Group 2b included 19 patients (90% men; mean age, 39 years) who had a structurally normal heart but idiopathic ventricular fibrillation. The indications for ICD placement were aborted sudden death in 12 patients, syncopal sustained polymorphic ventricular arrhythmia in 6 patients, and right bundle-branch block and a family history of sudden cardiac death in 1 patient. The number of shocks and the appropriateness of the shock were measured from the intracardiac electrograms or the R-R interval. Mean follow-up periods were 26 ± 18, 24 ± 21, and 39 ± 20 months in groups 1, 2a, and 2b, respectively.

Findings.—During follow-up, only 2 patients in group 1 received an appropriate shock. The calculated cumulative occurrence of appropriate shocks at 47 months in group 1 (21%) was significantly lower than the value predicted in groups 2a (68%) and 2b (65%). The frequency of inappropriate shocks did not differ in group 1 and group 2b (23% vs. 21%), but inappropriate therapy was significantly less frequent in group 2a (6%). During follow-up, patients in group 1 had a low incidence of ventricular tachycardia and fibrillation. None of the patients in groups 1 or 2b died, but 26 patients in group 2a died.

Conclusions.—The ICD was only used twice in patients in group 1, much less than use rates in group 2. These findings indicate that ventricular tachyarrhythmia may not always be the cause of syncope in patients with HCM. Thus, ICDs appear to be of limited value in patients with HCM.

▶ The data from this study were unexpected. Only 2 of 13 patients with HCM and ICD for the outlined reasons used the ICD during the study period. We clearly have much to learn about appropriate treatment of HCM. However, because we have no more sensitive indicators for ICD placement in these patients, I still find it hard to deny an ICD for the patients with HCM described in this study. A dilemma.

A.L. Waldo, M.D.

▶ The use of the ICD for patients who have HCM and either aborted sudden death or sustained ventricular tachycardia appears reasonable although potentially expensive. It is noteworthy that this study documented that ventricular tachyarrhythmias may not be the primary mechanism of syncope in sudden death in such patients. As noted by Borggrefe and Breithardt,[1] such therapy appears to be both a logical and cost-effective form of therapy.

R.C. Schlant, M.D.

Reference

1. Borggrefe M, Breithardt G: Is the implantable defibrillator indicated in patients with hypertrophic cardiomyopathy and aborted sudden death? (editorial) *J Am Coll Cardiol* 31:1086-1088, 1998.

Indications for Implantation of a Dual-Chamber Pacemaker Combined With an Implantable Cardioverter-Defibrillator
Higgins SL, Williams SK, Pak JP, et al (Scripps Mem Hosp, La Jolla, Calif)
Am J Cardiol 81:1360-1362, 1998   6–34

Introduction.—The dual-chamber pacemaker combined with a tiered therapy implantable cardioverter-defibrillator (ICD) became available in the United States in 1997. Its potential uses have been controversial. There have been no reports reviewing a modern ICD population in terms of associated indications for dual-chamber bradycardia pacemaker therapy. A series of 122 consecutive patients who received a new ICD or underwent ICD generator change were retrospectively reviewed to determine the incidence of conduction disease and the potential implications for dual-chamber pacing.

Methods.—Patient records were reviewed for: demographics, electrophysiologic studies, clinical history notes, procedure notes and forms, and indications for ICD implant or generator change. Indications for pacing were classified into: 1) group I, traditional pacemaker indications from the American College of Cardiology/American Heart Association Committee on Pacemaker Implantation; 2) other common indications prevalent since guideline publication; and 3) indications specific to an ICD population.

Results.—Of the 122 patients, 30 (24.6%) were females and 92 (75.4%) were males; mean age was 69 years. Mean ejection fraction was 34%. Most patients (72%) were in the New York Heart Association functional class II. Of 35 (28.7%) patients who met the published indications for pacemaker therapy, 10 already had implanted permanent dual-chamber pacemakers: 5 before, 3 concomitant with, and 2 after initial ICD implantation.

Conclusion.—Of 122 patients with single-chamber ICDs, 35 had traditional indications, 14 had other indications, and 18 had ICD-specific indications for the dual-chamber ICD. These findings suggest that over 50% of patients receiving an ICD are potential candidates for dual-chamber pacing support.

▶ This study confirms a long-held clinical impression that a large number of patients with an indication for an ICD would also benefit from or require a pacemaker system capable of pacing the atria. The combination of ICD and DDD pacing in a single device is a major advance.

A.L. Waldo, M.D.

Cardiac Death and Stored Electrograms in Patients With Third-Generation Implantable Cardioverter-Defibrillators

Grubman EM, Pavri BB, Shipman T, et al (Univ of Pennsylvania, Philadelphia; Ventritex Inc, Sunnyvale, Calif)
J Am Coll Cardiol 32:1056-1062, 1998   6–35

Introduction.—Cardiac death in patients with implantable cardioverter-defibrillators (ICDs) remains substantial despite the ability of these devices to terminate ventricular tachyarrhythmic episodes. Earlier generation ICDs were not able to provide data during terminal events. Third-generation ICDs can store intracardiac electrograms (EGMs). Stored EGMs from patients with third-generation ICDs who subsequently died were compared with clinical data and previously stored EGMs to evaluate modes of death and EGM characteristics associated with these deaths.

Methods.—Clinical data and stored EGMs from patients enrolled in the clinical trial of the Ventritex Cadence ICD were analyzed retrospectively. Of 1,729 patients enrolled, 119 died during a 6-year follow-up. Final recorded EGMs were analyzed. Postimplant EGMs and 50 control EGMs were used to determine normal EGM characteristics.

Results.—There were 36 (30%) and 83 (70%) noncardiac and cardiac events, respectively. In patients with cardiac deaths, 55 (66%) were non-sudden and 28 (34%) were sudden. There were no stored EGMs within 1 hour of death in 46 patients (55%), indicating that the deaths were not directly related to tachyarrhythmias. Stored EGMs were present within 1 hour of death in 37 cardiac deaths (18 nonsudden, 19 sudden). Thirty-three (89%) of 37 EGM recordings were wide (>158 msec). The wide EGMs were interpreted as ventricular tachycardia in 27 deaths and ventricular fibrillation in 6. Therapy was not delivered by 13 of 33 ICDs (39%); wide EGMs were incorrectly detected as a spontaneous termination of the arrhythmia. The EGMs recorded within 1 hour of death were significantly wider than those recorded from 1 to 48 hours before death.

Conclusion.—A stored EGM within 1 hour of death was available in only 37 patients (31%) who died after placement of an ICD. This suggests that most deaths were not the immediate result of a tachyarrhythmia. The EGMs that were recorded were wide in 89% of patients. These wide EGMs may represent intracardiac recordings of electromechanical dissociation. Of 119 deaths, 112 (94%) may not have been the immediate result of a tachyarrhythmia. The development of ICD systems that record additional physiologic variables may be helpful in determining pathophysiologic changes that occur at the time of death.

▶ These data support the growing appreciation that in patients with an ICD, cardiac death from factors other than ventricular tachyarrhythmia is common and is the usual cause of death. It also reinforces what has been demonstrated now in a series of clinical trials, namely that the ICD is the best prevention of sudden cardiac death from ventricular tachyarrhythmia.

A.L. Waldo, M.D.

The Cost-Effectiveness of Automatic Implantable Cardiac Defibrillators: Results From MADIT
Mushlin AI, for the MADIT Investigators (Univ of Rochester, NY)
Circulation 97:2129-2135, 1998   6–36

Background.—Patients with ventricular tachyrhythmias are at high risk of sudden cardiac death. The Multicenter Automatic Defibrillator Implantation Trial (MADIT) has shown that in patients at high risk of ventricular tachyrhythmia, placement of an implantable cardioverter-defibrillator (ICD) significantly reduces the all-cause mortality rates. However, whether these devices are cost-effective is not known. In this report, the MADIT investigators compared the cost-effectiveness of ICDs and of conventional therapy over 4 years in patients at high risk of ventricular arrhythmia.

Methods.—All patients had asymptomatic nonsustained ventricular tachycardia and an ejection fraction 35% or less and had previously suffered a myocardial infarction. In all patients, electrophysiologic testing induced a sustained ventricular tachycardia that could not be suppressed by procainamide. Patients received either a transthoracic (n = 92) or a transvenous ICD (n = 89). Over 4 years of follow-up, data were gathered regarding the patients' use of health care resources, including visits to a physician or emergency department, use of community services, drugs, tests, hospitalizations, and inpatient and outpatient procedures (including the cost of the ICD). These costs were then related to survival to determine incremental cost-effectiveness.

Findings.—Initially, the average costs were $18,900 in the conventionally treated group and $44,600 in the ICD group (mainly because of ICD-associated costs). However, after the initial 30 days, monthly costs tended to be lower in the ICD group ($1,384 vs. $1,915), especially for medications ($182 vs. $266). By 4 years, in the ICD group, the higher initial costs were offset by the lower monthly costs. Average survival over 4 years was significantly better in the ICD group (3.66 vs. 2.80). The incremental cost-effectiveness per life-year saved in the ICD group was $27,000. However, because patients in the ICD group lived longer, their accumulated net costs were higher ($97,560 vs. $75,980).

Conclusions.—ICDs are a cost-effective strategy to prevent death in selected patients at high risk of ventricular tachycardia. Use of the ICD added approximately 0.80 years to the patient's life. The associated incremental cost-effectiveness ratio ($27,000 per life-year saved) compares well with other health care costs, and should be reduced because virtually all ICDs are now placed transvenously rather than transthoracically.

▶ Without trying to be cynical, we can say death is always cheaper. This important corollary study to MADIT I shows that even when the authors include a large number of patients receiving a transthoracic placement of the ICD, the device is less expensive than many other accepted forms of therapy, including hemodialysis. In any event, this study provides us with some economic reality regarding this form of therapy.

A.L. Waldo, M.D.

Adverse Events With Transvenous Implantable Cardioverter-Defibrillators: A Prospective Multicenter Study
Rosenqvist M, Beyer T, Block M, et al (Karolinska Hosp, Stockholm; Ruprecht-Karls Univ, Heidelberg, Germany; Westfälische Wilhelms Universität, Münster, Germany; et al)
Circulation 98:663-670, 1998   6–37

Introduction.—It has become increasingly important to determine the risk for side effects of implantable cardioverter-defibrillator (ICD) devices, because of the suggestion that indications for these devices be expanded to include the prophylactic treatment of patients at high risk for ventricular arrhythmias. Described is an expanded version of the European Community and International Standards Organization classification system for adverse events related to the surgical procedure or function of ICDs. This expanded classification system was used to prospectively evaluate all adverse events observed during a multicenter clinical trial of a new ICD system implanted in 778 patients.

Methods.—All patients received either a Medtronic model 7,219 C (392 patients) or model 7,219 D (386 patients) Implantable Cardioverter-Defibrillator between March 1993 and November 1994. Patients underwent a predischarge test (induction of ventricular fibrillation) 3 to 7 days after implantation. Patients were evaluated at 1 month and for every 3 months thereafter or for adverse events. The ICD interrogation printouts were reviewed for unnoticed adverse events. Adverse effects were classified according to the definitions of the International Standards Organization 14,155 standard: severe and mild device-related and severe non–device-related. Events were also related to surgical procedure, treatment with the device, or cardiac function.

Results.—Average follow-up was 4.0 months (range, 0-21 months). There were 356 adverse events in 259 patients. Survival was 99%, 98%, and 97%, respectively, at 1, 3, and 12 months after ICD implantation; freedom from surgical intervention was 95%, 93%, and 92%, respectively; and freedom from adverse events was 79%, 68%, and 51%, respectively. Of 20 patient deaths, 6 were related to the surgical procedure, 12 were considered unrelated to ICD treatment, and 2 were of unknown causes. There were 111 nonlethal severe adverse device effects. Of these, 47 required surgical intervention, 19 for correction of a dislodged lead. Inappropriate delivery of therapy occurred 128 times in 111 patients. These events were usually resolved by reprogramming or drug adjustment. Nine patients had to be rehospitalized.

Conclusion.—Nearly 50% of patients who undergo ICD implantation experience an adverse event within the first year. The rate of inappropriate therapy highlights the need for improved detection algorithms and quality-of-life evaluations.

▶ The total number of events reported in a given study clearly depends on the authors' definition of an event. That in part explains the high (about 50%) incidence of adverse events reported from this study. However, to this editor, this incidence emphasizes the need for implantation and follow-up of ICD patients by appropriately trained physicians. Experience and expertise count.

A.L. Waldo, M.D.

New Technology in the Treatment of Disorders of Cardiac Rhythm and Conduction

Final Results From a Pilot Study With an Implantable Loop Recorder to Determine the Etiology of Syncope in Patients With Negative Noninvasive and Invasive Testing
Krahn AD, Klein GJ, Yee R, et al (Univ of Western Ontario, London, Canada)
Am J Cardiol 82:117-119, 1998   6–38

Introduction.—The etiology of syncope is difficult to determine when initial investigations are negative in patients with recurrent syncope. The sporadic and unpredictable nature of the underlying pathophysiologic mechanism results in the low diagnostic yield of most diagnostic approaches. To obtain a symptom-rhythm correlation in patients with infrequent symptoms, external and implantable loop recorder technology has helped to provide long-term ECG monitoring. A previous study found a high diagnostic yield for a prototype implantable loop recorder in 16 patients with negative tilt and electrophysiologic testing. The final outcome of patients who received the prototype device and the long-term follow-up are reported.

Methods.—Twenty-four patients with arrhythmia remained undiagnosed for syncope after clinical assessment, ambulatory or inpatient monitoring, myocardial imaging, tilt, and electrophysiologic testing. The device was implanted in the left pectoral region, using local anesthetic, in all 24 patients. It is an implantable loop recorder, a pacemaker-sized device, with 2 sensing electrodes 32 mm apart on the housing. If syncope did not recur after 2 years, the device was explanted.

Results.—Syncope or presyncope developed in 21 of the 24 patients (88%). Within 1 month of device insertion, 3 of the 21 patients had symptoms. In 11 of 21 patients (52%), syncope was arrhythmic. In 10 patients, the rhythm was sinus rhythm within physiologic rates that did not explain symptoms, and in 5 of these patients, vasodepressor syncope was suspected. Hypertrophic cardiomyopathy with outflow tract obstruction and sinus tachycardia during syncope was found in the remaining 5 patients. In the 18 patients who received a specific diagnosis, treatment was directed at the underlying condition, with 8 patients receiving a pacemaker. The patients with vasodepressor syncope and those with hypertrophic cardiomyopathy had β-blockers prescribed. Counseling was provided to the patient with psychogenic syncope. Over 40 ± 10 months of follow-up, syncope did not recur in 16 of the 18 treated patients. At 42 months after counseling, the patient with psychogenic syncope developed a recurrence. Three patients had the device explanted, and they did not have a recurrence after its removal.

Conclusion.—To diagnose syncope, the clinician would ideally obtain a correlation between symptoms and multiple physiologic parameters, such as blood pressure, heart rate, and brain function. The loop recorder technology is a step toward obtaining this gold standard.

▶ I believe that this implantable loop recorder is a very valuable tool for diagnosis of syncope in problematic patients. It fills a much-needed diagnostic role.

A.L. Waldo, M.D.

Prognostic Significance of Electrical Alternans Versus Signal Averaged Electrocardiography in Predicting the Outcome of Electrophysiological Testing and Arrhythmia-Free Survival

Armoundas AA, Rosenbaum DS, Ruskin JN, et al (Harvard Univ, Cambridge, Mass; Case Western Reserve Univ, Cleveland, Ohio; Massachusetts Gen Hosp, Boston)
Heart 80:251-256, 1998

6–39

Background.—A patient's susceptibility to ventricular tachyarrhythmias can be measured by several markers. One such marker is the presence of late potentials in the signal-averaged electrocardiogram (SAECG). Another is the presence of microvolt electrical alternans of the ST segment and the T wave (T-wave alternans). This study compared the accuracy of these 2 methods in predicting susceptibility to ventricular tachyarrhythmia during electrophysiologic testing and in predicting arrhythmia-free survival.

Methods.—The subjects were 43 patients (32 men and 11 women; mean age, 56 years) who underwent invasive electrophysiologic testing, SAECG testing, and T-wave alternans testing. None of the patients was taking class I or class III antiarrhythmic drugs at the time of testing. Additionally, 36 of these patients (24 men and 12 women; mean age, 54 years) were evaluated during a follow-up period (from 2.9 to 19.9 months) while they were not taking class I and class III antiarrhythmics. SAECGs were evaluated for 3 criteria: a filtered QRS duration greater than 114 msec, a low-amplitude signal duration greater than 38 msec, and a root mean square voltage of the last 40 msec less than 20 µv. Patients meeting 1 criterion were termed SAECG-I, and patients meeting 2 criteria were termed SAECG-II. The T-wave alternans test result was considered positive if the alternans ratio of the T wave was greater than 3.0. Arrhythmia-free survival while not taking class I or class III antiarrhythmic drugs was noted during follow-up and projected to 20 months.

Findings.—T-wave alternans testing was highly and significantly accurate (84%) in predicting the results of electrophysiologic testing. However, SAECG testing less accurately predicted electrophysiologic findings (accuracies of 60% for SAECG-I and 71% for SAECG-II). In the patients not using class I or class III antiarrhythmics during follow-up, 3 (8%) had ventricular tachycardia or fibrillation. Again, T-wave alternans testing was highly and significantly accurate (86%) in predicting arrhythmia-free survival, but SAECG testing was less accurate (accuracies of 65% for SAECG-I and 71% for SAECG-II).

Conclusions.—T-wave alternans testing was superior to SAECG testing and was highly accurate in predicting the outcomes of electrophysiologic testing and arrhythmia-free survival. An advantage of T-wave alternans testing is that it measures beat-to-beat variability rather than measuring variability against an average waveform during SAECG. Furthermore, T-wave alternans testing characterizes repolarization processes, whereas SAECG characterizes depolarization. Although prospective clinical trials are needed, these results suggest that T-wave alternans testing will be a valuable screening tool in patients at high risk of malignant ventricular arrhythmia.

▶ There is an important need to develop reliable markers in identifying patients at risk for ventricular tachyarrhythmia and sudden cardiac death. This study provides encouraging data that T-wave alternans has a high sensitivity and specificity for identifying the outcome of invasive electrophysiologic testing and arrhythmia-free survival. Moreover, the accuracy of T-wave alternans was slightly improved by combining the test with the SAECG. However, this was a retrospective study in a high-risk population: patients undergoing electrophysiologic testing who also had an SAECG and were not receiving either a class I or class III antiarrhythmic agent. The practical use of T-wave alternans must be demonstrated in a lower risk population more similar to that encountered in clinical practice where screening would be applied.

A.L. Waldo, M.D.

Use of a Three-Dimensional, Nonfluoroscopic Mapping System for Catheter Ablation of Typical Atrial Flutter

Nakagawa H, Jackman WM (Univ of Oklahoma, Oklahoma City; Dept of Veterans Affairs Med Ctr, Oklahoma City)
PACE 21:1279-1286, 1998

6–40

Background.—The typical atrial flutter (AFL) re-entrant circuit is now well known. It is confined to the right atrium, and one of its boundaries is the tricuspid annulus (TA). The creation of a complete line of conduction block is an isthmus of conduction between the TA and the eustachian ridge (ER) of the septum that will eliminate AFL. Fluoroscopy during mapping has been used to assist in achieving conduction block, but its lack of accuracy in localizing the anatomical boundaries and sites of previous radiofrequency (RF) ablation limits its usefulness. These authors used a 3-dimensional (3-D) nonfluoroscopic electroanatomical mapping system (CARTO) to localize the anatomical boundaries and allow the creation of a complete line of conduction block across the subeustachian isthmus.

Three-dimensional Mapping of the Right Atrium During Typical AFL.—The CARTO system uses 3 ultralow magnetic field emitters (at 3 different frequencies) positioned below the patient's table, 1 reference catheter, and 1 mapping/ablation catheter with a miniature magnetic field sensor at its tip to provide a 3-D view. 3-D mapping begins with the selection of the window of interest. The reference catheter is used to measure the AFL cycle length, and the window of interest should be 3 to 5 msec shorter. The reference atrial potential divides the window into 2 intervals. Atrial potentials recorded before the window of interest receive an early local activation time (and are red on the 3-D display). Later atrial potential receive progressively later activation times (and are colored according to a set sequence). Activation times between adjacent sites are interpolated. Then electrograms determine the local activation time at each mapping site. The ER and the crista terminalis are identified by their double atrial potentials (indicating their proximity to an area of blocked conduction).

Creation of the Conduction Block.—The block can be created either during coronary sinus pacing at a long cycle length (preferred) or during AFL. The subeustachian isthmus is mapped and the TA and ER are identified. The ablation electrode begins at the TA and delivers RF energy there for about 30 seconds. Then the electrode is drawn to the ER in 2- to 3-mm steps, applying RF continuously until transmural atrial necrosis occurs. The ablation line is marked on a right atrial map. Conduction block across the subeustachian isthmus is verified by further mapping, and mapping should continue for 1 hour or more to ensure persistent, complete block. Should conduction recur, the ablation line can be mapped to identify defects: a double atrial potential or no atrial potential indicates local conduction block, whereas a single atrial potential indicates that conduction is occurring and that further ablation is required to block conduction.

Conclusions.—The 3-D electroanatomical mapping system is useful in treating AFL with RF ablation. It aids greatly in precisely localizing the anatomical boundaries of the re-entrant circuit, and thereby helps to achieve complete conduction block in the critical isthmus of the AFL re-entrant circuit. This system can also be used to help localize and treat any defects in the ablation line.

▶ This article emphasizes the technical advances that we have now made in mapping, particularly with use of the CARTO system, and that really help us in many regards e ectrophysiologically. In particular, AFL is a very curable rhythm, provided we can achieve bidirectional block in the critical isthmus between the tricuspid valve and the eustachian ridge, which is part of the re-entrant circuit. This isthmus is a big area, varying from large to very large. It is also difficult to obtain a complete line of bidirectional block in this isthmus. The CARTO system adds another technological advantage in achieving this bidirectional block. The real message is that AFL should be a curable disease with RF ablation. Physicians should consider this a first-line treatment in patients in whom AFL is a problem.

A.L. Waldo, M.D.

New Method for Nonfluoroscopic Endocardial Mapping in Humans: Accuracy Assessment and First Clinical Results

Smeets JLRM, Ben-Haim SA, Rodriguez L-M, et al (Univ Hosp Maastricht, The Netherlands; Technion-Israel Inst of Technology, Haifa, Israel)
Circulation 97:2426-2432, 1998   6–41

Background.—For radiofrequency catheter ablation of a cardiac arrhythmia to be successful, the site of origin and the activation sequence must be accurately mapped. Endocardial catheter mapping allows the operator to associate the specific intracardiac recording with the underlying anatomy of the area of the heart from which the map is obtained; but current methods with standard fluoroscopic technique have poor reproducibility. These authors evaluated a new nonfluoroscopical mapping method (CARTO) that creates a real-time, 3-dimensional (3-D) electroanatomical activation map in patients undergoing radiofrequency ablation of arrhythmia.

Methods.—Fifteen patients (11 men and 4 women; mean age, 50 years) undergoing electrophysiologic studies in preparation for radiocatheter ablation of an arrhythmia were studied with the CARTO system. This system uses 3 ultralow magnetic field emitters (at 3 different frequencies) positioned below the patient's table, 1 reference catheter, and 1 mapping/ablation catheter with a miniature magnetic field sensor at its tip to provide a 3-D activation map. Fluoroscopy is needed only to position the mapping and reference catheters in the appropriate compartments of the heart. Mapping studies were performed in all 15 patients; additionally, 5 patients participated in an assessment of accuracy. In these 5 patients, two 9F sheaths were advanced into the inferior caval vein just below the right atrium. The reference catheter was placed in 1 sheath, then the mapping catheter was placed in the other sheath and advanced toward the femoral vein in 14 to 19 steps over a distance of 101.8 to 184.9 mm. The catheter shaft at the entrance of the sheath was marked each time the catheter was advanced, and the distance between marks was measured by 4 investigators and averaged.

Findings.—From the accuracy tests, the difference between the mapping system and the caliper measurements was 0.95 ± 0.8 mm (mean distance between steps, 8.73 ± 161 mm with mapping vs. 9.7 ± 1.8 mm with caliper measurements). The mapping system was used to record activation from the right atrium and the right or left ventricle during sinus rhythm. The system could also construct 3-D activation maps in patients with tachycardia (atrial and ventricular) and Wolff-Parkinson-White syndrome.

Conclusions.—The CARTO system provides an accurate geometric reconstruction of different compartments of the heart. With this system, the operator can maneuver the catheter in relation to the electroanatomical map in real time, thus improving reproducibility.

▶ This newly available mapping technique has added mightily to our ability to perform successful radiofrequency ablation of atrial flutter and atrial tachycardia. These are rhythms that now are best treated with radiofrequency ablation to obtain cure. Undoubtedly, it will also help in our assault on other tachyarrhythmias such as ventricular tachycardia.

A.L. Waldo, M.D.

Simultaneous Endocardial Mapping in the Human Left Ventricle Using a Noncontact Catheter: Comparison of Contact and Reconstructed Electrograms During Sinus Rhythm
Schilling RJ, Peters NS, Davies DW (St Mary's Hosp, London; Imperial College School of Medicine, London)
Circulation 98:887-898, 1998   6–42

Introduction.—The most frequent cause of ventricular tachycardia (VT) in coronary heart disease is re-entry. The chance to ablate VT with catheters is limited by the time required to adequately map endocardial activation using conventional sequential techniques. Thus, this technique has been limited to a subset of patients with hemodynamically stable VT. Reported is a noncontact multielectrode array (MEA) mapping system, used for the first time in humans, to detect far-field endocardial potentials from within a cardiac chamber. The timing and morphology of reconstructed unipolar electrograms were compared with those of contact unipolar electrograms from the same endocardial site.

Methods.—Thirteen consecutive patients underwent endocardial left ventricular mapping for catheter ablation of well-tolerated VT. Endocardial potentials detected from within the cardiac chamber were used to reconstruct unipolar endocardial electrograms at 3,360 points and to produce instantaneous endocardial isopotential maps on a computer-generated "virtual" endocardium. Contact electrograms were recorded at 76 points equatorial and 32 points nonequatorial to the MEA during sinus rhythm. using a catheter-locator signal to record the direction and distance from the MEA. Morphology (cross-correlation) and timing of maximum dV/dt of contact and reconstructed electrograms were compared, at varying distances from the MEA center to endocardium (M-E) and from the MEA equatorial plane.

Results.—The M-E was 32.12 mm; timing of reconstructed ECGs with respect to contact ECGs was −1.94 ms for M-E less than 34 mm and −14.16 msec at M-E greater than 34 msec (a significant difference). Cross-correlation of electrograms was 0.87 for M-E less than 34 mm and 0.76 for M-E greater than 34 mm. Mean nonequatorial points were 32.33 mm (range, 16.9-55.6 mm) from the MEA equatorial plane. There was an electrogram timing difference of −8.97 msec that was unrelated to this distance from the equator.

Conclusion.—The noncontact mapping system is accurately able to reconstruct endocardiograms in the human left ventricle during sinus rhythm. Accuracy of the reconstruction is dependent upon the distance between the endocardium and the center of the MEA. The consistent nature of the timing error indicates that the reconstruction of electrograms at an MEA-endocardial distance greater than 34 mm may be improved with refinements in the mathematical solution and in computer hardware.

▶ Technology has permitted so many advances in cardiology. This, of course, is also true for cardiac electrophysiology. The use of the so-called noncontact catheter for mapping all parts of the atria is a marvelous concept. These first reports of mapping using this virtual electrode from the ventricle are very encouraging, but we must await validation studies. In particular, this technology depends critically on both the anatomical confirmation of the ventricles and the accuracy of the mathematical formula for deriving the activation wave fronts. It will be an exciting future if this technique proves to be reliable. Our expectation is that it will.

A.L. Waldo, M.D.

High Perimeter Impedance Defibrillation Electrodes Reduce Skin Burns in Transthoracic Cardioversion

Garcia LA, Pagan-Carlo LA, Stone MS, et al (Univ of Iowa, Iowa City)
Am J Cardiol 82:1125-1127, 1998   6–43

Background.—Transthoracic cardioversion or defibrillation causes first-degree skin burns that are most severe at the edges of the electrode. This is because current preferentially flows to the edges of the electrode. If current flow could become more uniform across the electrode, then perhaps there would be less tissue injury at the electrode's edges. These authors used new defibrillation high-perimeter impedance (HPI) electrodes that reduce preferential current flow at the edges and report their findings regarding tissue injury.

Methods.—Elective cardioversion for atrial flutter or atrial fibrillation was performed on 26 patients. Conversion was accomplished with the HPI defibrillation electrodes in 15 patients and with standard defibrillation electrodes in 11 patients. With the HPI electrodes, the surface impedance at the edges is about 200 times that at the center of the electrode. The cardiologist selected the energy, number of shocks, and electrode position for each patient. Photographs and punch biopsy specimens from the most erythematous site along the edges were obtained within 12 to 24 hours of cardioversion. The degree of epidermal necrosis (on a scale of 0 to 2) and leukocyte infiltration (on a scale of 0 to 2) was determined by histologic examination.

Findings.—Some, but not all, of the patients who had been treated via the HPI defibrillation electrodes had a more uniform distribution of the erythema, but erythema varied considerably between patients. Damage scores, however, were significantly less with the HPI defibrillation electrodes (1.7 ± 0.3 U) than with the standard defibrillation electrodes (3.1 ± 0.4 U). Patients with whom standard defibrillation electrodes were used received a significantly higher peak delivered energy (289 ± 22 vs. 175 ± 28 J), but peak and cumulative currents did not differ between groups (between peaks of 35 and 38 amps and between cumulative values of 66 and 73 amps). Among the patients with whom HPI defibrillation electrodes were used, the damage scores did not differ between patients above and below the median peak and cumulative currents.

Conclusions.—The HPI defibrillation electrodes caused significantly less skin injury than standard defibrillation electrodes yet delivered the same peak and cumulative currents as standard defibrillation electrodes. The peak delivered energy with the standard defibrillation electrodes was significantly higher, which may account for the skin injury. However, the cause of skin injury after the application of defibrillator electrodes is believed to be transcutaneous current flow; if so, then defibrillation electrodes that deliver high impedance to the electrode's edges and thus better distribute current can reduce the skin injury after elective cardioversion.

▶ HPI electrodes hold promise of significantly reducing the all too prominent significant skin burns associated with use of currently available electrodes for DC cardioversion-defibrillation. We hope they will be commercially available soon.

A.L. Waldo, M.D.

Physiology: Insights Into Mechanism, Diagnosis, and Treatment

Cellular Basis for the Normal T Wave and the Electrocardiographic Manifestations of the Long-QT Syndrome

Yan G-X, Antzelevitch C (Masonic Med Research Lab, Utica, NY)
Circulation 98:1928-1936, 1998   6–44

Introduction.—ECG recordings have been an important diagnostic tool for almost a century. Yet correspondence between cellular events, particularly of intramural structures, and the various components of surface ECGs have not been well defined. The cellular basis for the T wave under baseline and long QT (LQT) conditions were evaluated with an arterially perfused canine left ventricular wedge preparation that allows direct temporal correlation of cellular transmembrane and ECG events to test the hypothesis that transmural voltage gradients prominently contribute to the T-wave and ECG manifestations of the LQT syndrome.

Methods.—Simultaneous recordings of transmembrane action potentials were obtained from epicardial, M-region (roughly the third to half of the ventricular wall), and endocardial sites or subendocardial Purkinje fibers with floating microelectrodes. This was synchronized with a transmural ECG recording.

Results.—Repolarization of the M cells was temporally aligned with the end of the T wave. Repolarization of the epicardial cells was coincident with the peak of the T wave. These findings were consistent in 20 of 20 preparations evaluated. The action potential duration of the longest M cells determined the QT interval. The T_{peak} to T_{end} interval acted as an index of transmural dispersion of repolarization. Repolarization of Purkinje fibers outlasted that of the M cell. This did not register on the ECG. Morphology of the T wave seemed to be caused by currents flowing down voltage gradients on either side of the M region during the second and third phase of the ventricular action potential. The interplay between these opposing forces defined the height of the T wave and the degree to which the ascending or descending limb of the T wave was interrupted. This allowed bifurcated T waves and "apparent T-U complexes" under LQT conditions. Spontaneous and stimulation-induced polymorphic ventricular tachycardia with characteristics of torsades de pointes was generated in the presence of dL-sotalol.

Conclusion.—These data offer the first evidence that opposing voltage gradients between epicardium and the M region and endocardium and the M region add greatly to the inscription of the ECG T wave under normal conditions and to the widened or bifurcated T wave and LQT interval seen under LQT conditions. The "pathophysiologic U" wave seen in acquired or congenital LQT syndrome might actually be a second component of an interrupted T wave. Thus, the term "T2" would be more appropriate than "U" to name this event.

▶ For decades, there has been much speculation about the cause of the U wave in the ECG. This study elegantly demonstrates that the U wave is part of ventricular repolarization and is generated by the longer (normal) or prolonged (abnormal) repolarization of the M region of the ventricular wall.

A.L. Waldo, M.D.

Cellular Basis for the ECG Features of the LQT1 Form of the Long-QT Syndrome: Effects of β-Adrenergic Agonists and Antagonists and Sodium Channel Blockers on Transmural Dispersion of Repolarization and Torsade de Pointes
Shimizu W, Antzelevitch C (Masonic Med Research Lab, Utica, NY)
Circulation 98:2314-2322, 1998   6–45

Background.—Four forms of congenital long QT syndrome (LQTS) have been identified. LQT1 is associated with a mutation on chromosome 11 that encodes for the slowly activating delayed rectifier potassium current (I_{Ks}). Patients with LQT1 syndrome typically have a phenotypic, broad-based, T-wave pattern; increased transmural dispersion of repolarization (TDR); and a predisposition to torsades de pointes (TDP). Previous studies have suggested that cardiac events in patients with LQT1 are associated with adrenergic factors. These authors developed an experimental model to evaluate the cellular basis for the phenotypic T waves, TDR, and TDP that occurs in LQT1 syndrome and examine the effects of β-adrenergic and sodium channel blockers on these characteristics.

Methods.—The basis for the model was an arterially perfused wedge of canine left ventricle. A transmural ECG and transmembrane action potentials were recorded simultaneously from 3 sites (epicardial cells, midmyocardial or M cells, endocardial cells). The defects in LQT1 syndrome were mimicked by adding incremental doses of chromanol 293B (a specific I_{Ks} blocker; 1 to 100 μmol/L) and isoproterenol (to mimic increased β-adrenergic tone; 10 to 100 nmol/L). After equilibrium had been reached, the action potential duration (APD) at 90% repolarization (APD_{90}), QT intervals, and T waves were examined.

Findings.—At doses of 10 μmol/L or greater, and in a dose-dependent manner, chromanol 293B significantly prolonged the QT interval and the APD_{90} of all 3 cell types. However, it had no affect on widening of the T wave, increased TDR, or TDP. The addition of isoproterenol at any dose to 30 μmol/L of chromanol 293B significantly reduced the APD_{90} of epicardial and endocardial cells, but not the M cells, causing a widening of the T wave, a marked increase in TDR, and spontaneous and induced (through electrical stimulation) TDP. The addition of the β-adrenergic blocker propranolol (0.5 to 1 μmol/L) to preparations treated with chromanol 293B and isoproterenol completely blocked the isoproterenol-induced increased TDR. Similarly, the addition of mexiletine (2 to 20 μmol/L) shortened the APD_{90} (particularly of M cells) and attenuated the isoproterenol-induced increase in TDR and induction of TDP.

Conclusions.—A deficiency in I_{Ks} does not by itself induce the characteristic changes seen in LQT1 syndrome. However, the addition of a β-adrenergic drug to the preparation significantly increased TDR, thus predisposing to TDP. Previous studies have shown that sodium channel blockade with class IB antiarrhythmic drugs can suppress TDP in other congenital types of LQTS (LQT2, LQT3); the current findings support the further use of these agents in patients with LQT1 syndrome.

▶ The congenital LQTS is a paradigm for understanding the mechanism of a cardiac arrhythmia at a molecular and genetic level. This study provides further understanding of the syndrome, in particular, LQTS. These data explain and reconfirm the importance of β-blocker therapy. They also indicate that mexiletine may work in this syndrome.

A.L. Waldo, M.D.

Influence of the Genotype of the Clinical Course of the Long-QT Syndrome

Zareba W, for the International Long-QT Syndrome Registry Research Group
(Univ of Rochester, NY; Univ of Milan, Italy; Univ of Pavia, Italy; et al)
N Engl J Med 339:960-965, 1998   6–46

Introduction.—The hereditary long QT syndrome is a familiar disorder characterized by prolonged ventricular repolarization on the ECG and a propensity for syncope, polymorphic ventricular tachycardia, and sudden death. The syndrome involves the LQT1, LQT2, and LQT3 loci, which are affected by cardiac potassium-channel genes and the sodium-channel gene. Distinct repolarization patterns on electrocardiography are seen with this syndrome. However, it is not known whether the clinical course of the disease is influenced by the genotype. The clinical course of the long QT syndrome on the basis of the genotype was studied.

Methods.—There were 38 families with 1,378 members enrolled in the International Long-QT Syndrome Registry, and of these individuals, 541 had their genotypes determined. There were 112 mutations at the LQT1 locus, 72 mutations at the LQT2 locus, and 62 mutations at the LQT3 locus. In the 246 gene carriers, and in all 1,378 members of the families studied, the cumulative probability and lethality of cardiac events—such as syncope, aborted cardiac arrest, or sudden death—occurring from birth through the age of 40 years were determined according to genotype.

Results.—Among patients with mutations at the LQT1 locus (63%) or the LQT2 locus (45%), the frequency of cardiac events was higher than among patients with mutations at the LQT3 locus (18%). Significant independent predictors of a first cardiac event were the genotype and the QT interval corrected for heart rate. There was a similar cumulative mortality through the age of 40 among members of the 3 groups of families. However, among families with mutations at the LQT3 locus (20%), the likelihood of dying during a cardiac event was significantly higher than among families with mutations at the LQT1 locus (4%) or the LQT2 locus (4%).

Conclusion.—The clinical course of the long QT syndrome is influenced by the genotype. Among patients with mutations at the LQT1 or LQT2 locus, the risk of cardiac events is significantly higher than among patients with mutations at the LQT3 locus. The percentage of cardiac events that are lethal is also significantly higher in families with mutations at the LQT3 locus, although cumulative mortality is similar across genotypes.

▶ We have made enormous advances in understanding the long QT syndrome. This study adds to that advance. The authors document how important it is to study members of families, and to understand as thoroughly as possible the abnormality families might manifest.

A.L. Waldo, M.D.

Physiology of the Escape Rhythm After Radiofrequency Atrioventricular Junctional Ablation
Shepard RK, Natale A, Stambler BS, et al (Med College of Virginia, Richmond; McGuire VA Med Ctr, Richmond, Va; Duke Univ Med Ctr, Durham, NC; et al)
PACE 21:1085-1092, 1998

6–47

Background.—Patients with atrial fibrillation whose condition does not respond to pharmacologic therapy have another option: radiofrequency ablation (RFA) of the atrioventricular junction (AVJ), which induces complete heart block. The AVJ has sympathetic and parasympathetic nerve fibers, and the proportions of these fibers vary along its course; thus, the location (proximal or distal) of the lesion produced by RFA may have an effect on the escape rhythms (ERs) that often develop after RFA. The electrophysiology and pharmacologic responsiveness of the ERs immediately after RFA of the AVJ were examined.

Methods.—Forty-eight patients (31 men and 17 women; mean age, 68 years) undergoing RFA of the AVJ because of refractory atrial fibrillation were studied. None of the patients had an ER that was less than 20 beats/min, and all were hemodynamically stable. Twelve-lead ECGs recorded the electrophysiologic characteristics at baseline and 15 minutes after the lesion was successfully created. Also, 1 minute of overdrive pacing (paced cycle lengths from 400 to 1,200 msec) was used to measure ER recovery times. The pharmacologic responsiveness of the ERs was measured by the administration of selected doses of adenosine (30 patients), lidocaine (28 patients), isoproterenol (23 patients), verapamil (19 patients), and atropine (7 patients).

Findings.—After RFA, 20 patients had a narrow ER QRS complex (<120 msec) and 28 patients had a wide ER QRS complex. Cycle lengths were similar in these 2 subgroups. Eleven of the 28 patients with a wide ER QRS complex developed new-onset bundle-branch block (right-sided in 9 and left-sided in 2). Recovery times after overdrive pacing were longer as the paced cycle lengths became faster. Pharmacologic responses were similar between the patients with wide and narrow ER QRS complexes. Isoproterenol and atropine significantly decreased the ER cycle length, lidocaine significantly increased the ER cycle length, and adenosine and verapamil had no appreciable effects on the ER cycle length.

Conclusions.—In patients undergoing RFA of the AVJ, ER may be stable even when the QRS complex is wide and bundle-branch block develops. The responses to overdrive pacing (increased recovery times at faster paced cycle lengths) and to isoproterenol and atropine (increased ER rate) support previous data indicating that the ER probably arises from the distal atrioventricular node or the proximal histidine bundle. Furthermore, the lack of response to verapamil but an increased response after lidocaine suggests that the ER is not sensitive to calcium channel blockade, but is sensitive to sodium channel blockers. Some patients may experience pacemaker failure or lead dislodgment after RFA of the AVJ. Should this occur, isoproterenol, or perhaps atropine, would be the best treatment until a temporary pacemaker can be inserted, and lidocaine should be avoided.

▶ The major new finding of this study is that patients undergoing RFA of the AVJ may have stable ERs even in the presence of pre-existing or new bundle-branch block. We still strive for the most proximal lesion to create complete heart block, as this will allow the fastest AVJ ER.

A.L. Waldo, M.D.

Acceleration of Typical Atrial Flutter Due to Double-Wave Reentry Induced by Programmed Electrical Stimulation

Cheng J, Scheinman MM (Univ of California, San Francisco)
Circulation 97:1589-1596, 1998

6–48

Background.—Re-entrant tachycardias, such as typical atrial flutter (AFL), can be accelerated by overdrive pacing, but the mechanism is not well understood. Patients with typical AFL were examined to determine the relationship between double-wave re-entry (DWR) and AFL.

Methods.—Twelve consecutive patients with typical AFL were studied between September 1996 and March 1997. Of the 12 participants, with an average age of 65.8 years, 11 were men. Electrode catheters were placed under fluoroscopic guidance. Pulse oximetry and vital signs were monitored. AFL cycle length was measured and the pacing threshold in the tricuspid annulus-eustachian ridge (TA-ER) isthmus was determined. A single atrial extrastimulus was delivered in the TA-ER isthmus. The timing was progressively decreased to scan the AFL cycle and the excitable gap was determined. Atrial overdrive pacing was performed to terminate AFL.

Findings.—In 5 patients, 27 episodes of AFL acceleration were induced by a single atrial extrastimulus delivered in the TA-ER isthmus and 1 episode was induced by rapid overdrive atrial pacing. Analysis indicated that the acceleration was caused by 2 successive activation wave fronts circulating in the same direction along the same re-entrant circuit (i.e.,

DWR). DWR was induced only 2 to 45 msec after the effective refractory period and was associated with unidirectional antidromic block of the paced impulse. Patients with DWR had a shorter effective refractory period and larger excitable gap than patients without inducible DWR. Most DWR episodes ended after 1 of the DWRs was blocked in the TA-ER isthmus.

Conclusions.—DWR is a mechanism that can cause programmed electrical stimulation-induced AFL acceleration. Induction requires a larger excitable gap and antidromic unidirectional block of the paced impulse in the TA-ER isthmus. The TA-ER isthmus is a common site of DWR termination.

▶ This very nice, neat article explains the well-recognized pacing acceleration of the AFL cycle length. Generally, this accelerated rhythm is unstable, returning to the basic AFL cycle length well before resulting in atrial fibrillation. We now have a good explanation for this phenomenon. It would not surprise this reviewer if the same turned out to be true for pacing acceleration of ventricular tachycardia. In fact, that is likely.

A.L. Waldo, M.D.

Anisotropic Conduction in the Triangle of Koch of Mammalian Hearts: Electrophysiologic and Anatomic Correlations

Hocini M, Loh P, Ho SY, et al (Hôpital Cardiologique du Haut-Lévèque, Pessac, France; Amsterdam and Interuniversity Cardiology Inst of The Netherlands; Imperial College School of Medicine, London)
J Am Coll Cardiol 31:629-636, 1998   6–49

Background.—Previous research has shown that in mammalian muscle fibers, conduction perpendicular to the orientation of the fibers is slower than conduction parallel to the fibers. These differences in velocity relative to fiber orientation (anisotropic conduction) could help to account for slow atrioventricular (AV) conduction in cardiac muscle. These authors performed electrophysiologic and anatomical studies of the triangle of Koch to characterize its anisotropic electrical properties.

Methods.—Atrial pacing from selected sites in isolated, blood-perfused porcine ($n = 9$) and canine ($n = 2$) hearts was used to determine the electrical activity within the triangle of Koch. Atrial pacing sites included the oval fossa, the high right atrium, and (in 7 hearts) a posterior and an anterior site within the triangle of Koch. After the electrophysiologic study, 7 porcine and 2 canine hearts underwent anatomical study.

Findings.—The superficial fibers histologically resembled ordinary atrial fibers. There were 2 patterns of fibers seen in the junctional area. Fibers in the posterior (from the coronary sinus ostium to the tricuspid valve annulus [TVA]) part of the triangle of Koch were oriented in the same direction as the TVA. However, toward the anterior portion of the triangle, the fibers began to change their orientation, and ultimately they were almost perpendicular to the TVA. Stimulation from anterior and posterior sites within the triangle produced electrical activity of high-conduction velocity (0.5 to 0.6 m/sec) that ran parallel to the TVA. Stimulation from the coronary sinus orifice, however, produced a very narrow zone of slow conduction in the posterior part of the triangle; the resultant isochronal lines were almost parallel to the TVA. Both above and below this zone, conduction was fast and ran parallel to the TVA. Stimulation increased the conduction delay in the triangle of Koch by up to 21 msec, but the arterial hypertension interval also increased by up to 210 msec.

Conclusions.—In these animal hearts, superficial myocardial fibers ran parallel to the TVA in the posterior part of the triangle of Koch and perpendicular to the TVA in the anterior portion. The electrical activity studies showed that high-velocity conduction occurred in fibers parallel to the TVA, and a narrow zone of slow conduction occurred in fibers perpendicular to the TVA. Thus, anisotropic conduction is evident in the triangle of Koch. However, the increased conduction delay in the AV junctional area could account for only a fraction of the large increase seen in the arterial hypertension interval. Thus, anisotropic conduction seems unlikely to be important in slow AV conduction.

▶ This study largely addresses questions relative to AV conduction, particularly, conduction in the region of the so-called slow pathway to the AV node. In that regard, the authors find little to support the notion of a slowly conducting pathway. However, this study is also of interest relative to atrial flutter, as a good part of the triangle of Koch includes this isthmus between the coronary sinus and the tricuspid valve annulus. This isthmus is thought to be the area of slow conduction during atrial flutter. The present study could be extrapolated logically to suggest that during atrial flutter, conduction in this region occurs parallel to muscle fiber orientation, and therefore should not be slow Unfortunately, conduction in this area was studied only at a pacing cycle length of 600 msec. It would have been of interest to study conduction at shorter cycle lengths, not only close to those of atrial flutter, but also close to those of AV nodal re-entrant tachycardia.

A.L. Waldo, M.D.

Subject Index

Propranolol
  for heart failure, severe congestive, in
      infants with left to right shunts, 89
  in long QT syndrome form 1 (in dog),
      410
Prostacyclin
  long-term, in severe pulmonary
      hypertension, 355
  in pulmonary hypertension, primary,
      pulmonary vascular resistance
      reduction with, 353
Prostaglandin
  long-term IV, in severe pulmonary
      hypertension, 355
Prosthesis
  bioprosthesis, stentless, aortic valve
      replacement with, 152
  St. Jude *vs.* Medtronic Hall, for mitral
      valve replacement, 168
  valve, anticoagulation, modern
      management of, 311
Protein
  C gene, cardiac myosin-binding, familial
      hypertrophic cardiomyopathy
      related to, clinical features and
      prognostic implications of, 322
  C-reactive, and coronary heart disease,
      254
  -losing enteropathy after Fontan
      operation, 107
Proximal flow convergence method
  to calculate effective regurgitant orifice
      area in aortic regurgitation, 301
PTFE
  expanded, sutures of, mitral valve repair
      for myxomatous disease with, long-
      term results, 172
Pulmonary
  anuli, geometric mismatch of aortic
      anuli and, in children undergoing
      Ross procedure, 91
  arterial tree, effects of modified and
      classic Blalock-Taussig shunts on,
      101
  arteries, effects of balloon dilatation in
      tetralogy of Fallot on, 122
  cardiopulmonary bypass (*see* Bypass,
      cardiopulmonary)
  cavopulmonary connection, superior,
      acute changes in preload, afterload,
      and systolic function after, 137
  edema, flash, as manifestation of
      renovascular disease, 72
  embolism in patients with proximal
      deep vein thrombosis, vena caval
      filters in prevention of, 352
  hypertension

primary, reduction in pulmonary
    vascular resistance with long-term
    epoprostenol in, 353
  severe, long-term IV prostaglandin in,
    355
regurgitation after repair for tetralogy
    of Fallot, MRI of biventricular
    systolic function and mass in
    children with, 108
valve replacement, autograft, pregnancy
    after, 158
vascular resistance reduction with long-
    term epoprostenol in primary
    pulmonary hypertension, 353
veins, ectopic beats originating in,
    spontaneous initiation of atrial
    fibrillation by, 375

Q

QT
  interval prolongation and sudden infant
      death syndrome, 126
  syndrome, long
    clinical course, influence of genotype
        on, 411
    electrocardiographic manifestations
        of, cellular basis for (in dog), 409
    LQT1 form, cellular basis for ECG
        features of (in dog), 410
Quality of life
  effect on doctors' decisions to
      anticoagulate patients with atrial
      fibrillation, 362
  after heart transplantation, 187
  after valve surgery in octogenarians,
      190
Quinapril
  therapy, long-term, in hypertension,
      time course of complete
      normalization of left ventricular
      hypertrophy during, 59
Q-wave
  myocardial infarction after thrombolytic
      therapy, 201

R

Race
  effect on antihypertensive efficacy of
      ACE inhibitor or calcium channel
      antagonist in salt-sensitive
      hypertensives, 55
Radial
  artery, intraoperative minimally invasive
      direct coronary bypass
      arteriography via, 175

S

Salt
  -sensitive hypertensives, ACE inhibitor
      or calcium channel antagonist in,
      55
  sensitivity and insulin resistance in
      essential hypertension, 40
Scintigraphy
  myocardial, dipyridamole-thallium, in
      Kawasaki disease, 83
Seasonal
  variation in myocardial infarction, 256
Secundum
  atrial septal defects, buttoned device
      occlusion of, intermediate-term
      results, 188
Septal
  defect *(see below)*
  myocardial ablation, percutaneous
      transluminal, in hypertrophic
      obstructive cardiomyopathy, 327
Septal defect
  atrial
      familial, reduced penetrance, variable
          expressivity, and genetic
          heterogeneity of, 134
      primum, in children, early results,
          risk factors, and freedom from
          reoperation, 96
      secundum, buttoned device occlusion
          of, intermediate-term results, 188
      ventricular, multiple, techniques and
          results in management of, 98
Septum
  (See also Septal)
  ventricular, intact, transposition of great
      arteries with, primary arterial
      switch operation in infants older
      than 21 days for, 94
Sestamibi
  technetium-99m, myocardial perfusion
      imaging with, prognostic value in
      patients with left bundle-branch
      block, 291
Shock
  cardiogenic, complicating myocardial
      infarction, systematic direct
      angioplasty and stent-supported
      direct angioplasty therapy for, 295
Shunt
  Blalock-Taussig, modified and classic,
      effects on pulmonary arterial tree,
      101
  left to right, beta-blocker therapy of
      severe congestive heart failure in
      infants with, 89

Sibrafiban
  after acute coronary syndrome, 227
Sick sinus syndrome
  follow-up, long-term, atrioventricular
      conduction during, 390
Single-photon emission tomography
  thallium
      dipyridamole-, in Kawasaki disease,
          83
      exercise-, after coronary bypass,
          prediction of death and myocardial
          infarction by, 270
Sinus
  node dysfunction
      devices for treatment, 386
      transient, after Cox-maze III
          procedure in patients with organic
          heart disease and chronic fixed
          atrial fibrillation, 393
  rhythm
      conversion of recent-onset atrial
          fibrillation to, effects of different
          drug protocols on, 383
      effect of amiodarone in heart failure
          and atrial fibrillation on, 382
      electrograms during, contact *vs.*
          reconstruction, 406
  sick sinus syndrome, atrioventricular
      conduction during long-term
      follow-up, 390
Skeletal
  muscle vasculature, depressor action of
      insulin on, as mechanism for
      postprandial hypotension, in
      elderly, 10
Skin
  burns in transthoracic cardioversion
      reduced by high perimeter
      impedance defibrillation electrodes,
      407
Sleep
  apnea, obstructive, prevalence in
      hypertensives, 74
Smooth muscle
  cell proliferation suppressed by ethanol
      in postprandial state, 42
Socioeconomic
  issues in coronary heart disease, 277
Sodium
  channel blocker effects on ECG features
      of long QT syndrome form 1 (in
      dog), 410
  channels, epithelial, T594M mutations
      in β subunit of, and hypertension,
      in black residents of London, 14
  intake, dietary, and mortality, 37
  reduction in hypertension treatment in
      older persons, 36

Author Index